Cochlear Implants and Other Implantable Hearing Devices

Cochlear Implants and Other Implantable Hearing Devices

EDITED BY
MICHAEL J. RUCKENSTEIN

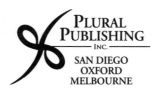

PLURAL
PUBLISHING
INC.

SAN DIEGO
OXFORD
MELBOURNE

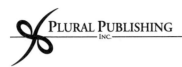

5521 Ruffin Road
San Diego, CA 92123

e-mail: info@pluralpublishing.com
Web site: http://www.pluralpublishing.com

49 Bath Street
Abingdon, Oxfordshire OX14 1EA
United Kingdom

Typeset in 10.5/13 Garamond Book by Flanagan's Publishing Services, Inc.
Printed in the United States of America by McNaughton & Gunn

Library of Congress Cataloging-in-Publication Data

Cochlear implants and other implantable hearing devices / [edited by] Michael J.
Ruckenstein.
      p. ; cm.
  Includes bibliographical references and index.
  ISBN-13: 978-1-59756-432-8 (alk. paper)
  ISBN-10: 1-59756-432-X (alk. paper)
  I. Ruckenstein, Michael J. (Michael Jay), 1960–
  [DNLM: 1. Cochlear Implants. 2. Auditory Brain Stem Implantation. 3. Auditory Brain
Stem Implants. 4. Cochlear Implantation. WV 274]
  LC Classification not assigned
  617.8'8220592—dc23
                                    2011047143

Contents

Preface

During my residency, I had the pleasure of attending several miniseminars dedicated to cochlear implants offered at the annual AAO-HNSF meeting. Cochlear implants had just been approved by the FDA, and as a young clinician-scientist with a background in auditory physiology, I was very excited to learn about these devices that restored hearing. Most of the speakers at the seminars provided detailed scientific data that documented the outcomes in patients who had received cochlear implants. One speaker, however, presented little science. He expounded on the wonder of restoring hearing, how it changed people's lives, how "miraculous" it was to participate in the process! At the time I remember dismissing this speaker's presentation as unscientific anecdotalism. However, as I have progressed through my career, I often hearken back to that early "anecdotal" talk. Although the necessity of scientific study is undisputed, it has become clear to me that the process of restoring hearing is somehow bigger than what the scientific data can convey. It is a true honor and privilege to be involved in the field of cochlear implantation, and it is from these feelings that this book emanates.

I have assembled a group of authors who are true experts in the field and I am truly grateful to each and every one of them for taking the time to contribute to this effort. The book is organized in what I hope is a logical way. The chapter topics were chosen to be practical, providing the student with the necessary background to understand, and hopefully one day contribute, to this exciting area of study. The recent advances in the field of middle ear implantable hearing devices are extremely exciting, and we attempt to provide readers with an introduction to this rapidly evolving field.

As always, I am very grateful to my editor, Judy Meyer, who manages to be extraordinarily pleasant and nice while she very effectively pushes for completion of a book! All the people at Plural are wonderful to work with, and I have enjoyed the process immensely.

Contributors

Robert B. A. Adamson, PhD
Assistant Professor
School of Biomedical Engineering
Dalhousie University
Halifax, Nova Scotia
Canada
Chapter 19

Manohar Bance, MBchB, MSc, FRCSC
Professor and Acting Head Division of
    Otolaryngology
Dalhousie University
Halifax, Nova Scotia
Canada
Chapter 19

D. C. Bigelow, MD
Associate Professor
Director of Otology and Neurotology
Department of Otolaryngology
University of Pennsylvania
Philadelphia, Pennsylvania
Chapter 7

Jason Brant, MA, MD
Resident Physician in Otorhinolaryngology
Hospital of the University of
    Pennsylvania
Philadelphia, Pennsylvania
Chapter 7

Craig A. Buchman, MD, FACS
Professor and Vice Chairman for Clinical
    Affairs
Chief Otology, Neurotology, and Skull
    Base Surgery
Department of Otolaryngology—Head
    and Neck Surgery
University of North Carolina
Chapel Hill, North Carolina
Chapter 17

Linda S. Burg, AuD, CCC-A
Coordinator, Koss Cochlear Implant
    Program
Department of Otolaryngology and
    Communication Sciences
Medical College of Wisconsin
Milwaukee, Wisconsin
Chapter 2

Joseph M. Chen, MD, FRCS(C)
Chief and Associate Professor
Department of Otolaryngology—Head
    and Neck Surgery
Sunnybrook Health Sciences Centre
University of Toronto
Toronto, Ontario
Canada
Chapter 15

Robert D. Cullen, MD
Otologic Center
Kansas City, MO
Chapter 17

Ross William Deas, PhD
Dalhousie University
Halifax, Nova Scotia
Canada
Chapter 19

Michael F. Dorman, PhD
Professor
Department of Speech and Hearing
    Science
Arizona State University
Tempe, Arizona
Chapter 4

Marc D. Eisen, MD, PhD
Medical Director, Hartford Hospital
    Hearing and Balance Center
Assistant Clinical Professor
Department of Surgery (Otolaryngology)
University of Connecticut Medical
    Center
Hartford, Connecticut
Chapter 1

David Friedland, MD, PhD
Associate Professor
Medical College of Wisconsin
Chief, Division of Research
Chief, Division of Otology and
    Neuro-otologic Skull Base Surgery
Milwaukee, Wisconsin
Chapter 2

Lendra M. Friesen, CCC-A, PhD
Associate Scientist
Sunnybrook Research Institute
Assisstant Professor
Department of Otolaryngology—Head
    and Neck Surgery
University of Toronto
Toronto, Canada
Chapter 15

René H. Gifford, PhD
Assistant Professor,
Vanderbilt University
Director, Cochlear Implant Research
    Laboratory
Vanderbilt University
Director, Cochlear Implant Program and
    Pediatric Audiology
Vanderbilt Bill Wilkerson Center
Nashville, Tennessee
Chapter 5

**Karen A. Gordon, PhD, CCC-A,
RegCASLPO**
Director of Research

Cochlear Implant Laboratory
Hospital for Sick Children
Toronto, Ontario
Canada
Chapter 14

David A. Gudis, MD
Department of Otorhinolaryngology—
    Head and Neck Surgery
University of Pennsylvania
Philadelphia, Pennsylvania
Chapter 20

**Barbara S. Herrmann, PhD,
CCC-A**
Assistant Professor
Department of Otology and Laryngology
Harvard Medical School
Clinical Associate
Department of Audiology
Massachusetts Eye and Ear Infirmary
Boston, Massachusetts
Chapter 18

Ellen G. Hoeffner, MD
Associate Professor
University of Michigan Health System
Department of Radiology
Division of Neuroradiology
Ann Arbor, Michigan
Chapter 6

**Yell Inverso, AuD, PhD, CCC-A/
FAAA**
Audiology Program Director
Nemours Alfred I. DuPont Hospital for
    Children
Assistant Professor
University of Pennsylvania School of
    Medicine
Department of Otorhinolaryngology—
    Head and Neck Surgery
Wilmington, Delaware
Chapter 16

Michael F. Jackson, MS, CCC-A
Senior Cochlear Implant Audiologist
Center for Childhood Communication
Children's Hospital of Philadelphia
Philadelphia, Pennsylvania
Chapter 13

Luv Javia, MD
Assistant Professor of Clinical
  Otorhinolaryngology—Head and
  Neck Surgery
University of Pennsylvania School of
  Medicine
Children's Hospital of Philadelphia
Pediatric Cochlear Implant Program
Philadelphia, Pennsylvania
Chapter 8

Jona Kronenberg, MD
Professor
Department of Otolaryngology—Head
  and Neck Surgery
Sheba Medical Center and
Tel Aviv University
Israel
Chapter 9

Jeffery J. Kuhn, MD, FACS
Department of Otolaryngology—Head
  and Neck Surgery
Naval Medical Center Portsmouth
Associate Professor of Clinical
  Otolaryngology—Head and Neck
  Surgery
Eastern Virginia Medical School
Portsmouth, Virginia
Chapter 21

Daniel J. Lee, MD FACS
Director, Wilson Auditory Brainstem
  Implant Program
Director, Pediatric Otology Center
Department of Otolaryngology
Massachusetts Eye and Ear Infirmary
Assistant Professor

Department of Otology and Laryngology
Harvard Medical School
Boston, Massachusetts
Chapter 18

Harrison W. Lin MD
Department of Otolaryngology
Massachusetts Eye and Ear Infirmary
Harvard Medical School
Boston, Massachusetts
Chapter 18

Laurie A. Loevner, MD
Professor of Radiology,
  Otorhinolaryngology: Head and Neck
  Surgery and Neurosurgery
Director of Head and Neck Imaging
Department of Radiology,
  Neuroradiology Section
Philadelphia, Pennsylvania
Chapter 6

Paul T. Mick, MD, FRCSC
Neurotology—Skull Base Surgery Fellow
University of Toronto
Toronto, Ontario
Canada
Chapter 15

Lela Migirov, MD
Professor, Chief of Cochlear Implant
  Service
Department of Otolaryngology—Head
  and Neck Surgery
Sheba Medical Center and
Tel Aviv University
Israel
Chapter 9

Suyash Mohan, MD, PDCC
Assistant Professor of Radiology
University of Pennsylvania School of
  Medicine
Philadelphia, Pennsylvania
Chapter 6

Michelle L. Montes, AuD, CCC-A
Clinical Audiologist
University of Pennsylvania Health
System
Philadelphia, Pennsylvania
Chapter 12

**Blake C. Papsin, MD, MSC,
FRCSC, FACS, FAAP**
Cochlear Americas Chair in Auditory
Development
Staff Otolaryngologist
Head and Neck Surgery
Hospital for Sick Children
Toronto, Ontario
Canada
Chapter 14

Robert R. Peters, MD
President, Dallas Ear Institute
President, Dallas Hearing Foundation
Dallas, Texas
Chapter 11

Sandra Prentiss, MA, CCC-A
Clinical Audiologist
Department of Otolaryngology—Head
and Neck Surgery
University of Kansas Medical Center
Kansas City, Kansas
Chapter 10

Peter S. Roland, MD
Professor and Chairman
Department of Otolaryngology—Head
and Neck Surgery
Professor Neurological Surgery
Chief of Pediatric Otology
UT Southwestern Medical Center
Dallas, Texas
Chapter 3

Jennifer Rotz, AuD
Clinical Specialist in Audiology
University of Pennsylvania Health System

Philadelphia, Pennsylvania
Chapter 12

**Michael J. Ruckenstein, MD, MSc,
FACS, FRCSC**
Professor, Vice Chairman
Residency Program Director
Department Otorhinolaryngology, Head
and Neck Surgery
University of Pennsylvania Health System
Philadelphia, Pennsylvania
Chapters 7 and 20

Christina Runge, PhD, CCC-A
Associate Professor
Director,
Koss Cochlear Implant Program
Department of Otolaryngology and
Communication Sciences
Medical College of Wisconsin
Milwaukee, Wisconsin
Chapter 2

**David B. Shipp, MA, FAAA, Reg
CASLPO**
Audiologist and Coordinator
Cochlear Implant Program
Assistant Professor
Department of Otolaryngology—Head
and Neck Surgery
University of Toronto
Toronto, Canada
Chapter 15

Hinrich Staecker, MD, PhD
David and Marilyn Zamierowski
Professor
University of Kansas School of Medicine
Kansas City, Kansas
Chapter 10

Blake S. Wilson
Co-Director, Duke Hearing Center
Adjunct Professor,
Department of Surgery

Division of Otolaryngology—Head and
  Neck Surgery
Adjunct Professor,
Department of Electrical and Computer
  Engineering
Duke University Medical Center (DUMC)
Durham, North Carolina
Chapter 4

Charles G. Wright, PhD
Adjunct Associate Professor
Department of Otolaryngology—Head &
  Neck Surgery
UT Southwestern Medical Center
Dallas, Texas
Chapter 3

*To Sean, Jennifer, and Laura—who bring
magic to my life on a daily basis!*

Chapter 1

History of Implantable Hearing Devices

MARC D. EISEN

INTRODUCTION

Generally, an implantable hearing device is designed to capture sound and present it to the auditory system to rehabilitate hearing, where at least part of the device is surgically implanted in the patient receiving it. In order to create a framework with which to systematically address the history of implantable hearing devices, we subdivide implantable by their invasiveness. Least invasive are bone-conduction aids. These function by oscillating the temporal bone and transmitting the vibration of sound directly to the cochlea. The bone-anchored hearing aid (Baha®) is the archetypal example of this technology. Next, is the group of aids whose sound transmission is through the middle ear anatomy. The implantable middle ear portion of the aid is driven either by an external microphone and processor (semi-implantable) or by an implantable microphone and processor (completely implantable). Finally, the cochlear implant bypasses the cochlea to stimulate the cochlear nerve fibers directly.

BONE-CONDUCTION DEVICES

The fact that sound can be conducted through the skull base to reach the cochlea, bypassing the middle ear, has been understood for millennia.[1] There are several very early descriptions of nonimplanted auditory prostheses that utilized the teeth as bone conductors. In 1812, J.M.G. Itard, for example, described a wooden rod that had a narrow and broader end. The speaker would speak with the narrow end between her teeth, and the listener held the broader end against the teeth.[1] *Implanted* bone-conduction prostheses had an unlikely precursor: Andrija Henry Karl Puharich (1918–1995) owned the patents to a "miniature tooth radio." Puharich was an eccentric who received his medical doctorate from Northwestern University, but spent little time practicing medicine. He proposed an "alternative" neural pathway that he called the "facial system," a theoretical pathway from the mandibular teeth through to the central auditory areas that bypasses the inner ear completely. Theoretically, stimulating the facial system with sound would give hearing to the deaf, and one entry point to the pathway was at the teeth. His U.S. Patent #2,995,633, "Means for Aiding Hearing," describes this parallel neural pathway as well as the receiver and piezoelectric stimulator implanted into a tooth.[2] A second patent[3] improves on the design of the implanted "miniature tooth radio," still claiming that it functioned as a neural stimulator. In reality, the miniature tooth radio could have functioned as an implanted bone-conduction device. The miniature tooth radio would have needed a microphone and transmitter, but this was not described in the patent. There is no evidence that the miniature tooth radio was ever manufactured.

Bone-conduction hearing aids play sound through the skin behind the ear to oscillate the temporal bone. An inherent inefficiency with this design is the damping effect of the skin and soft tissue, and the need to hold the device with pressure against the skin. The bone-*anchored* hearing aid was developed to overcome these two drawbacks of bone-conduction hearing aids by affixing the device to the skull. The technologic advancement that allowed this concept to be developed was the discovery that titanium integrates with bone without a connective tissue interface, which was described by Per-Ingvar Branemark in Sweden in the 1970s. Such integration led to the idea that the bone-conduction aid be attached to the titanium implant that penetrated through the skin, completely removing the damping effect of the skin. Anders Tjellstrom collaborated with Branemark and developed the first bone-anchored hearing aid, which was first implanted in a human in 1977.[4] With FDA approval in 2002 and subsequent acceptance by third-party payers, the Baha® gained wide acceptance and use.

J.V.D. Hough developed a semi-implantable bone conduction device initially for conductive loss, called the Audiant Bone Conductor. For this device, the implantable portion consisted of an assembly of a rare-earth magnet surrounded by a titanium screw unit. The titanium osseo-integrated. The external portion comprises a microphone and speech processing unit that drives the subcutaneously placed internal portion with electromagnetic induction. The FDA approved marketing for the Audiant in 1986. Although several thousand patients were implanted with the Audiant in the following decade, production of the device ended in the 1990s. Unlike the Baha®, the Audiant has no transcutaneous components. It was never covered by third-party payers, and it never reached the mainstream.

IMPLANTABLE MIDDLE EAR HEARING DEVICES

Implantable middle ear hearing devices are designed to drive the ossicular chain directly. The advantages of implantable middle ear hearing devices over conventional hearing aids, then, should be improved fidelity, freedom from feedback, more discrete or hidden hardware, and removal of the occlusion effect that conventional aids create. Goode[5] laid out these potential advantages in 1969. Several direct-drive designs emerged in the later part of the 20th century, which generally fall into two types: piezoelectric drivers and electromagnetic drivers. A piezoelectric driver contains a crystal that expands and contracts when an electrical field is passed across it. When one piezoelectric element is fixed, and one is free, either on the stapes superstructure or the footplate, the free element will transmit motion (ie, the vibration of sound) and stimulate the middle ear. One piezoelectric-based partially implantable device was developed at Ehime University in Japan, with the Rion and Sanyo Electric Companies. A prototype was available in 1983 whose ossicular vibrator (the Ehime [E]-type ossicular vibrator) was implanted through the mastoid. The external components stimulated the internal vibrator by transcutaneous induction. The complete device, the Rion Device E-type, was first implanted in a human in 1984.[6] After a number of complications with this initial device, a second-generation device was developed that improved on the first.[7] The device was implanted in about 100 patients until its manufacture ceased in 2005 due to lack of profitability.[8]

Electromagnetic designs of the ossocular driver involve rare earth magnets placed on the tympanic membrane or on the umbo and driven by coils placed in the ear canal.[9] One simple design was to implant a magnetic ossicular replacement (either a PORP or TORP) that could be driven via an ear canal electromagnet.[10,11] This driver's disadvantage was that it was worn in the ear canal, creating the occlusion effect. The magnetic element with this design is also relatively large compared to other middle ear magnets. J.V.D Hough was inspired by Aram Glorig[12] and Jack Vernon[13] to pursue implantable magnetic elements placed on an intact ossicular chain. Out of these efforts came the SOUNDTEC Direct Drive Hearing System. It consisted of a barrel-shaped magnet held by a collar on the incudostapedial joint. The microphone, processor, and power supply were contained in a behind-the-ear device, from which electrodes led

to a deeply placed canal coil. The coil created the oscillating magnetic field that drove the implanted element. Although the initial design[14] tended to break down in situ, results in clinical trials were favorable compared to conventional hearing aids.[15,16]

Richard Goode introduced a "floating mass transducer" that was developed by Jeff Ball and incorporated into the Symphonix Devices Corporation's Vibrant Soundbridge.[17] The Vibrant Soundbridge had the transducer and receiver both implanted, the transducer affixed to the stapes and the receiver into the mastoid.[18] The Food and Drug Administration approved the Vibrant Soundbridge for marketing and production in the United States in 2000.

The Otologics middle ear transducer ("MET") ossicular stimulator was developed by John Fredrickson at Washington University in St. Louis. The MET device consisted of an implanted receiver/transducer unit that is anchored to the mastoid and whose probe inserts into the incus directly. An external processor was worn behind the ear.[19,20] Direct-drive electromagnetic devices appear to have better fidelity and efficient energy transfer. Technical problems, a greater expense compared to conventional aids, and the need for surgical implantation are challenges that the implantable hearing aids have to overcome.

THE COCHLEAR IMPLANT

Many fields have contributed to the development of the cochlear implant over the course of the past half century. As a result of these efforts, we now have reliable, mass-produced devices expected to last a lifetime; we have a safe outpatient procedure to implant the device that is a routine part of otologic training programs; and we have rehabilitation and ongoing management of the cochlear implant by audiologists that is a routine part of the curriculum in audiology training programs. Individual contributions to the development of the cochlear implant cannot be considered in isolation, but this section highlights benchmarks in cochlear implant development by breaking them down into several categories. These categories include a proof of concept that electrical stimulation of the cochlea would yield audition, development of the hardware of the implant, development of the safety of the device, advances that allowed its mass production, advancement of speech processing strategies, and finally the relaxation of candidacy requirements.

PROOF OF CONCEPT— ELECTRICAL STIMULATION YIELDS AUDITION

Electrical stimulation of the auditory pathway has roots back to Alessandro Volta, who found that current passed across his own head created auditory sensations.[21] This and other similar attempts over the next 150 years to stimulate the auditory system electrically, however, did not systematically address which neuroanatomic structure in the auditory pathway was stimulated. Specific candidates included the organ of Corti and the auditory nerve fibers. Stevens had described in the 1930s that an intact organ of Corti will respond to electrical stimuli with a mechanical response, thus stimulating the normal release of neurotransmitter from cochlear hair cells onto fibers of the auditory nerve. This phenomenon was termed "electrophonic hearing,"[22] and required an intact, functioning organ of Corti. This type of stimulation would not be helpful in the deaf ear, where the organ of Corti is nonfunctional.

Stimulating the auditory nerve in a deaf patient to generate hearing was first demonstrated in Paris in the 1950s. André Djourno (1904–1996) and Charles Eyriès (1908–1996) collaborated in Paris in 1957 to implant the first auditory prosthesis. Djourno was a basic scientist, an electrophysiologist in the Department of Anatomy and Physiology at the Faculté de Medicine of Paris, with a special interest in developing implantable induction coils that stimulated nerves. Eyriès was a clinician, Chief of Otorhinolaryngology and Head and Neck Surgery at L'Institut Prophylactique (later L'Institut Arthur Vernes) in Paris, with a special interest in facial reanimation surgery. When Eyriès was consulted for facial reanimation in an unfortunate patient with bilateral deafness and facial paralysis after extensive cholesteatoma surgeries, Djourno convinced him to implant one of his induction coils during surgery to see whether the patient would hear. On February 25, 1957, Eyriès performed the surgery. The induction coil was implanted into the mastoid cavity, and a wire placed in close proximity to the cochlear nerve stump. Stimulation through the implant was tested intraoperatively and then postoperatively during testing sessions. The patient described auditory sensations, and the patient was able to discriminate lower frequency (described as "burlap tearing") from higher frequency (described as "silk ripping") stimuli. He appreciated environmental noises and several words, but could not understand speech.[23,24] The work of Djourno and

Eyriès was published only in French, and development of a commercial device was never pursued. Their work would likely have remained in obscurity were it not for a patient who brought the work to the attention of his otologist.

DEVELOPMENT OF THE HARDWARE OF THE IMPLANT

Around 1960 William F. House, MD, DDS, was in the earliest years of his practice with his half-brother Howard House, MD, at the Otologic Medical Group in Los Angeles. One of Bill House's patients brought him an article in the French lay press about the work of Djourno and Eyriès. Their work inspired House to pursue a cochlear implant of his own.[25] Over the ensuing year, he collaborated with two brothers, John (a neurosurgeon) and James Doyle (an electrical engineer), respectively, on developing a cochlear implant for human patients. The first two deaf volunteers received a simple gold wire electrode inserted through the round window and brought out through the skin.[26] Like the patient of Djourno and Eyriès, electrical stimulation generated hearing. These early results were encouraging, but were tempered by local infections that warranted early wire removal. One of the patients was re-implanted with a multielectrode wire array connected to an induction device seated underneath the skin, but again local tissue reaction forced Dr. House to remove the device for the concern of infection. Despite limited success at stimulating hearing and genuine concerns about biocompatibility raised by these two patients, the lay press made overly optimistic and premature claims of a pending artificial ear.[27,28] The

cochlear implant suffered from a lack of legitimacy among scientists and engineers involved in hearing science.

Two other otologists in the 1960s experimented with cochlear implants in human patients. F. Blair Simmons, then chairman of Otolaryngology at Stanford, implanted an electrode into the modiolus of a deaf patient in 1964. Following the procedure, the patient underwent auditory testing sessions to assess the implant's capabilities. Given the man's comorbidity of being blind, however, assessment of the subject's hearing generated by the device was exceedingly difficult.[29] Simmons's enthusiasm for the viability of the cochlear implant waned.[30] The other clinician who began experimenting with implants in the 1960s was Robin Michelson. The consummate tinkerer, Michelson began working on a cochlear implant on his own as a private practitioner in Redwood City, California. He moved to the University of California—San Francisco under the leadership of Francis Sooy. Michelson implanted several subjects with fully implantable single electrode devices and reported their experiences at national forums.[31,32]

DEVELOPMENT OF THE SAFETY OF THE DEVICE

The nascent efforts above were aimed at demonstrating proof of the concept that electrical direct stimulation of the auditory nerve in deaf patients could rehabilitate hearing. Manufacturing a viable, safe cochlear implant was a tremendous hurdle that then stood in the way. Societal pressures in the 1970s led to tighter regulation on device manufacturing. The emergence of much more stringent Food and Drug Administration (FDA) regulations of new devices in 1976 meant that efficacy and safety would have to be proven before a new device could be marketed.

The early 1970s brought more controversy to the cochlear implant than excitement. The basic science community in general adamantly opposed cochlear implantation on the grounds dictated by the current understanding of auditory physiology that cochlear implants would yield no useful hearing. Furthermore, they argued that before humans should be implanted, rigorous scientific method be applied and devices verified in animal models.

A turning point in the development of the cochlear implant came in 1975, when the NIH sponsored a thorough evaluation of the patients who had received cochlear implants up until that time. Thirteen subjects, all implanted with single-channel devices by either Robin Michelson or William House, volunteered to go to Pittsburgh for extensive psychoacoustic, audiologic, and vestibular testing led by Robert Bilger. The report concluded that single channel devices could not create speech understanding, but that patients' speech production, lip reading, and quality of life were all enhanced with the device.[33] The study and its report marks the first time that an objective evaluation of patients by the scientific mainstream was performed. Benefits from implants were evident, and the concept that electrical stimulation of the auditory nerve could yield useful hearing was finally confirmed.

Cochlear implant research gained a foothold in the scientific mainstream in the later part of the 1970s. Work on the implant emerged from legitimate, well-established academic centers, and funding to perpetuate the work increased. The group at the University of California — San Francisco, led by Michael Merzenich and Robert Schindler, addressed the safety and

feasibility of long term electrical stimulation of the auditory nerve in a cat model, showing that scala tympani electrodes inserted atraumatically could stimulate the auditory nerve chronically without dramatic neural degeneration.[34,35] The NIH contract mechanism pushed progress further by funding efforts to determine the most suitable materials for electrical biostimulation.[36] Two groups worked on the development of a multielectrode cochlear prosthesis — the UCSF group[34] and Graham Clark and his group at the University of Melbourne in Australia.[37] These groups made substantial improvements in miniaturization of the receiver/stimulator device and improved safety and durability of the electrode array. The work of these two groups resulted eventually in the production of the Advanced Bionics Clarion and the Cochlear Corporation's Nucleus devices. At the same time, William House and his engineer colleague Jack Urban continued to pursue the development of the single-channel device. Manufactured by the 3M Corporation, the House 3M single-channel implant was the first FDA-approved implant, and more than 1,000 were implanted from 1972 into the mid-1980s. FDA approval for the multichannel cochlear implant came in 1985 for adults and in 1990 for children as young as two years.

THE ADVANCEMENT OF SPEECH PROCESSING STRATEGIES

As the safety of the cochlear implant became well accepted, work on the cochlear implant focused on the understanding of speech. The superiority of multiple-channel devices over single-channel devices became clear, as demonstrated in large adult clinical trials.[38,39] A speech-processing scheme based on a high rate of alternating electrode stimuli was introduced by a collaboration between the UCSF group and the Research Triangle Institute, and was shown in 1991 to be a significant boost to speech recognition performance.[40]

RELAXATION OF CANDIDACY REQUIREMENTS

Candidacy was initially granted to adult patients with profound bilateral hearing loss (>100 dB thresholds) and no measurable open-set speech recognition with hearing aids. The 25 years that followed the initial FDA approval of the cochlear implant saw age requirements fall initially down to 2 years or older, and then 1 year or older in 2000. Through combined advances in universal newborn hearing screening and early diagnosis of deafness, education and rehabilitation of implantees, and greater acceptance of cochlear implantation by the deaf community, implantation of infants has become accepted and resulted in tremendous improvements in implant performance in these patients. Residual hearing requirements have also been liberalized to include patients with considerable residual hearing, both with pure tone threshold and with open-set speech recognition with hearing aids. As far as which ear is im-planted, initial thought was that residual hearing implied better neural element preservation, which would lead to better cochlear implant performance. A 2005 study from the Johns Hopkins cochlear implant center demonstrated that the degree of residual hearing did NOT correlate with the performance with the implant.[41]

CONCLUSIONS

The history of the development of implantable hearing devices closely follows the technologic advances of electronics, namely, miniaturization and sophistication of microcircuitry, materials, and sound processing. Although patient needs are the primary driving force behind implantable hearing devices, these concurrent technologic advancements borrowed from unrelated fields have been necessary to bring the vision of a few pioneering clinicians to fruition.

REFERENCES

1. Berger KW. *The Hearing Aid; Its Operation and Development*. Livonia, MI: National Hearing Aid Society; 1974.
2. Puharich AHK. Means for aiding hearing. United States; 1961.
3. Puharich AHK. Means for aiding hearing by electrical stimulation of the facial nerve system. United States; 1965.
4. Tjellstrom A, Hakansson B. The bone-anchored hearing aid. Design principles, indications, and long-term clinical results. *Otolaryngol Clin North Am*. 1995;28:53–72.
5. Goode R. An implantable hearing aid. *Trans Am Acad Ophth Otol*. 1969;74:128–139.
6. Yanagihara N, Aritomo H, Yamanaka N, Gyo K. Implantable hearing aid: report of the first human application. *Arch Otolaryngol Head Neck Surg*. 1987;113:869–872.
7. Yanagihara N, Sato H, Hinohira Y, Gyo K, Hori K. Long-term results using a piezoelectric semi-implantable middle ear hearing device: the rion device E-type. *Otolaryngol Clin North Am*. 2001;34:389–400.
8. Komori M, Yanagihara N, Hinohira Y, Hato N, Gyo K. Long-term results with the Rion E-type semi-implantable hearing aid. *Otolaryngol Head Neck Surg*. 2010;143:422–428.

9. Goode R, Glattke T. Audition via electromagnetic induction. *Arch Otolaryngol Head Neck Surg.* 1973;98:23–26.

10. Heide J, Tatge G, Sander T, et al. Middle ear implant: implantable hearing aids. In: Hoke M, ed. *Development of a Semi-immplantable Hearing Device.* Basel: Karger; 1988.

11. Tos M, Salomon G, Bonding P. Implantation of electromagnetic ossicular replacement device. *ENT J.* 1994;73:92–103.

12. Glorig A, Moushegian G, Bringewald R, Rupert AL, Gerken GM. Magnetically coupled stimulation of the ossicula chain: measures in kangaroo rat and man. *J Acoust Soc Am.* 1972;2:694–696.

13. Vernon J, Brummet R, Denniston R, Doyle P. Evaluation of an implantable type hearing aid by means of cochlear potentials. *Volta Review.* 1972;1:20–29.

14. Hough J, Vernon J, Johnson B, Dormer K, Himelick T. Experiences with implantable hearing devices and presentation of a new device. *Ann Otol Rhinol Laryngol.* 1986;95:60–65.

15. Hough J, Dyer K, Matthews P, Wood MW. Early clinical results: SOUNDTEC Implantable hearing device phase II study. *Laryngoscope.* 2001;111(1):1–8.

16. Roland PS, Shoup AG, Shea C, Richey HS, Jones DB. Verification of improved patient outcomes with a partially implantable hearing aid, the SOUNDTEC direct hearing system. *Laryngoscope.* 2001;111(10):1682–1686.

17. Gan RZ, Wood MW, Ball GR. Implantable hearing device performance measured by laser Doppler interferometry. *Ear Nose Throat J.* 1997;76:297–309.

18. Fraysse B, Lavieille J, Schmerber S, et al. A multicenter study of the vibrant soundbridge middle ear implant: early clinical results and experience. *Otol Neurotol.* 2001;22:952–961.

19. Kasic JF, Fredrickson JM. The otologics MET ossicular stimulator. *Otolaryngol Clin North Am.* 2001;34:501–513.

20. Jenkins HA, Niparko JK, Slattery WH, Neely JG, Fredrickson JM. Otologics middle ear transducer ossicular stimulator: performance results with varying degrees of sensorineural hearing loss. *Acta Otolaryngol.* 2004;124:391–394.

21. Volta A. On electricity excited by the mere contact of conducting substances of different kinds. *Phil Trans.* 1800.

22. Stevens SS. On hearing by electrical stimulation. *J Acoust Soc Am.* 1937;8:191–195.

23. Djourno A, Eyries C, Vallancien B. De l'excitation electrique du nerf cochleaire chez l'homme, par induction a distance, a l'aide d'un micro-bobinage inclus a demeure. *C R Soc Biol (Paris).* 1957;151: 423–425.

24. Eisen MD. Djourno, Eyries, and the first implanted electrical neural stimulator to restore hearing. *Otol Neurotol.* 2003;24: 500–506.

25. House WF. *Cochlear Implants: My Perspective.* Los Angeles, CA: World Wide Web, http://www.ears.com; 1995.

26. House WF. Cochlear implants: beginnings (1957–1961). *Otol Rhinol Laryngol.* 1976;1976:3–6.

27. Anonymous. California electronics firm readies "artificial ear" implant. *Space Age News.* 1961;3:1.

28. Anonymous. Electronics firm restores hearing with transistorized system in ear. *Space Age News.* 1961;21:1.

29. Simmons FB, Epley JM, Lummis RC, et al. Auditory nerve: electrical stimulation in man. *Science.* 1965;148:104–106.

30. Simmons FB. electrical stimulation of the auditory nerve in man. *Arch Otolaryngol Head Neck Surg.* 1966;84:2–54.

31. Michelson RP. The results of electrical stimulation of the cochlea in human sensory deafness. *Ann Otol Rhinol Laryngol.* 1971;80:914–919.

32. Michelson RP. Electrical stimulation of the human cochlea. *Arch Otolaryngol Head Neck Surg.* 1971;93:317–323.

33. Bilger RC, Black FO. Auditory prostheses in perspective. *Ann Otol Rhinol Laryngol.* 1977;86:3–10.

34. Schindler RA, Merzenich MM, White MW, Bjorkroth B. Multielectrode intracochlear implants. Nerve survival and stimulation

patterns. *Arch Otolaryngol Head Neck Surg.* 1977;103:691–699.

35. Schindler RA. The cochlear histopathology of chronic intracochlear implantation. *J Laryngol Otol.* 1976;90:445–457.

36. Hambrecht FT. In: Hambrecht FT, ed. *Functional Electrical Stimulation: Applicatons in Neural Prostheses.* New York, NY: Marcel Dekker Inc; 1977.

37. Clark GM, Black R, Dewhurst DJ, Forster IC, Patrick JF, Tong YC. A multiple-electrode hearing prosthesis for cochlea implantation in deaf patients. *Med Prog Technol.* 1977;15:127–140.

38. Cohen NL, Waltzman SB, Fisher SG. A prospective, randomized study of cochlear implants. The Department of Veterans Affairs Cochlear Implant Study Group. *N Engl J Med.* 1993;328:233–237.

39. Gantz BJ, Tyler RS, Knutson JF, et al. Evaluation of five different cochlear implant design: audiologic assessment and predictors of performance. *Laryngoscope.* 1988; 98:1100–1106.

40. Wilson BS, Finley CC, Lawson DT, Wolford RD, Eddington DK, Rabinowitz WM. Better speech recognition with cochlear implants. *Nature.* 1991;352:236–238.

41. Francis HW, Yeagle JD, Bowditch S, Niparko JK. Cochlear implant outcome is not influenced by the choice of ear. *Ear Hear.* 2005;26:7S–16S.

Chapter 2

Designing and Building a Cochlear Implant Program

LINDA S. BURG, DAVID FRIEDLAND, AND CHRISTINA RUNGE

INTRODUCTION

Over the past 30 years, cochlear implantation candidacy has significantly relaxed, from considering only patients with bilateral profound sensorineural hearing loss, to implanting patients with moderate to profound, and in some cases significantly asymmetric, hearing loss. This change has increased patient access to cochlear implants as a hearing rehabilitation option and placed greater demands on implant programs. Existing programs have seen patient volumes increase, and as a result programs are expanding rapidly as they aim to care for new patients in addition to the consistently increasing pool of already implanted patients. As such, starting a new cochlear implant program is a major endeavor for any facility or practitioner. Greater, and incrementally increasing, resources must be allocated to build these programs including financial support, physical plant space, and personnel. Further considerations include billing and insurance protocols, marketing, and ther-

apy services. Competing cochlear implant programs in the geographical area and the regional patient population are also important factors to consider.

This chapter serves as a guide to those deciding to start a cochlear implant program in their facility or office. Every practice and geographic location is different and the following information should be used as a guide, not an all-inclusive protocol.

GENERAL CONSIDERATIONS

Cochlear implants provide incredible benefit to those with hearing loss who have difficulty hearing despite using amplification. However, this benefit is not solely a product of the technology. Performance with a cochlear implant is reflective of the expertise of the implant team and involves appropriate preoperative evaluation, good surgical technique, and, most importantly, skilled programming and rehabilitation over long periods of time. Programs in which postimplant visits are limited to activation and perhaps one follow-up visit not only provide a disservice to the patient but are detrimental to the field. It is these patients that perpetuate a perception that implants "don't work well" and dissuade other patients and professionals from seeking implant services.

Without commitment to providing appropriate rehabilitation and programming services to patients after implantation, starting a program should be reconsidered. Likewise, an independent association between surgical and audiological services does not provide for optimal patient care. We strongly believe that an implant program needs to take an integrated team approach to patient care to ensure the best outcomes and maximize patient potential with the device.

PERSONNEL CONSIDERATIONS

A successful cochlear implant program is dependent on a team of professionals. Besides the implant surgeon and the audiologist, a program must include other professionals, and they should be experienced in working with the hearing-impaired population within their specialization. Deciding to have a cochlear implant is a lifelong commitment, and these patients will need care and services from the cochlear implant program staff for the remainder of their lives.

Team members will differ slightly depending on whether the program implants adults, children, or both. It is important to have the essential elements of the team in place before evaluating patients. Our program utilizes the following professionals:

Adult Implant Team

Surgeon

Audiologist

Speech-Language Pathologist

Nurse Practitioner

Psychologist

Pediatric Implant Team

Surgeon

Pediatric Audiologist

Audiology Technician (2nd tester)

Pediatric Speech-Language Pathologist

Pediatric Nurse Practitioner

Pediatric Psychologist

Social Worker

Educator

Audiologist

The audiologist is responsible for the cochlear implant evaluation, determining if the patient meets candidacy criteria, counseling the patient on potential outcomes, programming of the cochlear implant, and often performing aural rehabilitation. For children, the audiologist also supports the educational audiologist, as well as the educators. Depending on the size of the program, the audiologist may care for both adults and children.

Surgical support may also be the responsibility of the audiologist. Intraoperative measurement of electrode impedances, electrical compound action potentials, and electrical auditory brainstem responses may be performed to assist the surgeon in placement and to establish function of the device.

Speech-Language Pathologist

The speech-language pathologist is responsible for evaluating the patient's preimplant speech and language status, and often are the professionals who provide aural rehabilitation. For prelingual adult patients, the speech-language pathologist can also offer traditional SLP services.

For children, the speech-language pathologist evaluates the child before implantation, provides therapy to the child prior to surgery, and provides ongoing speech/language and often hearing therapy. The team speech-language pathologist also provides support to the school speech-language pathologist.

Nurse Practitioner

A nurse practitioner, or other physician extender, is another valuable team member. They can provide medical/postsurgical follow-up, respond to medical issues which may arise, and write prescriptions for replacement equipment (prescriptions are often required by insurance companies to replace broken components).

Psychologist

A psychologist is consulted for adults if unrealistic expectations are suspected. They may also be asked to evaluate the candidate if any other concerns arise during the evaluation process or if there is a history of psychological issues that may impact the postimplant performance.

For children, the psychological evaluation is often a mandatory part of the insurance protocol. The psychologist evaluates the child's developmental and emotional level, and provides support to the parents. The psychologist may also evaluate the family dynamic and parents' capacity

for providing the necessary home services needed after cochlear implantation.

Educator

Some insurance companies require an educator to be part of the team. The educator is responsible for any issues which may involve the child's classroom, teachers, school speech-language pathologist, and deaf educator. Some educators will perform school visits to determine if the child's needs are being met. Often, they will provide inservices to the school personnel to help in the child's transition from the hearing aid to the cochlear implant. The educator could be employed by the facility, or could be hired as a consultant.

Social Worker

A social worker provides support for families and patients. They assess the psychosocial functioning of patients and families. They connect families to necessary resources and support services in their community. They help families with financial and transportation issues that impact their health, and can also assist in some school-related issues.

Audiology Technician

An audiology technician can assist the implant audiologist in equipment troubleshooting, repairs and returns, device discussions, and can serve as the second tester for the pediatric implant audiologist when evaluating young children.

Administrative Assistant

A key component to a cochlear implant program is the administrative assistant, who is responsible for scheduling and coordinating patient appointments; triaging equipment and other patient issues; and facilitating communication between the patients, team members, and cochlear implant companies. As the initial point of contact for many prospective patients, this team member is the face of the cochlear implant program and interpersonal skills are important, as are organizational skills.

TEAM APPROACH SUMMARY

The integrated team approach is critical. All members on the team should be familiar with the roles of the other professionals. The counseling provided by individual team members should be consistent with the philosophy of the program. Patients and parents require a consistent message regarding all aspects of the implant and rehabilitative process. For many patients, hearing risks, benefits, and expectations consistently repeated by several team members is essential to ensuring compliance with the rigorous postimplant schedule and maximizing performance potential. We have found it is most effective to have regularly scheduled team meetings to discuss patient candidacy, troubleshoot complications, develop treatment plans, and evaluate program efficiency.

PHYSICAL PLANT

Specific space requirements are necessary to provide appropriate services. Sufficient space for an audiology booth is essential. The booth needs to be specially equipped to provide cochlear implant services. Although traditional audiological testing is completed under insert earphones, speech perception testing is completed

using speakers in a sound field (Fig 2–1A). For the pediatric population, the booth should also be equipped with a visual

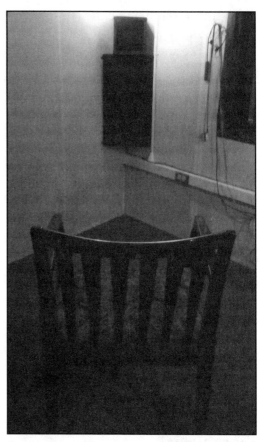

A

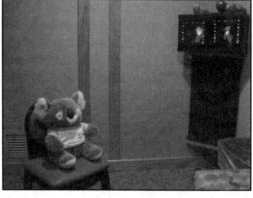

B

Figure 2–1. A. *Sound field configuration.* ***B.*** *Visual reinforcement system.*

reinforcement system (Fig 2–1B), and should be large enough to accommodate a high chair which can be very useful in testing younger children.

Postoperative programming of the cochlear implant should be in a quiet, car-

peted room equipped with a desk/table, a computer for the programming software, the interface boxes that connect the speech processor to the programming computer, and programming cables (Fig 2–2A). A carpeted room reduces ambient echo

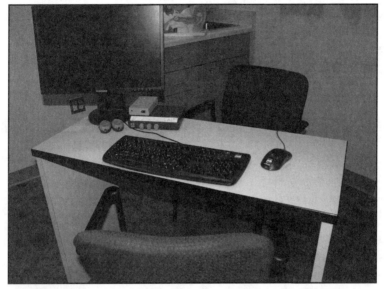

A

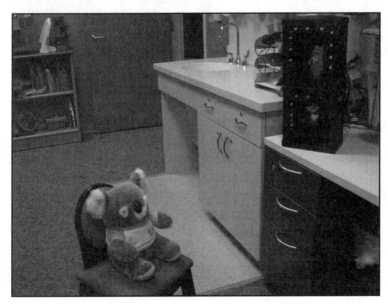

B

Figure 2–2. A. *Programming room configuration.* ***B.*** *Portable visual reinforcement system.*

and reverberation. Each implant manufacturer has designated software, designated interface boxes, and designated programming cables. Therefore, if offering more than one device, the space must be adequate to house all equipment and provide room for the audiologist, patient and family members. When programming young children outside of a sound room, you will need a portable visual reinforcement system (Fig 2–2B).

BUDGET CONSIDERATIONS

The startup budget for a new cochlear implant program should have sufficient funds to purchase the essential equipment for audiometric evaluation preimplantation and programming postimplantation (Table 2–1). Dedicated programming equipment for each manufacturer may be provided

Table 2–1. List of Basic Start-Up Equipment

Equipment	Purpose
2-Channel Audiometer	Hearing evaluation and speech perception testing
Tympanometer with Reflex Capability	Evaluate middle ear performance and perform electrical stapedial reflex measures following implantation
Auditory Brainstem Response with Electrical ABR capabilities	Objective hearing evaluation and electrical ABR testing
Otoacoustic Emissions	Evaluates outer hair cell function and useful to rule out Auditory Neuropathy Spectrum Disorder (ANSD)
Auditory Steady-State Response (optional)	Objective hearing evaluation in addition to the ABR
CD Player	Speech perception measures
Real-Ear System	Verification of hearing aids
Sound Level Meter	Calibration of equipment and CDs for speech perception measures
Visual Reinforcement System	For pediatric audiometry
Programming Computer	Programming of sound processors
Interface Boxes	Programming of sound processors
Troubleshooting Equipment	Troubleshooting of external implant equipment
Programming Cables	Programming of sound processors
Programmable Hearing Aids (2)	For cochlear implant evaluation process

by the company. It is also useful to have demonstration kits available for preoperative counseling and device selection discussions, and these are also typically provided by the companies (Figs 2–3A, 2–3B, 2–3C, and 2–3D).

INSURANCE CONSIDERATIONS

Coverage of cochlear implants varies with each insurance policy. Having an insurance/billing specialist available to the program is an asset. Often, the implant program will be associated with the same insurance providers contracting with the hospital, medical center, or private office from which they operate. Implant programs need to be aware of which insurance companies they are providers for and what types of services can be reimbursed. In some cases surgery may be covered but audiological services or equipment may be excluded.

INSURANCE COMPANIES AND PROVIDERS

Private Insurance

Many private insurance companies are managed care organizations (MCO) and include preferred provider organizations (PCOs) and health maintenance organizations (HMOs). Dependent on individual contracts with the provider, these organizations generally provide the highest reimbursement. Coverage varies, however, and is set up by the employer. As such, specific exclusions for cochlear implantation may be specified in the policy, and patients need to be counseled to read their policies carefully. Some private insurance may cover bilateral implants. When requesting bilateral implantation, it is often helpful to include a bibliography of resources which support bilateral cochlear implantation. One particularly relevant reference is the "International Consensus on Bilateral Cochlear Implants and Bimodal Stimulation" by Offeciers and colleagues.[1] We submit the following text and excerpt from the position statement to insurance companies when requesting approval for bilateral implantation:

> Binaural hearing is essential for understanding speech in the presence of background noise and under other listening conditions that are less than optimal such as speaker dialects, varying intensity levels, or varying acoustics. The International Consensus on Bilateral Cochlear Implants and Bimodal Stimulation states that, "binaural hearing allows listeners with normal hearing to understand speech better in silence and noisy conditions and is an essential requirement for spatial hearing and sound localization. Other benefits of binaural hearing are more natural hearing, reduced listening effort and an improved quality of life. It has been shown that binaural cochlear implantation restores fundamental aspects of binaural hearing and provides the binaural advantage experienced by normal hearing subjects."

Although some private insurance companies follow Medicare guidelines (see below), here is a general list of the information required for private insurance prior authorization:

➤ Cover letter describing a cochlear implant and the benefits
➤ Audiology report including the ear to be implanted
➤ Audiogram
➤ CT scan/MRI report

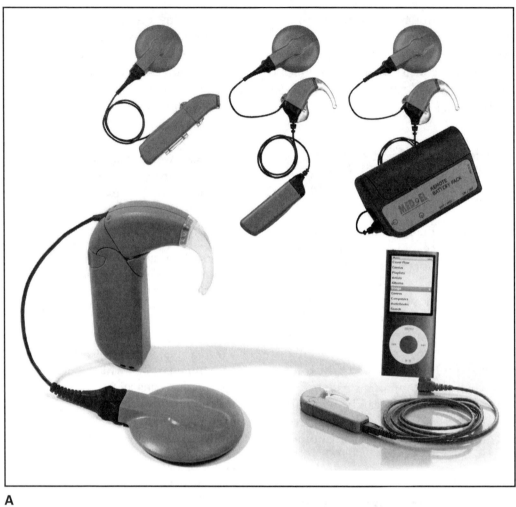

A

B

C

D

Figure 2–3. A. *MED-EL Demonstration Kit (Courtesy of MED-EL Corporation).* **B.** *Advanced Bionics Demonstration Equipment (Courtesy of Advanced Bionics).* **C** *and* **D.** *Cochlear Americas Demonstration Equipment (Courtesy of Cochlear Americas).*

➤ Physician report
➤ Cost estimate
➤ Speech-language report (if applicable)
➤ Social worker report (if applicable)
➤ Psychological report (if applicable)

Medicaid

Medicaid is a federal and state program for low income individuals.[2] A unique Medicaid provider number may be required, therefore this needs to be investigated with your state agency. Medicaid eligibility and coverage varies from state to state, as does the information required for cochlear implant approval. The following are Medicaid prior authorization guidelines:

➤ Specify which ear is to be implanted
➤ Submit the required standard forms
➤ Physician report
➤ Psychologist/social worker report— this is required by many states
➤ Audiologic report with audiogram
➤ Speech-language report
➤ Radiology report

All three cochlear implant manufacturers are Medicaid providers for some states. If your facility is not a DME (durable medical equipment) provider for Medicaid, the implant manufacturer may be able to provide the equipment and bill Medicaid on the patient's behalf if they are a Medicaid provider in your state.

In addition, there are State Children's Health Insurance Programs that are designed to provide insurance coverage for children whose families do not qualify for Medicaid, but who cannot afford private coverage.

Medicare

Medicare is a federal insurance program for persons 65 and older and Americans with severe disabilities.[3] As with Medi-

caid, all three implant manufacturers are Medicare DME providers and can bill insurance on the patient's behalf. Medicare reimburses audiologists for diagnostic services only, and does not reimburse audiologists for any therapy.

As of April 4, 2005, Medicare candidacy criteria were revised. Medicare coverage is provided only for those patients who meet all of the following selection guidelines[4]: Diagnosis of bilateral moderate-profound sensorineural hearing impairment with limited benefit, defined as open-set sentence recognition scores of less than or equal to 40% correct in the best-aided listening condition using prerecorded test materials with appropriate hearing (or vibrotactile) aids;

➤ Cognitive ability to use auditory clues and a willingness to undergo an extended program or rehabilitation;
➤ Freedom from middle ear infection, an accessible cochlear lumen that is structurally suited to implantation, and freedom from lesions in the auditory nerve and acoustic areas of the central nervous system;
➤ No contraindications to surgery; and
➤ The device must be used in accordance with the Food and Drug Administration (FDA)-approved labeling.

Note that if your patient has a Medicare replacement policy, the guidelines and coverage may be different (Table 2–2).

INSURANCE DENIALS

Some states have a mandatory law in effect that requires insurance companies to pay for cochlear implants for children 17 and under (Wisconsin) and up through age 21 (South Dakota).[5] However, self-funded insurance plans may be exempt

Table 2–2. Comparison of Insurance Coverage

	Coverage	Reimbursement	Exclusions	Manufacturer Billing
Private Insurance	Varies— Negotiated by the employer	Dependent on the contract between the insurance and the facility	May occur in the individual policies	External supplies may be billed by the manufacturer if the implant facility is not a DME provider. However, some private insurance will require the billing to be by the contracted facility. The manufacturer may be considered out of network
Medicaid	Varies between states	Generally low reimbursement	Varies between states	Consult the manufacturer regarding Medicaid Provider status
Medicare	Coverage is provided if they meet all the Medicare candidacy guidelines. Medicare will not provide prior authorization	Generally low reimbursement	None as long as the patient meets Medicare candidacy criteria	The manufacturers are Medicare DME providers

from these laws. If an exclusion exists, the patient may be able to negotiate an exception with the employer. If the denial states that the reason is experimental or not medically necessary, the patient should appeal and provide supporting documentation. If insurance denies coverage, and all appeals have been exhausted, consider exploring other options. Some procedures can be funded by local clubs (Lions, Lionesses) or through state funded programs such as the Division of Vocational Rehabilitation (Wisconsin).

Insurance coverage for the initial surgery and external equipment is only the first reimbursement obstacle to overcome when working with implant candidates. Throughout their entire life, patients will need to have their equipment replaced, repaired or upgraded. This equipment often falls under the DME category (Table 2–3). Patients must review their health insurance benefit or coverage of evidence book for information regarding coverage for DME.[6]

Once it is determined that DME is a covered benefit, the implant program submits to insurance for prior authorization. For this, most payors require a letter of medical necessity (LMN). The LMN would be written by the implant program, and would include the medical need for the requested equipment. Most equipment parts are considered medically necessary as long as they are needed for the sound processor to work. Some incidental parts

Table 2–3. Durable Medical Equipment (DME) Codes

Code	Equipment
L7510	Device Repair or replace minor parts
L8614	Cochlear Implant device all internal and external parts
L8615	Headset/Headpiece
L8616	Microphone
L8617	Transmitting Coil
L8618	Transmitter Cable
L8619	External speech processor and controller, integrated system
V5273	FM Assistive Listening Device, for use with CI
L8627	External speech processor, component, replacement
L8628	External controller, component, replacement
L8629	Transmitting coil and cable, integrated, for CI device, replacement
L8621	Zinc Air Batteries
L8622	Alkaline Batteries
L8623	Lithium Ion Batteries Body
L8624	Lithium Ion Batteries BTE

such as adaptor cables for personal listening devices may not meet the criteria for medical necessity and would have to be paid for by the patient.

Over the life of the implant, it is not uncommon for the external sound processor to become obsolete, thus no longer having parts available to maintain the device. When this occurs, the implant program would apply for a sound processor upgrade. As with most other items, each insurance plan differs as to when they will approve an upgrade for the patient. Some insurance plans have a 3- or 5-year rule, whereas others may require the obsolete processor to be broken before they will provide an upgrade for the patient. The patient or implant center would need to contact the individual insurance company to determine the current policy guidelines.

When working with Medicare, the state in which the manufacturer resides determines the upgrade criteria. Therefore, upgrade requirements will differ between the 3 manufacturers. MED-EL follows the rules in North Carolina, Cochlear Americas in Colorado, and Advanced Bionics in California.

CODING AND COCHLEAR IMPLANTS

All audiology, speech, and medical procedures have a corresponding CPT code. It is important to code correctly for preauthorization and services rendered to ensure reimbursement or approval. Provide the insurance company with a list of all of the procedures, codes, and fees. Codes for preimplant evaluation, the surgical procedure, programming over the first postoperative year, and further evaluations are noted in the accompanying tables (Tables 2–4 to 2–9).[3]

Table 2–4. Preimplant Evaluation Codes

Procedure	CPT Code
Comprehensive audiometry threshold evaluation and speech recognition	92557
Pure-tone audiometry threshold evaluation via air only	92552
Pure-tone audiometry threshold evaluation via air and bone	92553
Speech audiometry reception threshold evaluation	92555
Speech audiometry threshold evaluation with speech recognition	92556
Evoked otoacoustic emissions, limited	92587
Evoked otoacoustic emissions, diagnostic evaluation	92588
Tympanometry and reflex threshold measurements	92550
Acoustic immittance testing, includes tympanometry, acoustic reflex threshold testing and decay testing	92570
Tympanometry Only	92567
Acoustic Reflex Testing, threshold	92568
Auditory evoked potentials for evoked response audiometry and/or testing of the central nervous system; comprehensive	92585
Evaluation of auditory rehabilitation status, first hour	92626
Evaluation of auditory rehabilitation status, each additional 15 minutes	92627
Electroacoustic Evaluation/Binaural	92595
Hearing Aid Check/Binaural	92593
VRA-Visual Reinforcement Audiometry	92579
CPA-Conditioning Play Audiometry (threshold evaluation in children)	92582
Select Picture ID, threshold evaluation	92583
Speech-Language Evaluation—may only be provided by an SLP; Medicare will not pay audiologist for this code	92506
Otologic Evaluation	99244
CT Scan (facility fee)	70480
Radiologist's Fee	70480
Psychological Evaluation (2–3 hours)	90801/96101/ 96116/96118

Table 2–5. Surgical Codes

Procedure	CPT Code
Cochlear Device Implantation, with or without mastoidectomy	69930
Microsurgical techniques, requiring use of operating microscope	69990
Intraoperative neurophysiology testing, per hour	95920
Short latency somatosensory evoked potential study, simulation of any/all peripheral nerves or skin sites, recording from the central nervous system in the head	95927
Cochlear device, includes all internal and external components	L8614
Hospital Costs including anesthesia and operating room fees	

Table 2–6. First Year Postimplant Codes

Procedure	CPT Code/Pediatrics	CPT Code/Adults
Diagnostic analysis of cochlear implant, with programming	92601/92603*	92603
Diagnostic analysis of cochlear implant, subsequent reprogramming	92602/92604*	92604
Pure Tone Air/VRA/CPA; 2 wk, 1,2,3,6,9 month, and 1 year	92552/92579*/92582*	92552
Evaluation of auditory rehabilitation status, first hour; 1,3,6 month and 1 year	92626	92626
Evaluation of auditory rehabilitation status each additional 15 minutes, 1,3,6 month, and 1 year	92627	92627
Speech Threshold; 6 month and 1 year	92555	92555
Diagnostic analysis of cochlear implant, subsequent reprogramming; 2 wk, 1,2,3,6 month, and 1 year	92602/92604*	92604
Speech-Language Evaluation; 6 month and 1 year	92506	N/A
6 Month and 1 Year Otologic	99213	99213

*Codes/tests dependent on age and/or skill of child.

Table 2–7. Variable First Year Codes

Procedure	CPT Code	CPT Code/Adults
Auditory Rehabilitation Prelingual Hearing Loss, 60 minutes 5 sessions in the first year OR	92630*	92630*/92507
Auditory Rehabilitation Postlingual Hearing Loss, 60 minutes 5 sessions in the first year	92633*	92633*/92507

*Not payable by Medicare.

Table 2–8. Follow-Up Annual Evaluation and Programming Codes

Procedure	CPT Code
Evaluation of auditory rehabilitation status, 1st hour	92626
Evaluation of auditory rehabilitation status, ea additional 15 min	92627
Pure Tone Air/VRA/CPA	92552/92579*/ 92582*
Speech Threshold	92555
Programming	92602/92604*
Speech-Language Evaluation	92506
Otologic Evaluation	99213

*Codes/tests dependent on age and/or skill of child.

Coding Modifiers

Modifiers should be added to the code if the protocol for the procedure has not changed, but there were unusual circumstances. The most commonly used modifiers include[2]:

➤ 50 Bilateral procedure in the same operative session
➤ 51 Multiple procedure codes on the same claim
➤ 52 Reported CPT code is not fully performed or partially reduced
➤ 59 Two procedures are reported on the same date that are not typically performed together in a single visit

Payors have differing rules regarding the proper use of modifiers. You should consult individual payors to confirm their policies. Medicare has "edits" which do not allow specific code pairs to be billed on the same day. You should refer to the revised edits for cochlear implant programming on Medicare's Web site.

Table 2–9. Ongoing (After First Year) Codes

Procedure	CPT Code/Pediatrics	CPTCode/Adults
Auditory Rehabilitation Prelingual Hearing Loss, 60 minutes—OR	92630	92630*/92507
Auditory Rehabilitation Postlingual Hearing Loss, 60 minutes	92633	92633*/92507
Evaluation of auditory rehabilitation status, 1st hour	92626	92626
Evaluation of auditory rehabilitation status, ea additional 15 min	92627	92627
Pure Tone Air/VRA/CPA	92552/ 92579**/92582**	92552
Speech Threshold	92555	92555
Programming	92602/92604**	92604

*Not payable by Medicare.
**Codes/tests dependent on age and/or skill of child.

International Classification of Diseases, 10th Revision (ICD-10)

The implementation of the ICD-10 is set for October 1, 2013. This revision will replace the ICD-9 version currently used by speech/language pathologists, audiologists, physicians and other professionals for health care diagnosis. This revision will have additional codes. These additional codes will be available on the ICD Web site (http://www.cdc.gov/nchs/icd9.htm).[7]

MARKETING CONSIDERATIONS

Marketing plays an important role in the success of an implant program. Due to the uniqueness of cochlear implant candidacy, traditional marketing techniques such as broad audience advertising may not be effective. As patients may not be familiar with cochlear implants, marketing should primarily be geared toward professionals. Most patients are referred to a cochlear implant program by their own physician, an audiologist, a hearing aid specialist or an educator. Cochlear implant manufacturers dedicate most of their marketing resources to professionals.

When starting a program, attention should be given to local physicians, including internal medicine and family practice physicians, pediatricians and otolaryngologists. Host an open house, with a tour of the facility and an educational presentation. Discuss candidacy criteria.

Make arrangements to visit the area schools, and offer to provide an inservice to the teaching staff. Provide information on troubleshooting equipment, working with FM systems and give them aural rehabilitation ideas. Many educators have limited experience working with implanted children and welcome the guidance. Continuing to provide annual educational programs to the schools maintains the skills of the teaching staff, continues a positive relationship among professionals, and is therefore beneficial for the children.

Develop materials about your program to provide to the referral sources. Include the description of a cochlear implant, candidacy criteria, program highlights, team biographies, and information on how to make an appointment or contact the program. Include a map and directions.

A Web site including all pertinent information about your program is important, and is an ideal place to announce upcoming support groups, candidacy meetings, and other events. The program information packet and patient forms should be included and be easily downloadable. The Web site should be on page one for a local search. A professional Web designer is worth considering for Web site development. Other uses of Internet technology can also be useful such as social media Web sites, blogs, or chat groups. However, these need to be closely monitored by the implant team and must be in compliance with a facility's policies regarding use of these technologies.

Other marketing ideas include developing a professional brochure to distribute to referral sources; hosting a booth at a local conference; holding educational meetings for potential patients; and creating a newsletter directed toward current patients, potential patients, and professionals in your area. In addition, social events are an excellent way to support your current patients and to provide a forum for new candidates to meet current patients. Events could include picnics, coffee clubs or book clubs.

SUPPORT GROUP AND CANDIDACY MEETINGS

SUPPORT GROUPS

Adult and pediatric support group meetings provide a forum in which patients and families can interact with each other and with team members. Potential implant candidates and their family members can also attend, particularly if they are early in the discovery process and are seeking informal information and interactions with implant users. The format can include an invited guest speaker to cover a topic of interest before opening the session general discussion. Speakers may include professionals from the program or related specialties covering surgical, medical, educational, audiologic, and rehabilitation topics.

CANDIDACY MEETINGS

Candidacy meetings are somewhat more formal informational sessions directed at individuals who are considering cochlear implantation. The format for this meeting may begin with a brief presentation by team members that covers cochlear implant devices, surgery, recovery, programming, appropriate expectations, and specifics about the cochlear implant program. Following the presentation, a panel of current cochlear implant patients can share their individual stories of their implant experience, and then the floor opened for a question and answer period.

PATIENT EVALUATION PROTOCOL

The patient evaluation and treatment process requires a significant time commitment for both the patient and clinician. There are several preimplant visits and multiple postimplant visits, especially over the first year. A well-planned protocol is essential to maximizing efficiency for scheduling the audiologist's and other professional's time. This will allow for the most direct patient contact hours in each work day. It will also allow for scheduling of nonpatient contact hours for documentation and administrative duties.

In our program the typical adult pre- and postimplant evaluation and treatment protocol is described below.

SPEECH PERCEPTION TEST PROTOCOL FOR ADULTS

Create your test protocol to evaluate candidacy and to meet insurance requirements. Review standard test materials and determine which would work best for your program. The implant manufacturers provide CD's with current test materials. Keep abreast of candidacy changes, changes in test materials, and changes in test guidelines.

The recorded tests are presented in the soundfield at 60dB SPL(A) to represent loud but comfortable speech in quiet,[8] and at a +8 signal-to-noise ratio for the noise conditions. Preoperative testing

is completed with appropriately fit hearing aids for each ear individually and the binaural condition. Postoperative testing is performed for the cochlear implant and any other combination of bilateral or bimodal condition.

For adults who are unable to perform open-set tests, an alternative protocol should be developed to include closed set tests and less demanding open-set tests. These tests should be presented monitored live voice whenever possible.

FOLLOW-UP INTERVALS— ADULTS

Patients are seen at regular intervals for the first year. After the initial activation, patients are seen at 2 weeks, 1 month, 3 months, 6 months, 9 months, and 1 year. Speech perception testing is performed at all of the intervals after the 2-week programming session. A database with speech perception test scores helps track patients' progress over time. Following the 1st year, adults are seen annually with speech perception measures performed to monitor stability (Table 2–10).

SPEECH PERCEPTION TEST PROTOCOL FOR CHILDREN

As for adults, the pediatric tests are presented using recorded materials whenever possible and are presented at 60 dB SPL(A) in quiet[8] and a +8 S/N for noise conditions. Recorded materials may be difficult for young, inexperienced, or multiply involved children and speech perception testing may need to be performed using monitored live voice. Preoperative testing is completed with appropriately fit

Table 2–10. Adult Evaluation Protocol

	Preimplant	2 Weeks Post	1 Month Post	3 Months Post	6 Months Post	1 Year Post and Annually
Basic Comprehensive Audiometry	X					
Tympanometry and Reflex Testing	X					
Otoacoustic Emissions	X					
Auditory Brainstem Evaluation	X—as needed					
Audiogram		X				X
Speech Perception Hearing aid/s	X					
Speech Perception CI			X	X	X	X
Speech Perception CI + HA				X	X	X
CT Scan	X					
Medical/Surgical Evaluation/Consult	X			X		
Psychological Evaluation	X—as needed					

28

hearing aids for each ear individually and the binaural condition whenever possible. Postoperative testing is performed for the cochlear implant and any other combination of bilateral or bimodal condition.

FOLLOW-UP INTERVALS— CHILDREN

Children are seen at regular intervals for the first year. After the initial activation, children are seen at 2 weeks, 1 month, 3 months, 4 months, 6 months, 9 months, and 1 year. Outcome measures (questionnaires and speech perception tesing) are performed beginning at 3 months. Speech and language evaluations are also included at least annually or more often depending on the needs of the child. Children are seen twice a year up to 3 years of implant use, and annually thereafter. A database with speech perception and subjective auditory skill development scores tracks the child's progress over time (Table 2–11).

ASSISTIVE LISTENING DEVICES

The implant program should be equipped to provide patient and educators with information on how to use their sound processor with assistive listening devices. FM systems are compatible with current sound processors, but educators must be informed on each child's equipment needs. Phone devices are also very effective tools to use with sound processors. Guidelines and recommendations exist for all types of technology, including stethoscopes, Bluetooth devices, and music players (IPod, MP3) (Figs 2–4A, 2–4B, and 2–4C).

AURAL REHABILITATION

ADULT AR

Aural rehabilitation facilitates the adjustment to a cochlear implant and enhances the benefits. Hearing is maximized by providing listening tools, therapy techniques, and goals for hearing. An evaluation is performed to identify the patient's communication needs and communication difficulties. Expectations for improvement are also assessed. Hearing abilities are assessed with the cochlear implant in both an ideal quiet situation, and in more challenging noise environments. A treatment plan is developed based on the individual's skills and needs. The number of sessions is dependent on the treatment plan and patient logistics. Some patients will prefer a self-directed home program. This is especially useful for patients who live far from the clinic.

Care must be taken in deciding who will offer these services. Some insurances, such as Medicare will not reimburse aural rehabilitation services if performed by an audiologist (as of January 2011). If a speech pathologist offers the therapy, they should be experienced in working with the hearing impaired population.

PEDIATRIC AR

Aural rehabilitation is key in helping the child interpret the sounds in the environment and use the information in a meaningful way to understand and acquire spoken language. Aural rehabilitation will optimize the benefit the child receives from the cochlear implant through intensive therapy.

Table 2–11. Pediatric Evaluation Protocol

	Preimplant	2 Weeks Postactivation	1 Month Postactivation	3 Months Postactivation	6 Months Postactivation	1 Year Postactivation and Biannually for 3 Years Postimplant
Basic Comprehensive Audiometry	X					
Tympanometry and Reflex Testing	X					
Otoacoustic Emissions	X					
Auditory Brainstem Evaluation	X—as needed					
Speech/Language Evaluation	X					X
Audiogram		X				X
Speech Perception Hearing aid/s	X					
Speech Perception CI			X	X	X	X
Speech Perception CI + HA				X	X	X
MRI	X					
CT Scan	X					
Medical Evaluation/ Consult	X			X		
Social Work Consult	X					
Psychological Evaluation	X—as needed					

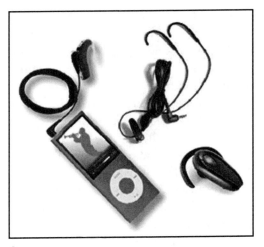

A

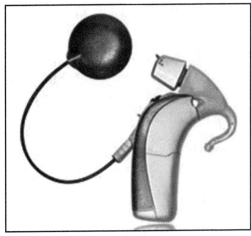

C

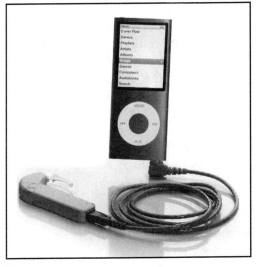

B

Figure 2–4. A. Cochlear Americas assistive listening device examples (Courtesy of Cochlear Americas). *B.* MED-EL Corporation assistive listening device example (Courtesy of MED-EL Corporation). *C.* Advanced Bionics assistive listening device example (Courtesy of Advanced Bionics).

The child's speech and language should be assessed prior to implantation to identify the child's communication needs, communication difficulties and the parent's expectations for improvement. The therapist should collaborate with the child's intervention and/or school staff to ensure that the child is receiving appropriate services before and after implantation. The therapist should also work with the family to determine which communication option and educational placement are best for the child. The team educational consultant should work with the family and school intervention staff to develop child-focused treatment plans. Therapy plans are individualized and vary from child to child.

Most pediatric AR is performed by the speech/language pathologist, but an audiologist could also perform this service. Attention should be given to the type of insurance and the requirements of the person performing the rehabilitation.

There are many resources for obtaining aural rehabilitation curriculums. The manufacturer Web sites offer thorough lesson plans that could be included in the therapy program.

Cochlear Americas Web site:

HOPE

HOPE "Notes" Music Program

Advanced Bionics Web site:

The Listening Room

Tune Ups Music Program

MED-EL Corporation:

Bridge to Better Communication

Soundscape: Interactive Listening Activities

MAXIMIZING EFFICIENCY

The preimplant audiologic evaluation typically requires 2 to 3 hours of testing. The audiogram, objective tests, and all speech perception testing are completed during this evaluation. For young children, 2 or more appointments may be needed to obtain all necessary information.

Postoperatively, the initial activation typically takes 2 to 3 hours for adults or children. Impedances are measured, and threshold and comfort levels are measured on most, if not all electrodes. External equipment must be reviewed.

After the initial activation, the follow up appointments can take anywhere from 1 to 2 hours, and include program-

ming and, at certain intervals, speech perception measures. Often, the implant audiologist is managing the contralateral hearing aid, and the patient may require optimization of the hearing aid.

As reimbursement for cochlear implant programming is typically poor, manufacturers have created programming protocols that expedite implant programming.[9] The streamlined approaches involve measuring only a few electrodes in an array, and interpolating for the rest of the electrodes.

Depending on the interval, programming may be completed alone, or programming and speech perception testing may be done. Again, to reduce time, measurements could be taken on certain electrodes and interpolated (over time, all the electrodes should be physically measured). Some clinics prefer to see patients for shorter time intervals, but over a course of 2 days (1 hour per day for 2 days). This may be more appropriate for young children who cannot sit for the longer sessions. Keep in mind that for very young children, 2 testers are needed: the pediatric audiologist, and a second tester such as another audiologist or an audiology technician.

Depending on your clinic's goals, speech perception testing may be limited to performance with implant alone. This would reduce the speech perception test time for adults to approximately 20 minutes, and if the patient is not having any problems, could limit the follow-up appointments to 1 to 1.5 hours. However, if the audiologist is also supporting the hearing aid, or if the patient is a bilateral implant user, the test time would be longer. In any case, be prepared to have longer audiologic appointment times for cochlear implant patients.

Acknowledgments. We thank Ryan Odorizzi for providing technologic assistance with the figures. This work was supported by NIDCD K23DC008837 (PI: Runge).

REFERENCES

1. Offeciers E, Morera C, Müller J, Huarte A, Shallop J, Cavallé L. International consensus on bilateral cochlear implants and bimodal stimulation. *Acta Otolaryngol.* 2005 Sep;125(9):918–919. Belgium. PMID: 16109670.

2. 2010 Application module for audiology/module six in the series of coding reimbursement, and advocacy modules. http://icohere-presentations.com/presentations/ASHA2010/06-ModuleSix/player.html

3. 2011 Medicare fee schedule and hospital outpatient prospective payment system for audiologists. Retrieved December 30, 2010 from http://www.asha.org/practice/reimbursement/medicare/feeschedule

4. CMS Web site. Retrieved from http://www.cms.hhs.gov/Transmittals/downloads/R601CP.pdf and http://www.cms.hhs.gov/Transmittals/downloads/R42NCD.pdf

5. Boswell S. (2009, July 14). Wisconsin passes insurance mandate: audiologists help win coverage for children's cochlear implants, hearing aids. *ASHA Leader.*

6. 2011 HCPCS: Level II National Codes.

7. ICD Web site at http://www.cdc.gov/nchs/icd9.htm

8. Firszt JB, Holden LK, Skinner MW, et al. Recognition of speech presented at soft to loud levels by adult cochlear implant recipients of three cochlear implant systems. *Ear Hear.* 2004;25:375–387.

9. Wolfe J, Schafer EC. *Programming Cochlear Implants—A Volume in the Core Clinical Concepts in Audiology Series.* San Diego, CA: Plural Publishing Inc; 2010.

Chapter 3

Electrode Design for Cochlear Implantation

CHARLES G. WRIGHT AND PETER S. ROLAND

INTRODUCTION

The multichannel electrode array is an essential component of present-day cochlear implant systems. These devices deliver electrical stimulation to spatially distinct neural structures inside the inner ear in a tonotopically appropriate manner. This is accomplished using a series of metal contacts linearly arranged on a flexible silicone carrier inserted along the cochlear spiral. The carrier also encloses fine wires connecting each of the contacts to a receiver/stimulator unit located outside the inner ear. The array thus provides an electrical interface between the electronics package of the implant and neural tissues of the cochlea. This chapter begins with a brief discussion of general principles relating to electrical stimulation using neural prostheses and then moves on to more specific consideration of contemporary electrode design.

ELECTRICAL STIMULATION AND COCHLEAR IMPLANTS

Extracellular neural stimulation has become a powerful technique for restoration of function in patients who have suffered sensory or motor loss. Neural prostheses affect sensory or motor activity by changing transmembrane potentials within targeted nerve cells, thereby affecting information transmission. Although stimulation paradigms must be adapted for use in specific organs, electrical stimulation generally operates by delivering a controlled amount of electrical charge via current or voltage generators to one or more metal electrodes located in the central or peripheral nervous system. Responses obtained from electrical stimulation depend in part on the biological properties of tissues between the electrodes and the targeted neurons and on the geometric disposition of the neural elements being stimulated. Current supplied by an active electrode will spread, taking various paths through tissue to the return electrode. For a given current strength, current spread will depend on the resistivity, homogeneity, and anisotropy of the conductive medium. (For example, current will flow preferentially through fluids rather than through bone or fibrous tissue.) The electrical stimulus tends to cause many neurons to fire synchronously. This is due in part to the fact that most electrodes are larger than the neural elements they are intended to stimulate, a factor particularly relevant to stimulation delivered by intracochlear electrode arrays.

In the case of devices designed for electrical stimulation of the cochlea, the term "electrode" is vague and can be used to refer to individual contacts on the array, the entire array, to the lead connecting the array to the receiver-stimulator unit or the combination of all three. The term "electrode array" refers to the distal part of the device that carries the electrode contacts and is inserted into the cochlea.

As used on an implant array, an electrode "contact" is a metal plate placed in an ionic fluid (ie, one containing charged particles or ions such as Na^+, Cl^-, K^+, etc.). When electric current is applied to the contact, it causes an ionic current to flow toward or away from the contact (depending on the polarity of the current). The current flow causes potential (voltage) changes within the immediate fluid environment of the electrode. In this case, the electrode acts as a transducer: it converts a current based on electron movements in the metal contact into an ionic current in the surrounding fluid. No transfer of electrons takes place between the contact and the fluid.

In order to drive a current (ionic in fluids or electrons in metallic structures) the active electrode must always have another electrode paired with it. The second paired electrode is referred to as a "ground," "return," "indifferent," or "neutral" electrode. The ground electrode is usually much larger and is preferably placed in a region where sensory tissues are absent (under the temporalis muscle, or example, or on top of the stimulator housing in typical cochlear implants). When current is applied to an electrode placed in the inner ear it flows across all tissue between it and the ground electrode, with the pattern of flow determined by the resistivity and other characteristics of the intervening tissues. An alternative arrangement is occasionally employed in which the ground electrode is another electrode on the cochlear array (in such cases, the electrodes on the array can function alternately as active or ground electrodes). Theoretically, such an arrangement would limit current flow to those tissues between the two electrodes and allow for more selective stimulation. In practice, however, this type of stimulation (called "bipolar stimulation") has not proven useful and is rarely employed. An electrode can also sense or detect a potential (voltage). Such potentials may be produced by an adjacent active electrode or they may be biologically generated in surrounding tissues. "Sensing" electrodes are now available on some cochlear implant arrays and are used to determine the stimulus threshold by detecting a neural response to stimulation.

Multichannel electrode arrays for cochlear stimulation are made using a medical grade silicone carrier that encloses thin (usually 25-micron bare diameter) Teflon or Parylene insulated platinum-iridium wires. Platinum is used because it is resistant to corrosion and iridium is added to increase tensile strength. The wires are welded to platinum plates (the electrode contacts) that are partially exposed to the cochlear fluids. Platinum is the best choice for electrostimulation in a biological medium because the metal is extremely inert. The relatively large surface area of the electrode contacts insures a low current density at each contact surface and also allows current to flow against less resistance, thus requiring less input from the stimulator. Partial isolation of the metal from body tissue is achieved by recessing the platinum contacts in the silicone carrier, resulting in any array without sharp edges and reduced friction during insertion into the cochlea. The metal contacts provide the necessary transduction of electronic current generated by the implant to ionic current that flows through surrounding fluid to depolarize adjacent neural structures, giving rise to action potentials in the cochlear nerve.

COCHLEAR IMPLANT ELECTRODE DESIGN

Commercially available electrode arrays differ in overall size and shape and in the number, spacing and size of electrical contacts positioned on the carrier. There has been increasing focus on details of array design in an effort to maximize effectiveness and efficiency of stimulation and to reduce insertional trauma during surgical placement. Design features intended to reduce the potential for trauma have become especially important given current emphasis on hearing preservation in patients who may be candidates for combined electrical and acoustic stimulation.

A major aspect of array design relates to how electrode contacts are positioned in relation to the modiolus. So-called perimodiolar arrays are fabricated in a pre-curved shape that permits placement of contacts near the modiolus where spiral ganglion cells are located. On the other hand, straight arrays are engineered to rest against the lateral wall of scala tympani immediately under the basilar membrane where their contacts are farther from the modiolar wall. Both approaches to electrode placement have their advantages and disadvantages as discussed below.

An important parameter of either type of array is the electrode extent, or distance between the first and last electrode contact. Typically, this distance may be anywhere from 15 to 27 millimeters. The total length of the array can be altered for lateral wall or perimodiolar placement inside scala tympani. Straight lateral wall arrays require a greater length for complete cochlear coverage and may be inserted up to 760 degrees. Perimodiolar arrays are shorter because placement along the medial wall of the cochlea is only possible for a maximum of 360 to 420 degrees; the modiolus becomes too thin above that point to accommodate an array without danger of fracturing and the spiral ganglion, which is the focus of stimulation, extends through only about 1¾ turns of the cochlea.

Along with the length of the array, the number of contacts defines the degree of contact separation. Wider contact spacing reduces channel interaction between adjacent electrodes, but also reduces the number of channels available. An array placed closer to the ganglion cells in the modiolus also reduces channel interaction. Contemporary electrode arrays offer both options: more numerous channels close to the modiolus over one cochlear turn, or fewer channels with greater contact separation over two turns. Both options work well with modern processing strategies. The interrelated parameters of electrode extent, contact separation and insertion depth relative to implant function have been discussed by Hochmair et al.[1]

Because of their closer proximity to the spiral ganglion, the contacts on perimodiolar arrays are theoretically more efficient and more selective for focused stimulation of ganglion cells, potentially providing lower current thresholds and reduced channel interaction for improved frequency discrimination. As lower current levels are possible with these devices, they may be more energy efficient and permit longer battery life.[2–4]

Perimodiolar arrays are molded to a curved shape so that they can coil around the modiolus. However, these arrays must be held straight during the initial phase of insertion to allow entry through the facial recess and a cochleostomy and to prevent inappropriate curling in the lower basal part of scala tympani. This is usually accomplished by use of a metal stylet. Prior to insertion, the malleable stylet is inserted into the silicone carrier in order to straighten the array at the time it is introduced into the cochlea. The array may then be fully inserted, after which the stylet is withdrawn to permit the precurved array to coil around the modiolus.[5] Alternatively, the stylet can be held immobile and the array "pushed off" the stylet. That is, after insertion of the array to the first major curvature of the basal turn, it is pushed off the stylet, allowing the array to regain its precurved shape and coil close to the modiolus as it moves upward in scala tympani. This "off the stylet" approach to insertion has been shown to facilitate reliable perimodiolar placement and reduce the incidence of intracochlear trauma associated with placement of these arrays.[6,7] Another

strategy for perimodiolar placement has been to utilize a space-occupying positioner which is usually inserted with the array that pushes the contacts toward the modiolus. These devices are, however, relatively large, require a larger cochleostomy, and can exert considerable pressure against the lateral wall, basilar membrane, and osseous lamina resulting in severe trauma.[8,9] Their use has also been associated with an increased incidence of otogenic meningitis.[10] They therefore are not in current use.

Overall size is also an issue with arrays requiring a stylet because the lumen necessary to accommodate the stylet inside the carrier increases the diameter of the array, making it more likely that there will be upward displacement and/or rupture of the basilar membrane or fracture of the osseous spiral lamina at some point during the insertion process.[11] The larger size of these arrays also makes them less suited for round window insertion because it is often more difficult to steer the array past the boney rim of the round window and into the midportion of scala tympani.[12] This difficulty can be overcome by drilling the anterior-inferior margin of the round window. However, drilling potentially increases the extent of trauma, compromising the theoretical advantage of a "pure" round window insertion for atraumatic electrode placement.

Our experience with perimodiolar electrode array insertion in human temporal bones has shown that electrode contacts along the length of the array are rarely at a uniform distance from the modiolus after insertion is complete. Often, a portion of the array lies against the lateral wall of scala tympani where contacts are relatively far from the modiolar wall. The probability that a portion of the array will "bow" outward to take a more lateral position is greater if the array is overinserted, past the recommended insertion depth. In areas of the cochlea where a relatively large, perimodiolar array is in direct contact with the lateral wall (Fig 3–1), it may compress the delicate tissues of the spiral ligament immediately beneath the basilar membrane, resulting in trauma and possible occlusion of venous blood vessels that drain the lateral wall structures[13] (Fig 3–2). In addition, during the initial phase of perimodiolar electrode insertion the array is held straight and is relatively rigid so that its tip may strike and injure the lateral wall or basilar membrane before the stylet is withdrawn (Fig 3–3). The basal turn of the normal human cochlea is variable in size[14,15] and, as shown by Rebscher et al,[16] accurate estimation of the appropriate depth of initial insertion is challenging due to sizable variations in the distance between the cochleostomy and the beginning of the first major curvature of the basal cochlear turn. (This distance varied between 4.6 and 8.2 mm in a series of 62 temporal bones included in their study.)

The possibility of modiolar injury is another risk associated with implantation of perimodiolar arrays. If the tip of the array impinges on the modiolar wall or if the body of the device is pushed into

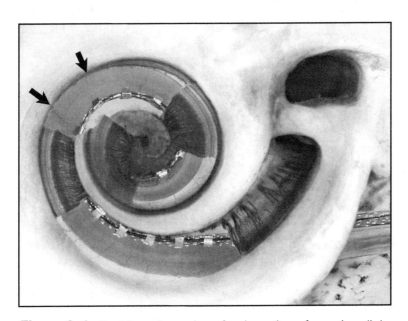

Figure 3–1. *Cochlear dissection after insertion of a perimodiolar electrode array. Portions of the osseous spiral lamina and basilar membrane have been removed to show the array inside scala tympani. The silicone carrier has been stained to improve contrast. The array shows close perimodiolar positioning in the basal turn. However, in the area indicated by arrows it is in direct contact with the lateral wall, potentially traumatizing the spiral ligament and/or basilar membrane. Reproduced with permission from Roland PS, Wright CG. Surgical aspects of cochlear implantation: mechanisms of insertional trauma. Adv Otorhinolaryngol. 2006;64:11–30.*

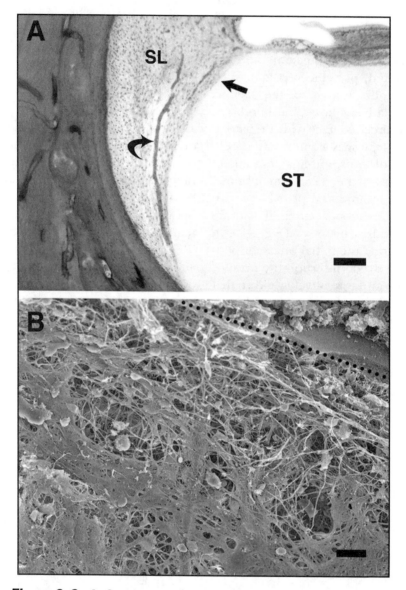

Figure 3–2. A. Cochlear cross-section showing the lower portion of the spiral ligament (SL) facing scala tympani (ST). The curved arrow indicates a venule coursing through the spiral ligament toward the floor of scala tympani. The straight arrow indicates the portion of the spiral ligament seen in B. The ligament and its vasculature are vulnerable to trauma by electrode arrays positioned against the lateral wall of scala tympani. Scale bar = 100 microns. **B.** Scanning electron micrograph of the surface of the spiral ligament in the area immediately below the attachment of the basilar membrane. The site of attachment of the basilar membrane to the lateral wall tissues is indicated by the dotted line. Note the highly porous, meshlike structure of the spiral ligament surface, which is susceptible to electrode array penetration and injury. Scale bar = 20 microns. Reproduced with permission from Roland PS, Wright CG. Surgical aspects of cochlear implantation: mechanisms of insertional trauma. Adv Otorhinolaryngol. 2006;64:11–30.

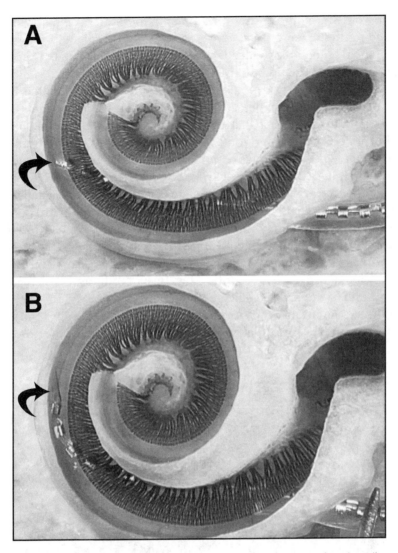

Figure 3–3. *Cochlear dissection showing initial phase of perimodiolar array insertion before withdrawal of the stylet. In this preparation the apical turn has been removed to provide an unobstructed view of the basal portion of the cochlea.* **A.** *After introduction into scala tympani the tip of the array (arrow) contacts the lateral wall immediately beneath the basilar membrane.* **B.** *As the array is advanced its tip impales the spiral ligament tissue (arrow) and pulls it inward, toward the modiolus. Continued advancement of the array may result in extensive damage of lateral wall tissues and blood vessels.*

contact with the modiolus by a positioner it may fracture the fragile bone overlying the spiral ganglion, resulting in ganglion cell injury and/or increased risk of meningitis due to wider communication between the perilymphatic and cerebrospinal fluid compartments as a result of the injury. Vascular injury can also occur because veins on the modiolar wall are often exposed to the lumen of scala tympani, making them vulnerable to mechanical trauma[13] (Fig 3–4). In addition, perimodiolar arrays may damage the modiolus should it be necessary to explant the devices. This is due to the fact that the array will be pulled into tighter contact with the modiolus as it is withdrawn from the inner ear. It might be noted, however, that when explantation is necessary months or years after initial placement, a connective tissue sheath may be present around the array that might reduce the probability of modiolar injury. On the other hand, precurved arrays require extra force to uncoil the shaped silicone carrier during explantation which could disrupt the fibrous sheath, so that reim-

plantation in the original sheath may not be possible. Explantation/reimplantation trauma is an especially important issue for children who may require multiple reimplantions over a lifetime. In those patients, intracochlear damage might preclude or limit the possible use of devices to be developed in the future or application of new therapies to encourage sensorineural regeneration in the inner ear. Finally, there is a potential for modiolar trauma associated with pulling a perimodiolar array back after insertion in order to draw the contacts closer to the modiolus, a procedure recently advocated by Basta, Todt, and colleagues[17]; such a maneuver must be done with caution.

Cochlear Ltd is currently developing a new perimodiolar electrode array (the

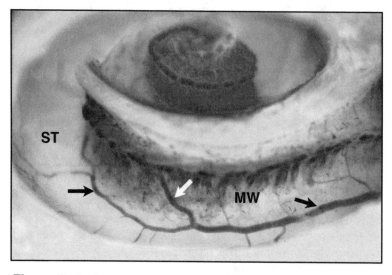

Figure 3–4. Cochlear dissection showing veins associated with the modiolus. The osseous lamina and basilar membrane have been removed to view the floor of scala tympani (ST) and modiolar wall (MW). The white arrow indicates a vein coursing down the modiolar wall to join the posterior spiral vein (black arrows). These superficially positioned vessels are vulnerable to injury by perimodiolar electrode arrays. Reproduced with permission from Roland PS, Wright CG. Surgical aspects of cochlear implantation: mechanisms of insertional trauma. Adv Otorhinolaryngol. 2006;64:11–30.

Modiolar Research Array or MRA) that does not require a stylet and is therefore thinner and more flexible, less likely to produce trauma, and potentially suitable for round window insertion.[18] Such new designs hold promise for significantly reducing intracochlear injury associated with this type of array.

Straight electrode arrays designed to track the lateral wall of scala tympani generally do not pose a risk to the modiolus or spiral ganglion. These arrays are also thinner and more flexible, making them less likely to rupture the basilar membrane or fracture the osseous spiral lamina. Some straight arrays, particularly those offered by MED-EL GmbH, are also longer, allowing them to reach apical regions of the cochlea for more effective stimulation of low-frequency neurons. There is, in fact, some evidence that more deeply inserted straight arrays positioned to selectively stimulate surviving dendrites in the osseous lamina of the apical cochlear turn may provide improved speech recognition.[1,19] This is because stimulation of the more apical dendrites that are arranged in a planar fashion in the osseous lamina theoretically offers more tonotopically specific neural activation than direct stimulation of the upper portion of the spiral ganglion where ganglion cells representing a wider frequency range are densely packed together, making it more difficult to selectively activate small numbers of cells that carry low frequency information. Ideally, a longer array with somewhat wider spacing of contacts distributed over the whole length of the cochlea should also provide better overall performance, including reduced channel interaction to provide improved frequency discrimination.[1,19,20] At present, however, there is ongoing discussion regarding the positive and negative

aspects of deep electrode insertion. Not all investigators are in agreement and the subject is a complex one, as documented in the recent review by Boyd.[21]

Longer arrays that track the lateral wall also carry with them a substantial risk of trauma. That is partly because a greater area of contact with the lateral wall is associated with higher frictional forces during deep insertion,[22] which can lead to bucking of the array in the lower basal turn, producing spiral lamina fractures and elevation and/or tearing of the basilar membrane (Fig 3–5).

Trauma to lateral wall structures is one of the most commonly reported types of implant insertional injury.[9,11,23] Although lateral wall trauma may occur with all types of arrays, it appears to be somewhat more common with those designed for lateral wall placement because of their more extensive contact with the outer wall of scala tympani. As the arrays are advanced during insertion, their tips may strike the spiral ligament beneath the basilar membrane and penetrate the ligament, dissecting their way upward immediately adjacent to the cochlear duct (Fig 3–6). This type of injury appears to be more likely in the upper cochlear turns where the volume of scala tympani decreases and the radius of curvature of the outer wall is such that the tip of an advancing array may strike at an angle that encourages soft-tissue penetration. Scanning electron microscopic studies have shown that the surface of the spiral ligament facing scala tympani is a delicate, porous meshwork of connective tissue that may be especially vulnerable to penetration by a fine-tipped electrode array[13] (see Fig 3–2B). Once an array enters that tissue, it tends to move upward and displace the cochlear duct toward the modiolus, often leading to

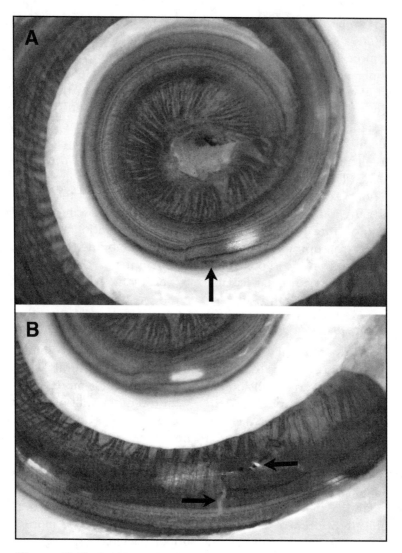

Figure 3–5. *Cochlear dissection showing an insertion in which the tip of the array met resistance in the middle turn and elevated the basilar membrane in the area indicated by the arrow in **A**. Although elevated, the basilar membrane remained intact. In this preparation the apical cochlear turn has been removed to provide an unobstructed view. Because the tip was blocked, continued effort to advance the array caused it to buckle in the lower basal turn, which fractured the osseous lamina in the area indicated by the arrows in **B**. Reproduced with permission from Roland PS, Wright CG. Surgical aspects of cochlear implantation: mechanisms of insertional trauma.* Adv Otorhinolaryngol. *2006;64:11–30.*

basilar membrane injury and tearing of Reissner's membrane, allowing intermixing of perilymph and endolymph. As mentioned above, spiral ligament trauma is also likely to injure and/or occlude blood vessels of the lateral cochlear wall, which

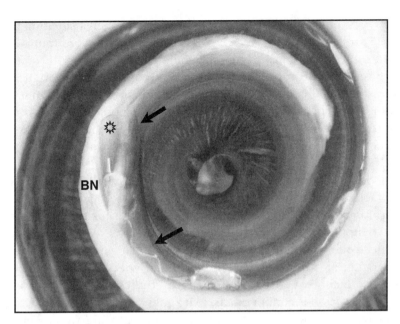

Figure 3–6. *Cochlear apex after an insertion in which the tip of an array (star) penetrated the spiral ligament below the basilar membrane and dissected its way between the ligament and surrounding otic capsule bone (BN) to reach a position above the basilar membrane and lateral to the cochlear duct. The array elevated the basilar membrane and displaced the cochlear duct toward the modiolus in the area between the arrows. Reproduced with permission from Roland PS, Wright CG. Surgical aspects of cochlear implantation: mechanisms of insertional trauma.* Adv Otorhinolaryngol. *2006;64:11–30.*

may compromise blood flow to the spiral ligament and stria vascularis, tissues that are of major significance for maintenance of cochlear fluid homeostasis.

New design modifications of straight electrode arrays continue to be developed and show promise for use in patients in whom hearing preservation is a primary goal. Examples are the Nucleus Hybrid L[24] and Straight Research Array (SRA)[25] from Cochlear Ltd., the FLEX [EAS] array from MED-EL GmbH,[26] and the Thin Lateral array from Advanced Bionics Corporation.[27] These arrays are thin and highly flexible and are suitable for a range of insertion depths using either a round window or cochleostomy approach. A design feature

for increasing the flexibility of electrode arrays, used particularly by MED-EL, is to fold the wires inside the silicone carrier into a zigzag or accordion-like pattern. Shaping the connecting wires in that manner significantly reduces the insertion force necessary for array placement, thereby reducing the potential for trauma.[20]

In recent years considerable effort has also focused on development of short arrays, specifically designed for limited basal turn placement in patients who may benefit from combined acoustic and electrical stimulation. These devices are intended to reduce trauma, making preservation of residual low-frequency hearing more likely while providing stimulation of high frequency neurons in the lower basal cochlear turn.[28,29]

The region of the first major curvature of the basal turn at approximately 180 degrees is especially susceptible to trauma from both perimodiolar and straight electrode arrays. Scala tympani of the human cochlea is three-dimensionally complex and is variable in its morphology between individuals. Because of a combination of factors involving curvature, variations in upward slope, and narrowing of scala tympani in the 180-degree region,[30,31] electrode arrays may deviate upward and penetrate the basilar membrane near its attachment to the spiral ligament. If the insertion is continued, the array will traverse the cochlear duct and enter scala vestibuli where it may twist or fold back on itself so that the tip of the array is oriented in a basal direction

(Fig 3–7). In such a situation the array not only produces severe trauma, but comes to lie in a position poorly suited for effective, frequency-appropriate stimulation of neural structures in either the osseous lamina or modiolus. As has been emphasized by Rebscher et al.[16] modifications of the mechanical properties of electrode arrays to limit "vertical" flexibility (ie, deviation toward the basilar membrane) appears to be beneficial for reducing the incidence of this type of trauma.

Research continues on efforts to define the ideal length of future arrays for optimal speech reception performance. The studies of Stakhovskaya and colleagues[32] have provided valuable information regarding frequency distribution along the length of the human spiral ganglion. These frequency mapping studies indicate that the tip of an ideal array

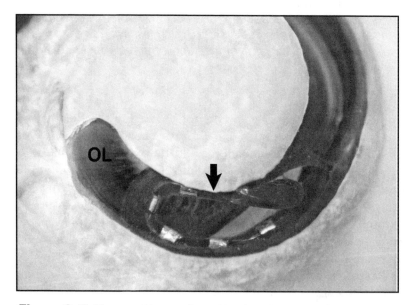

Figure 3–7. *Temporal bone dissection in which the basal cochlear turn has been opened to reveal a previously inserted electrode array. During insertion the array breached the basilar membrane/osseous lamina (OL), and moved upward, striking the bony roof of scala vestibuli (arrow) and then doubled back on itself.*

would need to be located at about 540 degrees around the cochlear spiral, or about 1.5 turns, in order to most effectively stimulate neurons responsible for the first formant frequencies of speech, which lie between 200 and 1200 Hz. Most arrays in current use do not reach that depth of insertion, which may compromise their performance due to mismatch between the frequency band locations assigned to each implant channel and the tonotopic organization of the spiral ganglion adjacent to the sites of electrical stimulation.[16] It is expected that as safer arrays are developed, electrode placements can be better optimized to match the tonotopic characteristics of cochlear neurons targeted for stimulation.

Thanks in large part to the introduction of new implant designs and improved surgical techniques for implantation, the population of patients for whom cochlear implantation is indicated continues to expand rapidly. This includes patients with ossified cochleas and those with various inner ear anomalies and malformations. Manufacturers such as MED-EL GmbH and Cochlear Ltd now offer double branch arrays for cases where ossification prevents insertion of a standard array and specially designed arrays for individuals with various cochlear malformations.[33]

In addition to performance improvements relating to stimulus delivery and hearing preservation, future arrays are likely to incorporate new features, such as the capability for intracochlear drug administration. Various design strategies for arrays capable of sustained drug delivery over a significant portion of the cochlear spiral are currently being explored.[20,34] These devices offer the possibility of delivering anti-apoptotic, anti-inflammatory, or neurotrophic agents in a controlled manner that may facilitate hearing preservation and

enable more effective interfacing of electrode contacts with neural structures.

As noted above, there are theoretical advantages to placing electrode contacts closer to dendrites or ganglion cells of the auditory nerve. Closer proximity to neural structures permits better stimulus selectivity and would allow more stimulus channels to be placed on an array because contact size can be smaller, limiting current spread and allowing stimulation of smaller numbers of neurons, thereby increasing frequency resolution. Efforts are underway to develop new approaches for reducing the distance between electrodes and target neurons without increased risk of trauma. One such strategy involves use of pharmacological agents to support the survival of existing dendrites in the osseous lamina or to promote regeneration of ganglion cell dendrites and guide them into direct contact with implanted electrode arrays.[35] As discussed by O'Leary et al,[4] formidable challenges must be resolved before such methods can be employed in the clinical setting, but they offer promise for significantly improved outcomes in future implant recipients.

REFERENCES

1. Hochmair I, Arnold W, Nopp P, Jolly C, Muller J, Roland P. Deep electrode insertion in cochlear implants: apical morphology, electrodes and speech perception results. *Acta Otolaryngol.* 2003;123:612–617.
2. Balkany TJ, Eshraghi AA, Yang N. Modiolar proximity of three perimodiolar cochlear implant electrodes. *Acta Otolaryngol.* 2002;122:363–369.
3. Wackym PA, Firszt JB, Gaggl W, Runge-Samuelson CL, Reeder RM, Raulie JC. Electrophysiologic effects of placing cochlear

implant electrodes in a perimodiolar position in young children. *Laryngoscope.* 2004;114:71–76.

4. O'Leary SJ, Richardson RR, McDermott HJ. Principles of design and biological approaches for improving the selectivity of cochlear implant electrodes. *J Neural Eng.* 2009;6:055002.

5. Briggs RJS, Tykocinski M, Saunders E, et al. Surgical implications of perimodiolar cochlear implant design: avoiding intracochlear damage and scala vestibuli insertion. *Cochlear Implants Int.* 2001;2: 135–149.

6. Stover T, Issing P, Graurock G, et al. Evaluation of the advance off-stylet insertion technique and the cochlear insertion tool in temporal bones. *Otol Neurotol.* 2005; 26:1161–1170.

7. Fraysse B, Ramos Macias A, Sterkers O, et al. Residual hearing conservation and electroacoustic stimulation with the Nucleus 24 Contour Advance cochlear implant. *Otol Neurotol.* 2006;27:624–633.

8. Tykocinski M, Cohen LT, Pyman BC, et al. Comparison of electrode position in the human cochlea using various perimodiolar electrode arrays. *Amer J Otol.* 2000;21: 205–211.

9. Wardrop P, Whinney D, Rebscher SJ, Luxford W, Leake P. A temporal bone study of insertion trauma and intracochlear position of cochlear implant electrodes. II: Comparison of Spiral Clarion™ and HiFocus II™ electrodes. *Hearing Res.* 2005;203: 54–67.

10. Reefhuis, J, Honein MA, Whitney CG, et al. Risk of bacterial meningitis in children with cochlear implants. *N Engl J Med.* 2003;349:435–445.

11. Wardrop P, Whinney D, Rebscher SJ, Roland JT, Luxford W, Leake PA. A temporal bone study of insertion trauma and intracochlear position of cochlear implant electrodes. I. comparison of Nucleus banded and Nucleus Contour™ electrodes. *Hearing Res.* 2005;203:54–67.

12. Souter MA, Briggs RJS, Wright CG, Roland, PS. Round window insertion of precurved perimodiolar electrode arrays: how successful is it? *Otol Neurotol.* 2010;32:58–63.

13. Roland PS, Wright CG. Surgical aspects of cochlear implantation: mechanisms of insertional trauma. *Adv Otorhinolaryngol.* 2006;64:11–30.

14. Escude B, James C, Deguine O, Cochard N, Eter E, Fraysse B. The size of the cochlea and predictions of insertion depth angles for cochlear implant electrodes. *Otol Neurotol.* 2006;11(suppl 1):27–33.

15. Erixon E, Hogstorp H, Wadin K, Rask-Andersen H. Variational anatomy of the human cochlea: implications for cochlear implantation. *Otol Neurotol.* 2009;30:14–22.

16. Rebscher SJ, Hetherington A, Bonham, B, Wardrop P, Whinney D, Leake PA. Considerations for design of future cochlear implant electrode arrays: electrode array stiffness, size, and depth of insertion. *J Rehab Res Dev.* 2008;45:731–748.

17. Basta D, Todt I, Ernst A. Audiological outcome of the pull-back technique in cochlear implantees. *Laryngoscope.* 2010; 120:1391–1396.

18. Briggs RJ, Plant KL, Tykocinski M, Risi F, Xu J, Cowan RS. *Insertion studies and clinical outcomes with the prototype Modiolar Research Array (MRA) cochlear implant.* Abstracts, 11th International Conference on Cochlear Implants and Other Implantable Auditory Technologies. Stockholm, Sweden, 2010.

19. Hamzavi J, Arnoldner C. Effect of deep insertion of the cochlear implant electrode array on pitch estimation and speech perception. *Acta Otolaryngol.* 2006;126:1182–1187.

20. Jolly C, Garnham C, Mizadeh H, et al. Electrode features for hearing preservation and drug delivery strategies. *Adv Otorhinolaryngol.* 2010;67:28–42.

21. Boyd PJ. Potential benefits from deeply inserted cochlear implant electrodes. *Ear Hear.* 2011;32(2)(Epub ahead of print.)

22. Adunka O, Kiefer J. Impact of electrode insertion depth on intracochlear trauma. *Otolaryngol-Head Neck Surg.* 2006;135: 374–382.

23. Nadol JB, Burgess BJ, Ketten DR, et al. Histopathology of cochlear implants in humans. *Ann Otol Rhinol Laryngol.* 2001; 110:883–891.

24. Lenarz T, Stover T, Buechner A, et al. Temporal bone results and hearing preservation with a new straight electrode. *Audiol Neurotol.* 2006;11(suppl 1):34–41.

25. Skarzynski H, Podskarbi-Fayette R. A new cochlear implant electrode design for preservation of residual hearing: a temporal bone study. *Acta Otolaryngol.* 2010; 130:435–442.

26. Adunka O, Kiefer J, Unkelbach MH, Lehnert T, Goesttner W. Development and evaluation of an improved cochlear implant electrode design for electric acoustic stimulation. *Laryngoscope.* 2004;114:1237–1241.

27. Wright CG, Roland PS, Kuzma J. Advanced Bionics Thin Lateral and Helix II electrodes: a temporal bone study. *Laryngoscope.* 2005;115:2041–2045.

28. Roland JT, Zeitler DM, Jethanamest D, Huang TC. Evaluation of the short hybrid electrode in human temporal bones. *Otol Neurotol.* 2008;29:482–488.

29. Woodson EA, Reiss LA, Turner CW, Gfeller K, Gantz BJ. The hybrid cochlear implant: a review. *Adv Otorhinolaryngol.* 2010;67: 125–134.

30. Verbist BM, Ferrarini L, Briaire JJ, et al. Anatomic considertions of cochlear morphology and its implications for insertion trauma in cochlear implant surgery. *Otol Neurotol.* 2009:30:471–477.

31. Biedron S. Prescher A, Ilgner J, Westhofen M. The internal dimensions of the cochlear scalae with special reference to cochlear electrode insertion trauma. *Otol Neurotol.* 2010;31:731–737.

32. Stakhovskaya O, Sridhar D, Bonham BH, Leake PA. Frequency map for the human cochlear spiral ganglion: implications for cochlear implants. *J Assoc Res Otolaryngol.* 2007;8:220–233.

33. Roland, JT, Huang TC, Fishman, AJ. Cochlear implant electrode history, choices, and insertion techniques. In: Roland JT, Waltzman SB, eds. *Cochlear implants.* 2nd ed. New York, NY: Thieme; 2006:110–125.

34. Hendricks JL, Chikar JA, Crumling MA, Raphael Y, Martin D. Localized cell and drug delivery for auditory prostheses. *Hearing Res.* 2008;242:117–131.

35. Evans AJ, Thompson BC, Wallace GG, et al. Promoting neurite outgrowth from spiral ganglion neuron explants using polypyrrole/BDNF-coated electrodes. *J Biomed Mater Res A.* 2009; 91:241–250.

Chapter 4

Signal Processing Strategies for Cochlear Implants

BLAKE S. WILSON AND MICHAEL F. DORMAN

INTRODUCTION

Three large steps were needed to produce the present-day cochlear implants (CIs): (1) the pioneering step to implant the first patients and to develop devices that were safe and had a life span of many years; (2) the development of devices that provided multiple sites of stimulation in the cochlea to take advantage of the tonotopic organization of the auditory system; and (3) the development of highly effective processing strategies that utilized the multiple sites of stimulation and supported for the first time high levels of speech recognition for most users of CIs. Findings from the now-classic "Bilger Study" in 1977[1]—and from the 1988 and 1995 NIH Consensus Statements on Cochlear Implants[2,3]—summarize the status of CIs at each of these steps. Principal conclusions from the Bilger study and the two consensus statements are presented in Table 4–1. As noted there, especially large gains in performance were obtained in step 3.

Today, most recipients of CIs can converse with ease in quiet acoustic environments and even using their cell phones.

The restoration of function possible with a present-day CI is remarkable and far surpasses that of any other neural prosthesis. The CI is now widely regarded as one of the major advances of modern medicine.

Despite this success, and despite further substantial gains in performance that have been achieved since the major step 3 in the list above, problems remain with CIs. Patients with the best results still do not hear as well as persons with normal hearing in all situations, such as speech presented in competition with noise or other talkers. Users of standard unilateral CIs do not have much access to music and other sounds that are more complex than speech. In addition and most importantly, a wide range of outcomes persists even with the current processing strategies and implant systems. That is, patients may score almost anywhere in the range of possible scores in tests of speech reception that are more difficult than high-context sentences presented in quiet conditions. Also, a small proportion of patients have low scores even for the relatively easy tests.

The primary aim of this chapter is to describe the designs of the processing strategies now in widespread use. In addition, speech reception and other data

Table 4–1. Major Indicators of Progress in the Development of Cochlear Implants

Persons or Event	Year	Comment or Outcome
Bilger et al	1977	"Although the subjects could not understand speech through their prostheses, they did score significantly higher on tests of lipreading and recognition of environmental sounds with their prostheses activated than without them." (This was an NIH-funded study of all 13 implant patients in the United States at the time.)
First NIH Consensus Statement	1988	Suggested that multichannel implants were more likely to be effective than single-channel implants, and indicated that about 1 in 20 patients could carry out a normal conversation without lipreading. (The world population of implant recipients was about 3,000 in 1988.)
Second NIH Consensus Statement	1995	"A majority of those individuals with the latest speech processors for their implants will score above 80% correct on high-context sentences, even without visual cues." (The number of implant recipients approximated 12,000 in 1995, and the number exceeded 220,000 in early 2011.)

are presented to indicate strengths and weaknesses of the present approaches. Possibilities for improvements in processing strategies also are presented. In broad terms, great progress has been made in the development of processing strategies for CIs, but at the same time considerable room remains for improvement.

PROCESSING STRATEGIES FOR UNILATERAL COCHLEAR IMPLANTS

All CI systems now in widespread use include multiple channels of sound processing and multiple sites of stimulation along the length of the cochlea. The aim of these systems is to mimic at least to some extent the "place" or "tonotopic" representation of frequencies in the normal cochlea, that is, by stimulating electrodes near the basal end of the cochlea to indicate the presence of sound components at high frequencies and by stimulating electrodes closer to the apical end to indicate the presence of sound components at lower frequencies.

At present, the largest manufacturers of implant devices include Advanced Bionics Corp of Valencia, California, USA; Cochlear Ltd of Lane Cove, Australia; and MED-EL GmbH of Innsbruck, Austria. Together these three have more than 99% of market share for CIs.

The processing strategies used in conjunction with each of these devices are listed in Table 4–2. The strategies include the continuous interleaved sampling (CIS),[4]

Table 4–2. Processing Strategies in Current Widespread Use*

Manufacturer	CIS	CIS+	HDCIS	n-of-m	FSP	ACE	SPEAK	HiRes	HiRes 120
MED-EL GmbH	•	•	•	•	•				
Cochlear Ltd	•					•	•		
Advanced Bionics Corp	•							•	•

*Manufacturers are shown in the left column and the processing strategies used in their implant systems are shown in the remaining columns. The full names of the strategies are presented in the text.

CIS+,[5,6] "high definition" CIS (HDCIS),[6,7] *n*-of-*m*,[8] advanced combination encoder (ACE),[9] spectral peak (SPEAK),[10] HiResolution (HiRes),[11] HiRes with the Fidelity 120 option (HiRes 120),[12,13] and fine structure processing (FSP)[14] strategies. As shown in Table 4–2, each manufacturer offers multiple strategies. Among these choices, FSP recently supplanted CIS+ or HDCIS as the default strategy for the MED-EL devices (CIS+ and HDCIS are implemented with different hardware "platforms," as explained below); HiRes and HiRes 120 are each used frequently with the Advanced Bionics devices; and ACE is the default choice for the Cochlear Ltd devices.

In the remainder of this section, we describe the principal features of these various strategies. Further detailed (but in some cases somewhat less current) information about the strategies is presented in comprehensive reviews by Loizou,[15] Wilson,[16,17] Wilson and Dorman,[18] and Zeng et al.[19] These reviews also present information about prior strategies, potential new strategies on the horizon, and other parts of CI systems including the transcutaneous transmission link, the implanted receiver/stimulator, and the implanted electrode array. As emphasized in several of the reviews, all parts of the system are important and the processing strategy functions (or fails to function well) in the context of the other parts.

CIS, CIS+, HDCIS, AND HIRES

One of the simpler and most effective approaches for representing speech and other sounds with the present-day CIs is illustrated in Figure 4–1. This is the CIS strategy, which is used as a processing option for all of the implant systems now in widespread use and is the basis for other strategies, as described later in this chapter.

The CIS strategy filters input sounds into bands of frequencies with a bank of bandpass filters. Envelope variations in the different bands are represented at corresponding electrodes in the cochlea with modulated trains of biphasic electrical pulses. The envelope signals may be extracted from the bandpass filters using a rectifier followed by a low-pass filter (or by other means; see below). The signals are compressed with a nonlinear mapping function prior to the modulation, to map the wide dynamic range of audible sounds in the environment (about 100 dB) into the much narrower dynamic range of electrically evoked hearing (stimulus levels needed for eliciting loud percepts with electrical pulses typically are only 10 dB higher than the levels needed for eliciting threshold percepts). The output of each bandpass channel is directed to a single electrode, with channels with low-to-high center frequencies assigned to apical-to-basal electrodes, to mimic at least the order, if not the precise locations, of frequency mapping in the normal cochlea. The pulse trains are interleaved in time, so that the pulses across channels and the associated electrodes are nonsimultaneous. This eliminates a principal component of electrode interaction, which otherwise would be produced by direct vector summation of the electric fields from different (simultaneously stimulated) electrodes. (Other interaction components are not eliminated with the interleaving, but those components are generally much lower in magnitude than the principal component that results from the summation of the electric fields.[20]) The corner or "cutoff" frequency of the

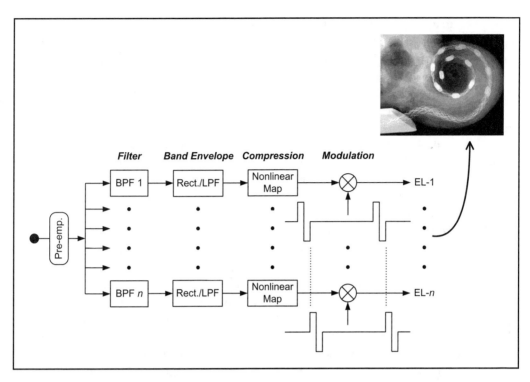

Figure 4–1. *Block diagram of the continuous interleaved sampling (CIS) strategy. The input is indicated by the filled circle in the left-most part of the diagram. This input can be provided by a microphone or alternative sources. Following the input, a pre-emphasis filter (Pre-emp.) is used to attenuate strong components in speech below 1.2 kHz. This filter is followed by multiple channels of processing. Each channel includes stages of bandpass filtering (BPF), envelope detection, compression, and modulation. The envelope detectors generally use a full-wave or half-wave rectifier (Rect.) followed by a low-pass filter (LPF). A Hilbert Transform or a half-wave rectifier without the LPF also may be used. Carrier waveforms for two of the modulators are shown immediately below the two corresponding multiplier blocks (circles with an "X" mark within them). The outputs of the multipliers are directed to intracochlear electrodes (EL-1 to EL-n), via a transcutaneous link or a percutaneous connector. The inset shows an X-ray micrograph of the implanted cochlea, to which the outputs of the speech processor are directed. (Block diagram is adapted with permission from Wilson BS, Finley CC, Lawson DT, Wolford RD, Eddington DK, Rabinowitz WM. Better speech recognition with cochlear implants. Nature. 1991;352:236–238. Copyright 1991 Nature Publishing Group. Inset is reproduced with permission from Hüttenbrink KB, Zahnert T, Jolly C, Hofmann G. Movements of cochlear implant electrodes inside the cochlea during insertion: an x-ray microscopy study. Otol Neurotol. 2002;23:187–191. Copyright 2002 Lippincott Williams & Wilkins.)*

low-pass filter in each envelope detector usually is set at 200 Hz or higher, so that the fundamental frequencies of voiced speech and other periodic sounds are represented in the modulation waveforms. The frequency range spanned by the bandpass filters typically begins at a frequency near or slightly above the cutoff frequency of the low-pass filters in the envelope detectors and ends at a frequency near or somewhat above the highest frequencies included in speech. The idea is that extension of the lower boundary to lower frequencies is unnecessary and indeed possibly redundant, because those lower frequencies already are represented in the timing variations of the modulation waveforms. In one implementation of CIS, for example, 12 bandpass filters span the range from 250 to 8500 Hz, and the frequency boundaries (and the center frequencies) for the filters are distributed along a logarithmic scale, which mimics the logarithmic mapping of frequencies for most of the extent of the cochlear partition in normal hearing.

Pulse rates in CIS processors typically approximate or exceed 1000 pulses/s/electrode, for an adequate "sampling" of the highest frequencies in the modulation waveforms (a "four times" oversampling rule usually is applied, for example, for a 200-Hz cutoff frequency for the low-pass filters in the envelope detectors, a pulse rate of at least 800 pulses/s/electrode is used[21-23]). CIS gets its name from the continuous sampling of the (compressed) envelope signals by rapidly presented pulses that are interleaved across electrodes. As many as 22 channels and associated stimulus sites have been used in CIS implementations to date, although speech reception scores generally do not increase with increases in the number of channels beyond 4 to 8, for the CIS and the other strategies in current widespread use.[21,24-27]

The CIS+, HDCIS, and HiRes strategies are close variations of CIS. The CIS+ strategy is implemented in the MED-EL TEMPO+ processor, and the HDCIS strategy is implemented in the newer MED-EL OPUS 1 and OPUS 2 processors. Each of these strategies use a Hilbert transform to derive the envelope signals for each bandpass channel, instead of a rectifier

followed by a low-pass filter. The Hilbert transform may provide a better representation of the envelope variations in the band.[5] In addition, the CIS+ and HDCIS strategies use bandpass filters with bell-shaped response patterns in the frequency domain, with substantial overlaps in responses between filters with adjacent center frequencies. These patterns differ from other implementations of CIS, in that other implementations use bandpass filters or Fast Fourier Transform (FFT) processing with relatively sharp cutoffs beyond the corner frequencies and with less overlap in responses between adjacent filters. The filters with the bell-shaped (or, more ideally, triangular shaped) frequency responses may produce a more uniform magnitude of the summed outputs of adjacent filters (and channels) when the frequency of a sinusoidal input is varied between the center frequencies of the filters. This in turn may provide a "smoother" and more salient representation of the intermediate frequencies compared with filters with sharp cutoffs and little overlap in responses between adjacent filters, as discussed in detail by Nobbe et al[6] and as discussed further in the subsection below on the FSP strategy.

The HDCIS strategy differs from the CIS+ strategy in two respects. First, a refined design is used for the "front end" processing in the OPUS 1 and OPUS 2 hardware platforms, prior to the pre-emphasis filter in the block diagram of Figure 4–1. The design includes a substantially larger dynamic range of the amplifiers and other electronics in the input stages (providing an input dynamic range of 75 dB), and improvements in the (dual loop) automatic gain control for bringing the analog input signal into the best range for the subsequent digital processing. Thus, HDCIS may have a better input signal to "work with" compared to

CIS+ and most likely other implementations of CIS that use different hardware and therefore different input processing.

In addition, the OPUS 1 and OPUS 2 processors in conjunction with the implant systems that utilize them support aggregate rates of stimulation across electrodes up to 50,704 pulses/s, whereas the TEMPO+ processor and the earlier MED-EL COMBI 40+ system support rates up to 18,180 pulses/s. Thus, a further potential advantage of HDCIS over CIS+ is that HDCIS may use much higher stimulation rates.

HiRes is a CIS strategy that uses relatively high rates of stimulation and up to 16 processing channels and associated stimulus sites. For nonsimultaneous stimulation across 16 electrodes, the rate at each electrode can be as high as about 2900 pulses/s (producing an aggregate rate of about 46,400 pulses/s). In addition, the HiRes strategy uses the averaged output of a half-wave rectifier for envelope detection, instead of a rectifier and low-pass filter. The averaging operation produces a signal that is similar to the signal that would be produced with a low-pass filter. The HiRes strategy is identical in overall design compared with other implementations of CIS, but uses a somewhat different approach for envelope detection (which produces outputs that are highly similar to those produced with a half-wave rectifier followed by a low-pass filter) and can support in some instances a higher maximum rate of stimulation or a higher maximum number of channels and associated stimulus sites compared with the other implementations.

In general, implementations of CIS can vary widely among and even within implant systems. Some of the differences among implementations include: (1) the quality of the front-end processing; (2) the quality of the current source(s) in the implanted receiver/stimulator; (3) the range and res-olution of the current outputs; (4) how the bandpass filtering is accomplished, either with FFT processing or with discrete filters; (5) the characteristics of the frequency response for each of the bandpass filters, for example, the spacing of the center frequencies for the filters and whether each filter has a rectangular or bell-shaped response; (6) the quality of the filter implementations as determined by the digital word length and other factors; (7) the way in which the envelope signals are derived; (8) the exact shape and range of the nonlinear mapping function; (9) the rate of stimulation at each electrode; (10) the number of channels and electrodes; (11) the order in which the electrodes are stimulated for each frame of stimulation; and (12) the positions of the electrodes within the cochlea, including the extent of the cochlear "tonotopic map" spanned by the electrodes, the interelectrode spacing, and the proximity of the electrodes to excitable tissue. Additional differences specific to comparisons of CIS as implemented in the Cochlear Ltd devices versus CIS as implemented with other devices are presented and discussed in Kiefer et al.[9] Those authors emphasize that "as implementations (eg, for CIS) can vary considerably between different implant systems, the present results can be interpreted only in relation to the Nucleus CI 24M cochlear implant system." (Kiefer et al compared the performances of the CIS, ACE, and SPEAK strategies, as implemented in Cochlear Ltd's Nucleus CI 24M cochlear implant system.) Any of the aforementioned differences among implementations may affect performance. Thus, great caution should be used when interpreting results from various comparisons of CIS versus other (basic) strategies, or from comparisons of CIS or CIS-like strategies between different implant systems or even within systems but using different parameter values or filtering approaches. Indeed, as Kiefer et al suggest, comparisons in some cases are not warranted at all because the implementations are so very different. Conservative approaches in comparing processing strategies for CIs are either to: (1) attend to comparisons between or among strategies implemented on the same hardware and holding everything constant beyond the strategy changes, or (2) choose the best results among the various implementations of each of the comparison strategies as representative of each strategy's true potential.

N-OF-M, ACE, AND SPEAK

The *n*-of-*m*, ACE, and SPEAK strategies derive stimulus pulses in the same way as the CIS strategies, that is, each channel of processing includes a bandpass filter, an envelope detector (or its equivalent), a nonlinear mapping function, and a multiplier (or modulator). In addition, all the strategies use nonsimultaneous pulses for the stimuli.

The principal difference between the *n*-of-*m*, ACE, and SPEAK strategies on the one hand, and the CIS strategies on the other hand, is that the former strategies each use a channel selection scheme in which the envelope signals are "scanned" prior to each frame of stimulation across the intracochlear electrodes, to identify the signals with the *n*-highest amplitudes from among *m* processing channels and their associated electrodes. The parameter *n* is fixed in the *n*-of-*m* and ACE strategies; that parameter can vary from frame to frame in the SPEAK strategy, depending on the level and spectral composition of the signal from the microphone or other input source. Stimulus rates typically approximate or exceed 1000 pulses/s/ selected electrode in the *n*-of-*m* and ACE

strategies, and they approximate 250 pulses/s/selected electrode in the SPEAK strategy. (This choice was initially guided by the fact that the transcutaneous transmission link of the implant system initially used with SPEAK could not support rates of stimulation much higher than 250 pulses/s/electrode, for six electrodes in each stimulus frame.) The basic designs of the *n*-of-*m* and ACE strategies are identical, although the details of the implementations vary among implant systems. In addition, these strategies are quite similar to CIS except for the channel selection feature. The SPEAK strategy uses much lower rates of stimulation and an adaptive *n*, as noted above. Perhaps somewhat curiously, the strategy retains the 200 Hz cutoff frequency for the low-pass filters in the envelope detectors, even though the pulse rates at each of the selected electrodes approximate 250 pulses/s. This combination breaks the "4 times" rule and is likely to produce distortions in the representations of the modulation waveforms (see the final paragraph in this subsection for a discussion of speech recognition with the ACE and SPEAK strategies).

The channel selection or "spectral peak picking" scheme used in the *n*-of-*m*, ACE, and SPEAK strategies is designed in part to reduce the density of stimulation while still representing the most important aspects of the acoustic environment. The exclusion of channels with low-amplitude envelope signals for each frame of stimulation may reduce the overall level of masking or interference across electrodes and excitation regions in the cochlea. To the extent that the excluded channels do not contain significant information, such "unmasking" may improve the perception of the input signal by the patient. In addition, for positive speech-to-noise ratios (S/Ns), selection of the channels with the highest envelope signals in each frame may emphasize the primary speech signal with respect to the noise.

A further potential advantage of the spectral peak picking strategies is that the reduced number of pulses per frame of stimulation (compared with the CIS and CIS-like strategies) may allow higher pulse rates, use of broader duration pulses, savings in power consumption (by holding the rate constant and thereby reducing the number of pulses presented per unit of time), or some combination of these possible attributes. The use of broader duration pulses may be especially helpful among these options as such use can: (1) reduce the upper limit of voltages needed in the implanted receiver/stimulator for effective stimulation and (2) increase the dynamic range of electrical stimulation from threshold to comfortably loud percepts.[28] The reduction in the upper limit of voltages needed for the receiver/stimulator can produce a further substantial savings in power consumption.

A possible problem with the *n*-of-*m*, ACE, and SPEAK strategies is that all of the perceptually important peaks in the short-term spectra of an input sound may not be represented. That is, two or more adjacent channels may be selected in any frame for an intense or broad peak, because the criterion for selection is the amplitudes of the envelope signals and not the shapes of the spectra, including the peak locations. Thus, for a fixed *n*, "clusters" of adjacent channels typically are selected for the most prominent peak or two peaks, and this clustering: (1) exhausts the opportunity for representing other peaks which also may be important and (2) may exacerbate deleterious masking effects with the selections of adjacent channels.

This clustering problem might be addressed by changing the selection algorithm, as has been recently suggested by Kals et al[28] and Nogueira et al,[29] among others. In addition, application of techniques developed at the Bell Laboratories decades ago for the analogous "peak picking" vocoders (vocoder is an acronym for "voice coder") might be helpful. (These techniques are reviewed in Flanagan's classic book on "Speech Analysis, Synthesis and Perception," published in 1972.[30]) For example, one such technique involves a statistical analysis to identify the most significant peaks in the short-term spectra and then to transmit information about the frequency locations and amplitudes of those peaks only, to the exclusion of everything else including the amplitudes and positions of adjacent frequency locations. Quite possibly, selection of all perceptually important peaks, and a reduction or elimination of clustering for any single peak, could lead to improvements in performance for the *n*-of-*m* class of processing strategies for CIs, or could lead to a reduction in *n* (with its attendant advantages) while still maintaining performance that is on a par with standard implementations of *n*-of-*m*. Indeed, the latter has been achieved with the approaches suggested by Kals et al and Nogueira et al. Further progress is certainly possible.

In broad terms, the performance of the higher rate *n*-of-*m* strategies (called *n*-of-*m* in the MED-EL GmbH systems and ACE in the Cochlear Ltd systems) is on a par with or somewhat better than that of the CIS strategy, depending on the hardware implementations of the strategies.[9,31,32] The best implementations of the *n*-of-*m* strategies on the one hand, and of the CIS strategy on the other hand, produce results that are statistically indistinguishable. In contrast, comparisons between SPEAK and ACE generally have indicated a clear superiority of the latter.[9,33–35] Those strategies have been implemented using the same hardware and choices for filter designs, so the difference must be due to some other factor or factors. Possible contributors to the lower performance with SPEAK include its relatively low rate of stimulation, the departure from the "four times" oversampling rule, the particular channel selection algorithm used with SPEAK, or some combination of these factors.

HIRES 120

The representation of frequencies may be coarse with the CIS, n-of-m, and the related strategies described in the two preceding subsections. In particular, those strategies present stimuli to a maximum of 22 intracochlear electrodes, whereas the number of stimulus sites in normal hearing approximates 3500, corresponding to the number of rows of sensory hair cells distributed along the length of the cochlea. In addition, the number of effective sites of stimulation with the present-day CIs is far below the maximum of 22 electrodes, as mentioned previously. The number of effective sites or channels also is far below the number of "equivalent rectangular bandwidths" (ERBs) in normal hearing,[36] which for the range of frequencies in speech is approximately 28 ERBs. (The number for the full range of audible frequencies is around 39 ERBs.) The ERBs correspond to independent channels of perception and processing in normal hearing for a wide variety of tasks including speech reception.

In an attempt to increase the number of effective sites of stimulation for CI users, and possibly the number of effective channels as well, Wilson et al developed a variation of CIS in the early 1990s that used simultaneous stimulation of pairs of adjacent electrodes to "shift" or "steer"

the electric fields to positions in between the positions produced with stimulation of either electrode alone.[37–40] The idea was that the perceived pitches elicited by the simultaneous stimulation would be intermediate to the pitches elicited by stimulation of either electrode in the pair. Thus, with the inclusion of simultaneous stimulation of pairs of electrodes in the (otherwise) nonsimultaneous update sequence in a CIS-like strategy, additional discriminable pitches might be produced, beyond the number of electrodes in the implant. The intermediate sites of stimulation could be controlled with separate and additional channels of processing that also would include bandpass filtering, envelope detection, nonlinear mapping, and modulation, just like the channels in a conventional CIS strategy. These additional channels were called "virtual channels," and the processors that used them were called "virtual channel interleaved sampling" (VCIS) processors. In one implementation of VCIS processors, simultaneous stimulation of adjacent pairs of electrodes was alternated with stimulation of a single electrode only. Thus, the nonsimultaneous update sequence for the implementation included stimulation of the apical-most electrode only, then simultaneous stimulation of the apical-most electrode and the electrode just basal to it, then stimulation of that latter electrode only, and so on until all of the electrodes in the array had been stimulated and all of the channels had been updated. This arrangement utilized almost twice as many processing channels compared with a conventional CIS strategy, for example, for six electrodes in the implant, 11 processing channels were used, with six of the channels controlling stimuli for the single electrodes with five of the channels controlling the five pairs of electrodes receiving the simultaneous stimulation at different times in the update sequence. If the intermediate sites and associated pitches corresponded to separate channels of information, then the VCIS strategy might have the potential to support a higher number of effective channels than the CIS or other related strategies that used nonsimultaneous stimulation of electrodes only.

A series of diagrams illustrating the construction of virtual channels is presented in Figure 4–2. With virtual channels, adjacent electrodes may be stimulated simultaneously to shift the perceived pitch in any direction with respect to the percepts elicited with stimulation of either of the electrodes only. Results from studies with implant subjects indicate that pitch can be manipulated through various choices of simultaneous and single-electrode conditions.[38,40] If, for instance, the apical-most electrode in an array of electrodes is stimulated alone (electrode 1, panel *a*), subjects have reported a low pitch. If the next electrode in the array is stimulated alone (electrode 2, panel *b*), a higher pitch is reported. An intermediate pitch can be produced for the great majority of subjects studied to date by stimulating the two electrodes together with identical, in-phase pulses (panel *c*). The pitch elicited by stimulation of a single electrode can also be shifted by presentation of an opposite-polarity pulse to a neighboring electrode. For example, a pitch lower than that elicited by stimulation of electrode 1 only can be produced by simultaneous presentation of a (generally smaller) pulse of opposite polarity at electrode 2 (panel *d*). (The stimulus paradigm illustrated in panel *d* and involving the presentation of pulses of opposite polarities at neighboring electrodes has been described as the "phantom electrode" technique in a recent paper by Saoji and Litvak.[41]) The availability of pitches other than those elicited with stimulation of single electrodes only may provide additional discriminable sites along (and beyond) the length of the electrode array. Such additional sites may (or may not) support a higher number of effective information channels with implants, compared with stimulation that is restricted to single electrodes only.

The concept of virtual channels can be extended to include a quite-high number of sites and corresponding pitches, using different ratios of the currents delivered between simultaneously-stimulated electrodes. This possibility is illustrated in Figure 4–3, in which stimulus site 1 is produced by stimulation of electrode 1 only, stimulus site 2 by simultaneous stimulation of electrodes 1 and 2 with a pulse amplitude of 75% for electrode 1 and of 25% for electrode 2, and so on. The total number of sites and corresponding pitches that might be produced for a good subject in the illustrated case is 21, with six intracochlear electrodes. (A subject was tested with this arrangement and indeed obtained 21 discriminable pitches.[42]) Other ratios of currents may produce additional pitches. Results from several recent studies have indicated that a high number of discriminable pitches can be created with this general approach, eg, Koch et al[43] found an average of 93 (range 8 to 466) discriminable pitches for a large population of subjects using either of two versions of the Advanced Bionics electrode array, both of which include 16 physical intracochlear electrodes spaced approximately 1 mm apart. (Some of the subjects did not perceive pitch differences even with stimulation of adjacent or more distant electrodes in isolation, producing a number of discriminable pitches that was less than the number of physical electrodes.)

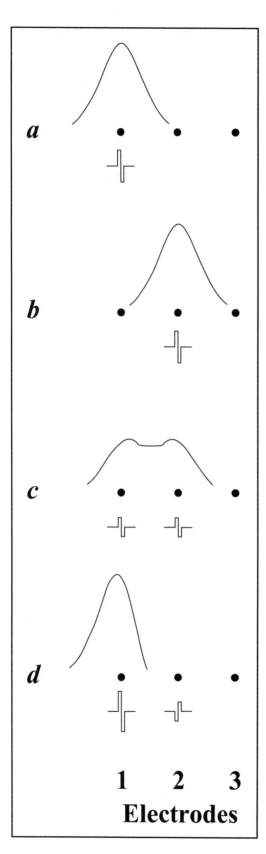

Figure 4–2. *Schematic illustrations of neural responses for various conditions of stimulation with single and multiple electrodes. The top curve in each panel is a hypothetical sketch of the number of neural responses, as a function of position along length of cochlea for a given condition of stimulation. The condition is indicated by the pulse waveform(s) beneath one or more of the dots, which represent the positions of three adjacent intracochlear electrodes. These different conditions of stimulation elicit distinct pitches for implant patients, as described in the text. (Reproduced with permission from Wilson BS, Schatzer R, Lopez-Poveda EA. Possibilities for a closer mimicking of normal auditory functions with cochlear implants. In: Waltzman SB, Roland JT Jr, eds.* Cochlear Implants. *2nd ed. New York, NY: Thieme; 2006:48–56.)*

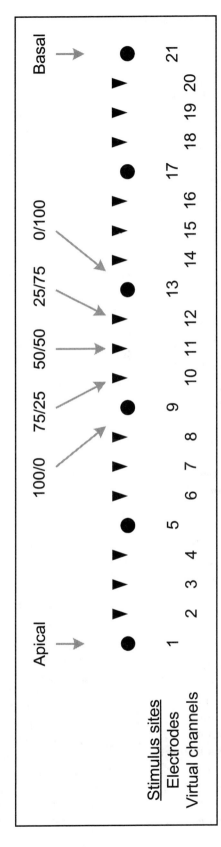

Figure 4-3. *Diagram of stimulus sites used in virtual channel interleaved sampling (VCIS) processors and other similar processors that followed them. The filled circles represent sites of stimulation at each of six intracochlear electrodes. The inverted triangles represent additional sites produced with simultaneous stimulation of adjacent electrodes, at the indicated ratios of pulse amplitudes for the two electrodes. Thus, in this arrangement 21 sites may be produced, including the six electrodes and including the 15 "virtual" sites, between simultaneously stimulated electrodes. More electrodes may be used, and more sites may be formed between adjacent electrodes, for example, as in the 120 sites produced with the HiRes 120 strategy. Some patients are able to discriminate a high number of sites on the basis of pitch as described in the text. (Reproduced with permission from Wilson BS, Schatzer R, Lopez-Poveda EA. Possibilities for a closer mimicking of normal auditory functions with cochlear implants. In: Waltzman SB, Roland JT Jr, eds. Cochlear Implants. 2nd ed. New York, NY: Thieme; 2006:48–56.)*

The original implementations of the VCIS strategy only used stimuli like those illustrated in panels *a* through *c* in Figure 4–2, that is, stimulation of single electrodes was alternated with simultaneous stimulation of pairs of electrodes using identical pulses for the pairs. The update sequence for an eleven-channel VCIS strategy is shown in Figure 4–4. As mentioned previously, this particular implementation of the VCIS strategy might produce nearly twice as many discriminable pitches and associated channels of information compared with a CIS strategy using the same number of intracochlear electrodes.

However, within-subjects comparisons between VCIS and CIS strategies using the same number of electrodes and other aspects of processing (eg, envelope detection, rate of stimulation, filter shapes, etc.) did not demonstrate a speech reception advantage of this implementation of VCIS.[39,40] Some of the subjects commented that VCIS sounded "better," or "fuller," or "more natural" than CIS, but the scores for a variety of speech tests in quiet were not statistically different between the strategies for any of the tests. Possibly, tests with more subjects, or tests with the speech materials presented in competition with noise or other talkers, may have demonstrated a difference. In the administered tests, though, no difference was found. This was a disappointing outcome.

Later implementations of VCIS included more virtual sites of stimulation between the simultaneously stimulated electrodes,[42,44,45] by using multiple ratios of currents for the simultaneously stimulated electrodes as illustrated in Figure 4–3. Those later implementations were first tested in 2003.[44] The results were not different in kind from the prior results, ie, scores with the VCIS processor were not significantly different from the scores

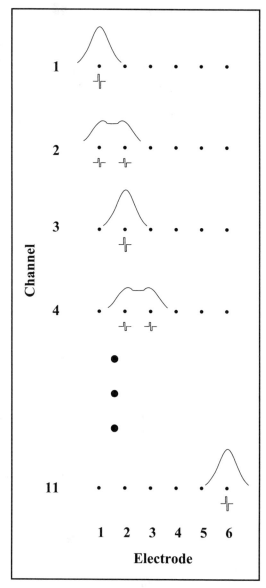

Figure 4–4. *Construction of an 11-channel virtual channel interleaved sampling (VCIS) processor. The organization of the panels is the same as that in Figure 4–2. (Reproduced from Wilson BS, Lawson DT, Zerbi M. Speech processors for auditory prostheses: evaluation of VCIS processors. Sixth Quarterly Progress Report, NIH project N01-DC-2-2401. Bethesda, MD: Neural Prosthesis Program, National Institutes of Health; 1994; permission is not required for reproduction of figures from NIH Progress Reports.)*

obtained with a control CIS processor using the same number of intracochlear electrodes.[42,44] (In these later studies, the tests included identification of consonants presented in competition with speech-spectrum noise at the S/N of +5 dB.)

Most recently, another variation of the VCIS approach has been developed by the Advanced Bionics Corp. This is the HiRes 120 strategy, which "targets" sites for stimulation according to the frequency of the predominant component detected in each of 15 bandpass ranges.[12,46-48] One among eight possible sites are selected for each range in each frame of stimulation across all of the ranges. In addition, an envelope signal is derived via a Hilbert transform for each bandpass range, as in implementations of the CIS, *n*-of-*m*, and other related strategies. Two adjacent electrodes are assigned to each bandpass range, and the electrodes are at corresponding tonotopic or frequency positions along the length of the cochlea, that is, the apical-most electrodes 1 and 2 are assigned to the bandpass range with the lowest center frequency, electrodes 2 and 3 are assigned to the range with the next highest center frequency, and so on, up to electrodes 15 and 16, which are assigned to the range with the highest center frequency. (The Advanced Bionics electrode array includes 16 intracochlear electrodes.) At the time of stimulation for each pair of electrodes, either the apical member of the pair is stimulated alone, or both electrodes are stimulated concurrently with one of seven possible ratios of currents for the electrodes. A predominant frequency in the lowest eighth of the frequency range invokes stimulation of the apical electrode only, and a higher predominant frequency in the range invokes stimulation of both electrodes with the current ratio and associated virtual site of stimulation that most closely corresponds to the predominant frequency. This procedure is repeated for each of the 15 bandpass ranges, involving 120 possible sites of stimulation (15 sites produced with stimulation of single electrodes plus 105 virtual sites produced with simultaneous stimulation of pairs of adjacent electrodes). The overall energy in each bandpass range (the envelope signal) is mapped onto the dynamic range of electrically evoked hearing using a nonlinear mapping function, as in the standard CIS strategy (see Fig 4–1). That mapped amplitude then is distributed to the two electrodes assigned to the range, according to the previously determined ratio of currents. For the one case among the eight in which only one electrode is stimulated, that electrode receives all of the current.

As in the prior implementations of the VCIS strategy, the stimuli for each of the bandpass ranges are sequenced across ranges, so that the pulse(s) for any one bandpass range do not overlap the pulse(s) for any other bandpass range. This sequencing eliminates direct summation of the electric fields produced by the stimuli for the different bandpass ranges.

The preceding description of the HiRes 120 strategy is only a brief overview. A detailed description is presented in section 2.2 of the excellent paper by Nogueira et al.[48]

Comparisons between HiRes and HiRes 120 have been published by Brendel et al,[49] Donaldson et al,[50] Drennan et al,[51] and Firszt et al.[13] In addition, comparisons between HiRes and research versions of HiRes 120 have been published by Berenstein et al,[52] Buechner et al,[46] and Nogueira et al.[48]

In broad terms, the results from these studies are consistent with the results from the earlier comparisons between CIS and

VCIS, that is, in some cases preferences are expressed by the subjects in favor of HiRes 120, but the gains in speech reception are small or nonexistent. Indeed, when the HiRes and HiRes 120 strategies are implemented on the same hardware (either the "Platinum Sound Processor" or "Harmony" hardware), results from all of the studies cited in the preceding paragraph except the study by Firszt et al demonstrate a statistical equivalence between the two strategies; in particular, no significant differences were found across multiple tests for each of the studies, including tests of speech reception in quiet, speech reception in noise, and speech reception in competition with another talker or other talkers. The results from the study by First et al show small but statistically significant differences in favor of HiRes 120 for some of the administered tests including recognition of monosyllabic words in quiet and two tests of sentence recognition in noise. However, scores for the other administered tests are statistically indistinguishable. Those other tests included a third test of sentence recognition in noise and two tests of sentence recognition in quiet, with easy sentences in one of the tests and difficult sentences in the other of the tests.

Preference questionnaires were administered in all of the studies except the study by Drennan et al. The questionnaires included questions about speech quality in all cases, and the questionnaires included questions about music quality in the studies by Firszt et al and Nogueira et al. The mean of the preference measures for HiRes 120 and the Harmony hardware was significantly higher than the mean for HiRes in the study by Brendel et al. However, because the judgments were between HiRes 120 as implemented in the Harmony hardware, versus HiRes as implemented in the earlier "Auria" or "CII" hardware, the preference may have resulted from the change in hardware as opposed to the change in strategy. (The Harmony hardware includes better front-end circuitry and processing compared with the Auria or CII hardware.) The measures from all of the remaining studies except the study by Firszt et al are statistically identical for the two strategies, that is, no preference was expressed for either of the strategies, either for speech quality[46,48,50,52] or music quality.[48] The measures from the study by Firszt et al indicated a significant preference for HiRes 120 for music quality. (The music ratings for HiRes 120 were about 10 percentage points higher than the ratings for HiRes.) However, the measures for speech quality were not significantly different for the two strategies.

The great preponderance of the results reported to date indicates that the HiRes and HiRes 120 strategies are equivalent in terms of speech reception performance. Results from some of the tests in one among the seven studies conducted to date have indicated a small advantage of HiRes 120. However, results from other tests in that study, and all of the results from all of the other studies, indicate a statistical equivalence between the two strategies. Any differences if present between the strategies are small and apparently difficult to detect.

Although the concept of virtual channels is appealing, at least three plausible explanations have emerged as to why the various applications of the concept have failed to produce large gains in performance. The first explanation is that an apparent disconnect exists between the number of discriminable sites and the number of effective channels with implants. A patient can have a high number of discriminable sites when stimuli are delivered to different sites in isolation, one at a time and with long periods between sequential stimuli for the different sites. For example, many patients implanted with electrode arrays having 22 sites of stimulation can discriminate all 22 sites in ranking or same/different tasks with the stimuli presented in isolation as just described. However, no patient tested to date has more than about eight effective channels, including patients using the 22-electrode array and other arrays, and also including multiple processing strategies. The relatively low number of effective channels may be due to a combination of broad overlaps in the electric fields for the different electrodes and substantial masking across those electrode positions when dynamic (time-varying) stimuli are presented rapidly and continuously, as in a speech processor context. The masking could be at the periphery, or within the central auditory system, or both. In addition, the masking could arise even with nonsimultaneous stimulation across channels and their associated electrodes, as is used in all present-day CI systems.

Regardless of the mechanism, the number of effective channels may not be increased at all by simply increasing the number of discriminable sites. For example, a patient might have more than 400 discriminable sites using virtual channels,[43,53] but this high number does not guarantee that the number of effective channels will be any higher than with a far lower number of discriminable sites. To date, none of the tested processing strategies, electrode arrays, or combinations of strategies and arrays, have produced an increase in the number of effective channels. The same may be true for virtual channel processors. (This hypothesis should be evaluated.)

The second explanation is that we may well have had virtual channels all along and just did not realize it until recently. In particular, McDermott and McKay[54] and others[6,55] have shown that intermediate pitches also are produced when closely spaced electrodes are stimulated in a rapid sequence, as compared with the pitches that are produced when each of the electrodes is stimulated separately. The pitch elicited with the rapid sequential stimulation of two electrodes in isolation varies according to the ratio of the currents delivered to the electrodes, just as with the intermediate pitches produced with simultaneous stimulation of the electrodes. Indeed, the numbers of discriminable pitches that can be produced with nonsimultaneous versus simultaneous stimulation are not significantly different.[6,55] Thus, a fully nonsimultaneous strategy such as CIS may produce the same number of pitches (and discriminable sites) as a virtual channel strategy that stimulates pairs of electrodes simultaneously in the update sequence. If so, little or no difference in performance would be expected between the two types of strategy.

The third explanation has been offered by Drennan et al.[51] They have suggested that any gain in the number of discriminable sites or pitches produced with HiRes 120 may be offset by the temporal "smearing" imposed by the FFT processing used in HiRes 120 but not HiRes. Thus, an increase in spatial or spectral resolution may be traded for a decrement in temporal resolution and the net result is zero or close to it.

Each of these explanations is highly plausible. Finding the correct explanation could lead to a major insight. At present, our knowledge is largely limited to the observation that the VCIS and HiRes 120 strategies have not produced large gains in the performance of CIs.

FSP

The term "fine structure" refers to small frequency differences in a signal or, equivalently, to fine temporal variations in a signal. The representation of frequencies with CIs may be coarse, as discussed previously. Some additional detail may be provided with the virtual channel approaches, but the increment may be small if present at all compared with CIS and other strategies that present nonsimultaneous stimuli only. As mentioned in the preceding subsection, the numbers of discriminable frequencies produced with CIS and the related strategies may be just as high as the numbers produced with the virtual channel strategies involving simultaneous stimulation of pairs of electrodes.

Fine structure information has been shown to be important for music reception, speech reception in noise, word (or lexical) distinctions in tonal languages, and lateralization of sound sources in the horizontal plane.[56–58] An increment in the amount or quality of this information that is presented and perceived with implants could be helpful for music and speech reception using either a unilateral CI or bilateral CIs, or for sound lateralization using bilateral CIs.

An alternative to the virtual channel approaches for presenting fine structure information is the FSP strategy recently introduced by MED-EL GmbH. This strategy also is a variation of CIS. The FSP strategy is designed to represent frequency variations within bandpass channels by initiating short groups of pulses at the positive zero crossings in the bandpass output(s) for the apical 1 to 4 channels. (If all four channels are used, the strategy is called the "FS4" strategy.) This temporal code may be more robust than the representation of temporal information with the envelope signals only,[14,59] which is used in all other strategies reviewed thus far.

In addition, the range of frequencies spanned by the bandpass filters is extended downward in the FSP strategy compared to the range used in standard implementations of the CIS strategy. A typical range for the FSP strategy is 70 to 8500 Hz, whereas a typical range for the CIS strategy is 250 to 8500 Hz. The range for the FSP strategy includes the fundamental frequencies for male, female, and child talkers, and the downward extension of the range compared to CIS allows the presentation of time-locked bursts of pulses at rates as low as about 70 bursts/s.

The combination in the FSP strategy of: (1) the downward extension of the frequency range spanned by the bandpass filters and (2) the presentation of time-locked stimuli at low rates might improve frequency discrimination at low frequencies compared to the CIS and the other strategies reviewed thus far. In fact, Krenmayr et al[60] recently evaluated this hypothesis in a comparison between the FSP and CIS strategies and found that the range of distinct pitches elicited with complex periodic sounds with varying fundamental frequencies is indeed extended to lower fundamental frequencies with the FSP strategy.

The temporal representation of fine structure information that is presented at one or more of the apical electrodes with the FSP strategy may be effective only up to frequencies of about 300 Hz for most implant patients and up to about 1000 Hz for exceptional patients. That is, pitch increases with the rate or frequency of stimulation at single electrodes for implant patients only up to these values.[61] Higher rates or frequencies do not produce higher pitches. Instead, the pitch remains the same as at the asymptotic point, sometimes called the "pitch saturation limit," for implant patients. Thus, variations in the temporal patterns of stimulation provided by the FSP strategy will be perceived only for the bandpass channels that include frequencies below the pitch saturation limit.

For this reason, the remaining (higher frequency) channels present conventional CIS stimuli. (The pitch saturation limit also guided the choice for the cutoff frequencies of the envelope detectors in the CIS and related strategies; that is, cutoff frequencies between 200 and 400 Hz restrict envelope variations to those upper limits, which do not generally exceed the pitch saturation limit.) The lowest or lower channels thus represent the "temporal fine structure" at the outputs of the corresponding bandpass filters by "marking" the positive zero crossings with stimulus presentations, and the higher channels represent the envelope variations with CIS stimuli. As mentioned above, those envelope variations also may convey fine-timing information up to the cutoff frequency of the envelope detectors. However, the salience of that representation may be less than the salience of the time-locked stimulus bursts presented to the apical electrode(s).

The FSP, CIS+, and HDCIS strategies all use bandpass filters with bell-shaped responses. As noted previously, this design may produce a smooth transition from one filter to the next when a sinusoidal input is "swept" between the center frequencies of the filters. Such smooth transitions may enhance the "channel balance" cue obtained with sequential stimulation of adjacent electrodes. In particular, frequencies in the input that are intermediate to the center frequencies of the bandpass filters will produce an output from both filters, and the ratio of the outputs from the filters will vary almost linearly as a function of the input frequency. Thus, a good approximation of the input frequency is represented in the ratio of the bandpass outputs, for all frequencies between the center frequencies of the filters. Many different ratios may be perceived as different pitches, and thus the channel balance cue in conjunction with the bell-shaped responses for the filters may be another way to convey fine structure information to implant patients. (The situation for multiple components with different frequencies in the input to any two adjacent filters is considerably more complex.)

Alternative filter designs also may be effective in this regard, for example, the filters with the more rectangular responses that are used in other implementations of the CIS and other strategies. However, filters with the bell-shaped responses would be expected to maximize the transmission of fine structure information using the channel balance cues. (This hypothesis remains to be demonstrated.) The FSP, CIS+, and HDCIS strategies may convey fine structure information at relatively high frequencies with the channel balance cues produced with nonsimultaneous stimulation and with the bandpass filters with the bell-shaped responses. In addition, these strategies may convey information about the fundamental frequency through temporal variations in the modulation waveforms for the channels. The FSP strategy may augment this latter representation, and may convey further fine structure information at low frequencies (ie, frequencies below the pitch saturation limit), with the stimulus bursts that are time locked to the positive zero crossings in the bandpass outputs.

As in the CIS and other strategies, stimulus magnitudes for the apical channel(s) in the FSP strategy are determined with an envelope detector and nonlinear mapping function for each of the channels. Thus, channel balance cues are provided for all channels including the apical channels. Such cues may reinforce the temporal code provided with the time-locked stimuli for the apical channels, or indeed may be as important or even more important in conveying the fine structure information at the low frequencies that are included in the apical channels.

We note that the FSP strategy is similar in design to a strategy described by Wilson et al in 1991,[62] called the "peak picker/CIS" (PP/CIS) strategy. The principal difference between the FSP and PP/CIS strategies is that single pulses are presented at the peaks in the bandpass filter outputs in the PP/CIS strategy, whereas groups of pulses (including the possibility of a single pulse) are presented at the positive zero crossings in the FSP strategy. Two additional differences are that: (1) bandpass filters with bell-shaped responses are used in the FSP strategy, whereas filters with more-rectangular responses (Butterworth responses) are used in the PP/CIS strategy, and (2) the range of frequencies spanned by the bandpass filters is not extended downward in the PP/CIS strategy. (The FSP approach may possibly be better as a result of either or both of these latter two differences.) Subjects noted that the PP/CIS strategy sounded more natural and lower in overall pitch than the control CIS strategy, but the results from tests of open-set speech recognition in quiet were not statistically different between the two strategies.

Comparisons between the CIS+ and FSP strategies have been published by Arnoldner et al,[59] Riss et al,[63,64] and Vermeire et al.[65] In addition, comparisons between HDCIS and FSP have been published by Riss et al,[66] and Magnusson.[67] Comparisons among CIS+, HDCIS, and FSP also have been published by Lorens et al[7] and presented by Brill et al.[68] Furthermore, comparisons between research versions of CIS and FSP implemented with the same processor hardware have

been published by Schatzer et al.[69] All studies included measures of speech reception, and the studies of Arnoldner et al, Brill et al, Lorens et al, Magnusson, and Vermeire et al also included questionnaires for the subjects. Most of the questionnaires related to speech quality and strategy preferences. The questionnaires in the studies of Lorens et al and of Magnusson also related to judged differences in music quality between or among the tested strategies.

In broad terms, significant differences are found between CIS+ and FSP in the objective scores on speech tests (especially speech recognition in noise or in competition with other talkers) and in the responses to the questionnaires, in favor of FSP. These differences could be the result of the previously described differences between the TEMPO+ versus the OPUS 1 or OPUS 2 hardware; the use of the time-locked stimuli for the apical channel(s) in FSP; the difference between the frequency range spanned by the bandpass filters for CIS+ versus the range for FSP; or some combination of these factors.

In contrast, small or no differences are found between CIS and FSP when the two strategies are implemented with the same hardware. In particular: (1) the speech reception results reported by Brill et al did not favor HDCIS over FSP or vice versa, with both strategies implemented with the OPUS hardware; (2) the speech reception results reported by Mangusson et al did not show any statistically significant differences between HDCIS and FSP; (3) the speech reception results reported from the 2008 study by Riss et al comparing CIS and FSP with each using 2, 3, 5, 8, or 12 channels of processing and stimulation and with each implemented with the same hardware did not show any statistically significant differences between the strategies, including the standard 12-channel versions of the strategies; and (4) the speech and tone reception results reported by Schatzer et al did not show any statistically significant differences between research versions of the CIS and FSP strategies, as implemented using the same processor hardware and as tested with Cantonese materials and native Cantonese speakers. (Cantonese is a tone language whose reception might be significantly enhanced with a better representation of fine structure information at low frequencies, which is exactly what the FSP strategy is designed to provide.) Lorens et al found a small advantage of FSP over HDCIS for a speech reception measure in quiet but not for the same measure in noise. In addition, the responses to the questionnaires in that study indicated a preference for FSP versus HDCIS for listening to speech ($p = 0.048$) but no preference between the two strategies for listening to music. The preference for listening to speech was small and just attained statistical significance. The responses to the questionnaires in the study of Magnusson did not indicate a strategy preference for either speech or music reception.

The data to date indicate advantages of FSP over CIS+. In addition, the data indicate either a small advantage of FSP over HDCIS or a full equivalence between the two strategies. Most of the studies conducted thus far did not include a crossover design or other experimental controls for possible learning effects, which may have favored FSP in some of the comparisons. FSP is a promising approach, but more studies are needed to establish the magnitude of the benefit and whether the benefit may vary among different populations of patients or different listening situations, for example, speech in quiet versus speech in noise, or speech versus music reception. Such studies also

could help identify beneficial aspects of the hardware changes incorporated in the OPUS processors. Those changes could possibly support better results with a variety of implemented strategies, including the CIS and FSP strategies.

PERFORMANCE WITH UNILATERAL IMPLANTS

Representative findings from evaluations of the speech reception performance of unilateral CIs are presented in Figure 4-5, which shows scores for 55 users of the MED-EL COMBI 40 CI system and the CIS processing strategy as implemented with that system.[70] The subjects were postlingually deafened adults. Scores for recognition of the Hochmair-Schultz-Moser sentences are presented in Figure 4-5, panel *a*, and scores for recognition of the Freiburger monosyllabic words are presented in panel *b*. The sentences and words were presented in quiet without any interfering sounds. Results for five measurement intervals are shown, ranging from one month to 2 years following the initial fitting of the external speech processor. The solid line in each panel shows the mean of the individual scores. The fittings for most of the subjects included eight channels of processing and associated sites of stimulation and a pulse rate of about 1500/s/electrode. The fittings for some of the subjects included a lower number of channels and a proportionately higher rate. All fittings used the maximum overall pulse rate supported by the COMBI 40 implant, 12,120 pulses/s. The presented data are a superset of those reported in Helms et al[70] that include scores for additional subjects at various test intervals, as reported in Wilson.[17]

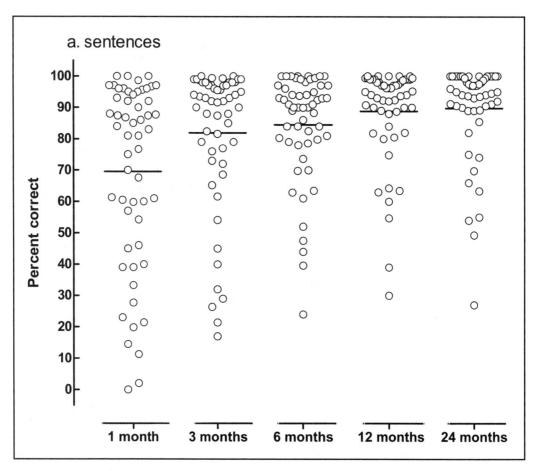

Figure 4–5. *Percent correct scores for 55 users of the COMBI 40 cochlear implant and the continuous interleaved sampling (CIS) processing strategy. Scores for recognition of the Hochmair-Schultz-Moser sentences are presented in panel a, and scores for recognition of the Freiburger monosyllabic words are presented in panel b. Results for each of five test intervals following the initial fitting of the speech processor for each subject are shown. The horizontal line in each panel indicates the mean of the scores for that interval and test. (The great majority of the data are from Helms J, Müller J, Schön F, Moser L, Arnold W, et al. Evaluation of performance with the COMBI40 cochlear implant in adults: a multicentric clinical study.* ORL J Otorhinolaryngol Relat Spec. *1997;59:23–35, with an update reported in Wilson BS. Speech processing strategies. In: Cooper HR, Craddock LC, eds.* Cochlear Implants: A Practical Guide. *2nd ed. Hoboken, NJ: John Wiley & Sons; 2006:21–69. Figure is adapted from Dorman MF, Spahr AJ. Speech perception by adults with multichannel cochlear implants. In: Waltzman SB, Roland JT Jr, eds.* Cochlear Implants. *2nd ed. New York, NY: Thieme Medical Publishers; 2006:193–204, and is used here with the permission of Thieme Medical Publishers.) continues*

Figure 4–5 shows broad distributions of scores for both tests. However, ceiling effects are encountered for the sentence test for many of the subjects, especially at the later test intervals. At 24 months, 46 of the 55 subjects score above 80% cor-

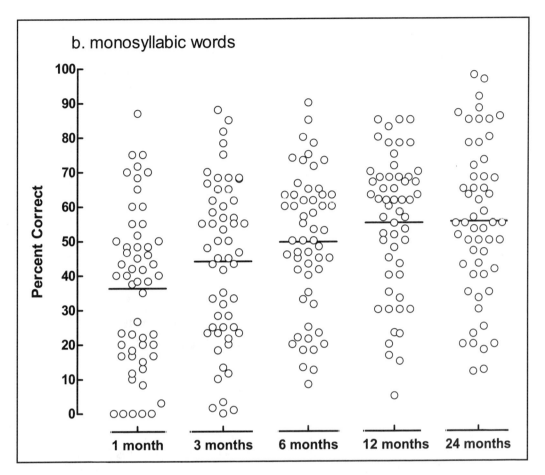

Figure 4–5. continued

rect, consistent with the conclusion from the 1995 NIH Consensus Statement on Cochlear Implants[3] that is presented in Table 4–1. Scores for the recognition of the monosyllabic words are much more broadly distributed. For example, at the 24-month interval only nine of the 55 subjects have scores above 80% correct, and the distribution of scores from about 10% correct to nearly 100% correct is almost perfectly uniform.

An interesting aspect of the results presented in Figure 4–5 is the improvement in performance over time. This improvement is even easier to see in Figure 4–6, which shows the means and standard errors of the means (SEMs) for these same data and for the additional intervals that were included for the sentence test. The means of the scores increase for both the sentence and word tests out to 12 months and then plateau thereafter. The means for the sentence test asymptote at about 90% correct, and the means for the word test asymptote at about 55% correct. The long-term course needed to attain the asymptotic performances indicates a role of the brain in determining outcomes with CIs. In particular, the time course far exceeds that of any possible changes at the periphery and must instead reflect plastic changes in brain organization and

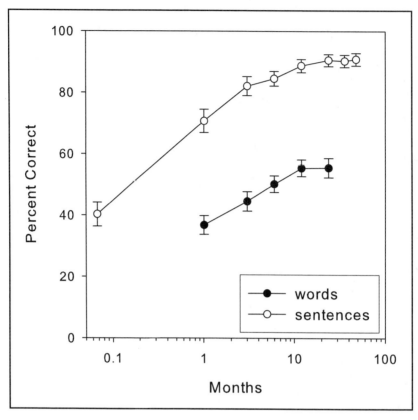

Figure 4–6. *Means and standard errors of the means for the data and subjects in Figure 4–5. Note that the time scale along the x-axis is logarithmic. (Reproduced with permission from Wilson BS. Speech processing strategies. In: Cooper HR, Craddock LC, eds. Cochlear Implants: A Practical Guide. 2nd ed. Hoboken, NJ: John Wiley & Sons; 2006:21–69.)*

function, as the brain "reconfigures" itself over the months to make progressively better use of the decidedly sparse and unnatural input from the periphery, as produced with the stimuli provided by the CI.

The results presented in Figures 4–5 and 4–6 typify performances with the best of the contemporary CI systems and unilateral stimulation. This fact is illustrated in Figure 4–7, which compares results from the Helms et al study, conducted in the mid-1990s and reported in 1997, with results from the subjects in Group 5 in the study of Krueger et al,[71] who received their unilateral CIs in the mid-2000s and whose results were reported in 2008. Group 5 included 310 subjects who used the newest devices of the time, including the CII or HiRes90K implant devices from Advanced Bionics Corp, the Freedom implant device from Cochlear Ltd, or the COMBI 40+ or Pulsar implant devices from MED-EL GmbH. The processing strategies implemented with these various devices included the CIS, CIS+, *n*-of-*m*, ACE, and HiRes strategies. Means of the scores for the recognition of the Freiburger monosyllabic

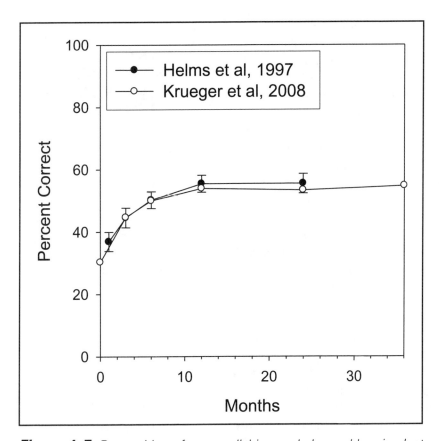

Figure 4–7. *Recognition of monosyllabic words by cochlear implant subjects in the study of Helms et al (closed symbols) and in Group 5 in the study of Kruger et al (open symbols). The Freiburger test was used in both studies. The means of the scores are shown for both studies and the standard errors of the means (SEMs) are shown for the Helms et al study. The SEMs for the Kruger et al study are infinitesimally small due to the high number of subjects in Group 5 in the study (310 subjects). The x-axis indicates the time in months at and following the first fitting of the external sound processor for the subjects. (Data are from Helms J, Müller J, Schön F, Moser L, Arnold W, et al. Evaluation of performance with the COMBI40 cochlear implant in adults: a multicentric clinical study. ORL J Otorhinolaryngol Relat Spec. 1997;59:23–35, and from Krueger B, Joseph G, Rost U, Strauss-Schier A, Lenarz T, Buechner A. Performance groups in adult cochlear implant users: speech perception results from 1984 until today. Otol Neurotol. 2008;29:509–512.)*

words in quiet are shown for the 55 subjects in the Helms et al study and the 310 subjects in Group 5 in the Krueger et al study. In addition, SEMs are shown for the subjects in the Helms et al study. (The SEMs for the subjects in the Krueger et al study are much smaller due to the large number of subjects.)

The comparison presented in Figure 4–7 shows a complete overlap in the results for unilateral CIs that were reported in 1997 and 2008. That is, the scores for the recognition of monosyllabic words are statistically indistinguishable between the groups of subjects at all test intervals out to 24 months following the initial fitting of the external speech processor. In addition, for this relatively difficult test, the scores and the means of the scores do not exhibit even the slightest hint of ceiling effects that might reduce the statistical power for detecting any differences between the groups.

This remarkable correspondence in the scores across the decade indicates that the large step forward with the introduction of CIS into widespread clinical use in the mid 1990s was not surpassed at least until the late 2000s. Indeed, as reviewed in the preceding major section on processing strategies for unilateral CIs, no processing strategy since the late 2000s has surpassed CIS and the related strategies with the possible exception of the FSP strategy for some tests. That latter possibility needs further evaluation, as also noted in the preceding section.

The results reviewed above generally apply to postlingually deafened patients. Results for prelingually deafened patients may be different, depending on the age of implantation. If the implant occurs at an early age, for example, 18 months or less, then the results for the prelingually deafened population are as good as the better outcomes for the postlingually deafened population.[72,73] In contrast, implantations after the second or third birthday for the prelingual (or perilingually deafened) patients are associated with outcomes that are usually worse than those for the postlingual patients, and the odds for a good outcome are very poor for prelingually deafened persons implanted after 4 to 6 years of age.

STIMULATION IN ADDITION TO THAT PROVIDED WITH UNILATERAL IMPLANTS

The stimulation provided with unilateral CIs may be augmented by electrical stimulation on the contralateral side with another CI, or with acoustic stimulation for persons who have at least some residual hearing in either or both ears. Either mode of the additional stimulation can produce large improvements in speech reception, especially for speech presented in competition with noise or other talkers. For the cases in which both ears are stimulated, sound localization abilities also may be reinstated at least to some extent. Such abilities can restore a sense of fullness in auditory percepts and a sense of "living in a three-dimensional world," as has been stated by many patients. The abilities also can confer further benefits in attending to a primary speaker or other source of sound in typical acoustic environments with multiple interfering sounds at other locations. The combination of electric plus acoustic stimulation (combined EAS) can improve the reception of music and tonal languages substantially, whether or not both ears are stimulated. These benefits of bilateral electrical stimulation and of combined EAS are described in detail in recent reviews by Dorman and Gifford[74] and by Wilson and Dorman.[18,75]

Some of the aforementioned benefits are illustrated in Figure 4–8, which shows differences in percent correct scores between unilateral stimulation with one CI and either: (1) bilateral electrical stimulation with a CI on both sides or (2) combined EAS, with stimulation of one ear with a CI and the other ear with acoustic stimuli.

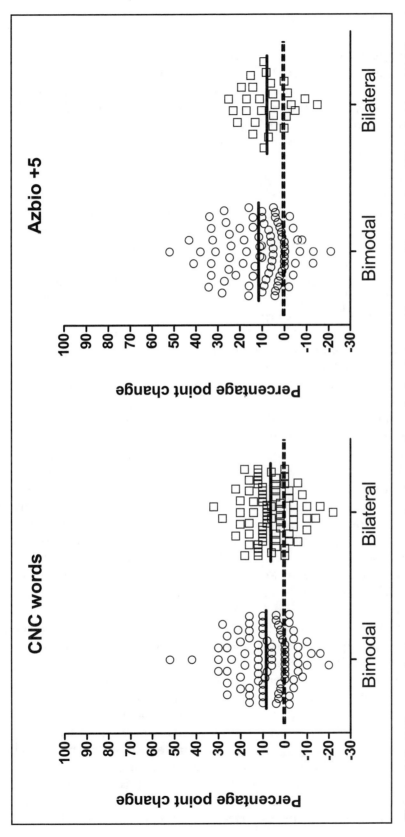

Figure 4–8. Differences in percent correct scores between unilateral stimulation with one cochlear implant (CI) and either: (1) bilateral electrical stimulation, with two CIs and with one on each side, or (2) combined electric and acoustic stimulation (bimodal stimulation), with stimulation of one ear with a CI and the other ear with acoustic stimuli. The tests included recognition of consonant-nucleus-consonant (CNC) monosyllabic words presented in quiet, and recognition of the Arizona Biomedical Institute (Azbio) sentences presented in competition with a four-talker speech babble noise at the speech-to-noise ratio of +5 dB. Additional details about the conditions of the tests and the sources of the data are presented in the text.

This latter condition is labeled "bimodal" in the figure. The comparisons for the bimodal subjects are between stimulation with the unilateral CI only versus stimulation of that CI plus acoustic stimulation of the contralateral ear. The comparisons for the bilateral subjects are between stimulation of the unilateral CI producing the better speech reception scores for each subject versus stimulation with both CIs. The bimodal subjects are from a cohort described in Dorman and Gifford, and the bilateral subjects are from participants in the clinical trials of bilateral implants in the United States. These latter subjects used either an Advanced Bionics Corp CI on both sides, a Cochlear Ltd CI on both sides, or a MED-EL GmbH CI on both sides. The tests included recognition of consonant-nucleus-consonant (CNC) monosyllabic words presented in quiet for all subjects in both groups of subjects, and recognition of the relatively difficult Arizona Biomedical Institute (Azbio) sentences[76] presented in competition with a four-talker speech babble noise at the S/N of +5 dB for subsets of the subjects. Recognition of the CNC words was measured with 83 bimodal subjects and 80 bilateral subjects. Recognition of the Azbio sentences in noise was measured with 80 bimodal subjects and 29 bilateral subjects. The scores presented in Figure 4–8 are referenced to the mean scores for the CI only for the bimodal subjects and the better of the two CIs for the bilateral subjects. Those mean scores for the bimodal subjects were 58 and 32% correct for the CNC word and Azbio sentence tests, respectively. The mean scores for the bilateral subjects were both 55% correct for the two tests.

The data presented in Figure 4–8 indicate that large gains in speech reception may be obtained with either intervention. That is, the numbers of subjects whose scores are higher than the baseline for either test with either intervention far outweigh the numbers of subjects whose scores are lower than the baseline. In addition, the mean scores increase up to about 10 percentage points with the stimulation in addition to the unilateral CI for both tests and for both types of additional stimulation. Between the two types of additional stimulation, combined EAS (bimodal) may provide the possibility of larger gains for speech reception in noise than bilateral CIs. The overall improvements for either mode of additional stimulation are substantial.

Although the gains can be substantial, not all prospective patients will be able to take advantage of the possibilities offered by bilateral CIs or combined EAS. For example, national health care plans or third-party insurers do not always cover the additional cost of the second implant for bilateral CIs. In addition, some candidates for a CI do not have any useful residual hearing that could be stimulated effectively with the acoustic stimulation part of combined EAS. Thus, a need remains to improve the performance of unilateral CIs for many patients. That need also is evident in the remaining variability in outcomes even with bilateral CIs or combined EAS (see Fig 4–8). The scores with these interventions are higher on average than the scores obtained with unilateral CIs, but the results across patients are still highly variable and much room remains for improvements in the mean scores and most especially in the scores for individuals that are below the mean. A better contribution from each unilateral CI could exert a salutary effect on the performance of bilateral CIs, and a better contribution from the CI could produce substantially better results with the combination of electric plus acoustic stimulation.

POSSIBILITIES FOR IMPROVEMENT

Fortunately, there are many promising possibilities for improvement in the design and performance of unilateral CIs. Some of the possibilities are described in two recent reviews by Wilson and Dorman,[18,75] and include: (1) a closer mimicking of the intricate processing in the normal cochlea; (2) continued development of approaches to represent fine structure information with implants, including representations of the first several harmonics for periodic sounds, which are so very important for pitch and music perception; (3) an increase in the number of effective channels with implants, for example, with new electrode designs or placements, optical rather than electrical stimulation, or directed growth of neurites toward intracochlear electrodes as promoted by various neurotrophic drugs; (4) a "top down" or "cognitive neuroscience" approach to the design of CIs and other neural prostheses that takes differences in brain function among users into account; and (5) identifying the cause or causes of the apparent disconnect between the number of discriminable sites of stimulation versus the number of effective channels with implants, and then acting on that knowledge to bring the latter number closer to the former number. Of course, possibilities 3 and 5 may be related. Further detailed information about the "closer mimicking" and "top down" approaches to CI designs is presented in several recent papers by Wilson et al,[42,45,77,78] and further detailed information about the importance of representing the harmonic structure of periodic sounds is presented in a seminal paper by Oxenham et al.[79] Realization of any of the listed possibilities could produce another breakthrough, akin to the advent of multichannel processing and multiple sites of stimulation in the early 1980s, and akin to the advent of the CIS and related processing strategies in the late 1980s and early 1990s.

CONCLUDING REMARKS

We as a community have come a long way indeed in the development of CIs and processing strategies for them, but much room remains for further improvements. Fortunately, there are multiple promising possibilities for such improvements. Changes in processing strategies have produced large gains in performance in the past and may well do so in the future.

Acknowledgments. Parts of this chapter are drawn or adapted from prior publications, including Wilson and Dorman[18,75,80] and Wilson et al.[78] Author BSW is a consultant for MED-EL GmbH of Innsbruck, Austria, and author MFD is a consultant for Advanced Bionics Corp of Valencia, California, USA. None of the statements in this chapter favor either of those companies or any other company.

REFERENCES

1. Bilger RC, Black FO, Hopkinson NT, et al. Evaluation of subjects presently fitted with implanted auditory prostheses. *Ann Otol Rhinol Laryngol.* 1977;86(suppl 38, no 3, pt 2):1–176.
2. National Institutes of Health. Cochlear implants. *NIH Consensus Statements.* 1988; 7(2):1–9. (This statement also is available

in *Arch Otolaryngol Head Neck Surg.* 1988;115:31–36.)

3. National Institutes of Health. Cochlear implants in adults and children. *NIH Consensus Statements.* 1995;13(2):130. (This statement also is available in *JAMA.* 1995; 274:1955–1961.)

4. Wilson BS, Finley CC, Lawson DT, Wolford RD, Eddington DK, Rabinowitz WM. Better speech recognition with cochlear implants. *Nature.* 1991;352:236–238.

5. Helms J, Müller J, Schön F, Winkler F, Moser L, et al. Comparison of the TEMPO+ ear-level speech processor and the CIS PRO+ body-worn processor in adult MED-EL cochlear implant users. *ORL J Otorhinolaryngol Relat Spec.* 2001;63:31–40.

6. Nobbe A, Schleich P, Zierhofer C, Nopp P. Frequency discrimination with sequential or simultaneous stimulation in MED-EL cochlear implants. *Acta Otolaryngol.* 2007;127:1266–1272.

7. Lorens A, Zgoda M, Obrycka A, Skarzynski H. Fine structure processing improves speech perception as well as objective and subjective benefits in pediatric MED-EL COMBI 40+ users. *Int J Pediatr Otorhinolaryngol.* 2010;74:1372–1378.

8. Wilson BS, Finley CC, Farmer JC Jr, et al. Comparative studies of speech processing strategies for cochlear implants. *Laryngoscope.* 1988;98:1069–1077.

9. Kiefer J, Hohl S, Sturzebecher E, Pfennigdorff T, Gstoettner W. Comparison of speech recognition with different speech coding strategies (SPEAK, CIS, and ACE) and their relationship to telemetric measures of compound action potentials in the Nucleus CI 24M cochlear implant system. *Audiology.* 2001;40:32–42.

10. Skinner MW, Clark GM, Whitford LA, et al. Evaluation of a new spectral peak (SPEAK) coding strategy for the Nucleus 22 channel cochlear implant system. *Am J Otol.* 1994;15(suppl 2):15–27.

11. Koch DB, Osberger MJ, Segal P, Kessler D. HiResolution and conventional sound processing in the HiResolution Bionic Ear:

using appropriate outcome measures to assess speech-recognition ability. *Audiol Neurootol.* 2004;9:214–223.

12. Trautwein, P. HiRes with Fidelity™ 120 sound processing: implementing active current steering for increased spectral resolution in CII BionicEar® and HiRes90K users. Advanced Bionics Corporation, Valencia, CA, 2006. (This report is presented at http://www.bionicear.com/userfiles/File/ HiRes_Fidelity120_Sound_Processing.pdf and was retrieved on April 19, 2011.)

13. Firszt JB, Holden LK, Reeder RM, Skinner MW. Speech recognition in cochlear implant recipients: comparison of standard HiRes and HiRes 120 sound processing. *Otol Neurotol.* 2009;30:146–152.

14. Hochmair I, Nopp P, Jolly C, Schmidt M, Schösser H, Garnham C, Anderson I. MED-EL cochlear implants: state of the art and a glimpse into the future. *Trends Amplif.* 2006;10:201–219.

15. Loizou P. Speech processing in vocoder-centric cochlear implants. In: Moller A, ed. *Cochlear and Brainstem Implants.* Basel: Karger; 2006:109–143. (An alternative citation for this reference is *Adv Otorhinolaryngol.* 2006;64:109–143.)

16. Wilson BS. Engineering design of cochlear implant systems. In: Zeng F-G, Popper AN, Fay RR, eds. *Auditory Prostheses: Cochlear Implants and Beyond.* New York, NY: Springer-Verlag; 2004:14–52.

17. Wilson BS. Speech processing strategies. In: Cooper HR, Craddock LC, eds. *Cochlear Implants: A Practical Guide.* 2nd ed. Hoboken, NJ: John Wiley & Sons; 2006:21–69.

18. Wilson BS, Dorman MF. The design of cochlear implants. In: Niparko JK, Kirk KI, Mellon NK, Robbins AM, Tucci DL, Wilson BS, eds. *Cochlear Implants: Principles and Practices.* 2nd ed. Philadelphia, PA: Lippincott Williams & Wilkins; 2009:95–135.

19. Zeng FG, Rebscher S, Harrison WV, Sun X, Feng H. Cochlear implants: system design, integration and evaluation. *IEEE Rev Biomed Eng.* 2008;1:115–142.

20. Favre E, Pelizzone M. Channel interactions in patients using the Ineraid multichannel cochlear implant. *Hear Res.* 1993; 66:150–156.

21. Wilson BS. The future of cochlear implants. *Brit J Audiol.* 1997;31:205–225.

22. Busby PA, Tong YC, Clark GM. The perception of temporal modulations by cochlear implant patients. *J Acoust Soc Am.* 1993; 94:124–131.

23. Wilson BS, Finley CC, Lawson DT, Zerbi M. Temporal representations with cochlear implants. *Am J Otol.* 1997;18:S30–S34.

24. Fishman KE, Shannon RV, Slattery WH. Speech recognition as a function of the number of electrodes used in the SPEAK cochlear implant speech processor. *J Speech Lang Hear Res.* 1997;40:1201–1215.

25. Friesen LM, Shannon RV, Baskent D, Wang X. Speech recognition in noise as a function of the number of spectral channels: comparison of acoustic hearing and cochlear implants. *J Acoust Soc Am.* 2001; 110:1150–1163.

26. Garnham C, O'Driscol M, Ramsden R, Saeed S. Speech understanding in noise with a Med-El COMBI 40+ cochlear implant using reduced channel sets. *Ear Hear.* 2002;23:540–552.

27. Dorman MF, Spahr AJ. Speech perception by adults with multichannel cochlear implants. In: Waltzman SB, Roland JT Jr, eds. *Cochlear Implants.* 2nd ed. New York, NY: Thieme Medical Publishers; 2006:193–204.

28. Kals M, Schatzer R, Krenmayr A, et al. Results with a cochlear implant channel-picking strategy based on "Selected Groups." *Hear Res.* 2010;260:63–69.

29. Nogueira W, Büchner A, Lenarz T, Edler B. A psychoacoustic "NofM"-type speech coding strategy for cochlear implants. *EURASIP J Appl Signal Processing.* 2005; 2005:3044–3059.

30. Flanagan JL. *Speech Analysis, Synthesis and Perception.* 2nd ed. New York, NY: Springer-Verlag; 1972.

31. Ziese M, Stützel A, von Specht H, et al. Speech understanding with the CIS and the n-of-m strategy in the MED-EL COMBI 40+ system. *ORL J Otorhinolaryngol Relat Spec.* 2000;62:321–329.

32. Lawson DT, Wilson BS, Zerbi M, Finley CC. Speech processors for auditory prostheses: 22 electrode percutaneous study—results for the first five subjects. *Third Quarterly Progress Report*, NIH project N01-DC-5-2103. Bethesda, MD: Neural Prosthesis Program, National Institutes of Health; 1996.

33. Pasanisi E, Bacciu A, Vincenti V, Guida M, Berghenti MT, Barbot A, Panu F, Bacciu S. Comparison of speech perception benefits with SPEAK and ACE coding strategies in pediatric Nucleus CI24M cochlear implant recipients. *Int J Pediatr Otorhinolaryngol.* 2002;64:159–163.

34. Skinner MW, Holden LK, Whitford LA, Plant KL, Psarros C, Holden TA. Speech recognition with the nucleus 24 SPEAK, ACE, and CIS speech coding strategies in newly implanted adults. *Ear Hear.* 2002; 23:207–223.

35. David EE, Ostroff JM, Shipp D, Nedzelski JM, Chen JM, Parnes LS, Zimmerman K, Schramm D, Seguin C. Speech coding strategies and revised cochlear implant candidacy: an analysis of post-implant performance. *Otol Neurotol.* 2003;24:228–233.

36. Glasberg BR, Moore BC. Derivation of auditory filter shapes from notched-noise data. *Hear Res.* 1990;47:103–138.

37. Wilson BS, Lawson DT, Zerbi M, Finley CC. Speech processors for auditory prostheses: virtual channel interleaved sampling (VCIS) processors—initial studies with subject SR2. *First Quarterly Progress Report*, NIH project N01-DC-2-2401. Bethesda, MD: Neural Prosthesis Program, National Institutes of Health; 1992.

38. Wilson BS, Zerbi M, Lawson DT. Speech processors for auditory prostheses: identification of virtual channels on the basis of pitch. *Third Quarterly Progress Report*, NIH project N01-DC-2-2401. Bethesda, MD: Neural Prosthesis Program, National Institutes of Health; 1993.

39. Wilson BS, Lawson DT, Zerbi M. Speech processors for auditory prostheses: evaluation of VCIS processors. *Sixth Quarterly Progress Report*, NIH project N01-DC-2-2401. Bethesda, MD: Neural Prosthesis Program, National Institutes of Health; 1994.

40. Wilson BS, Lawson DT, Zerbi M, Finley CC. Recent developments with the CIS strategies. In: Hochmair-Desoyer IJ, Hochmair ES, eds. *Advances in Cochlear Implants*. Vienna: Manz; 1994:103–112.

41. Saoji AA, Litvak LM. Use of "phantom electrode" technique to extend the range of pitches available through a cochlear implant. *Ear Hear*. 2010;31:693–701. Erratum in: *Ear Hear*. 2011;32:143.

42. Wilson BS, Schatzer R, Lopez-Poveda EA. Possibilities for a closer mimicking of normal auditory functions with cochlear implants. In: Waltzman SB, Roland JT Jr, eds. *Cochlear Implants*. 2nd ed. New York, NY: Thieme Medical Publishers; 2006: 48–56.

43. Koch DB, Downing M, Osberger MJ, Litvak L. Using current steering to increase spectral resolution in CII and HiRes 90K users. *Ear Hear*. 2007;28(suppl):39S–41S.

44. Wilson BS, Wolford D, Schatzer R, Sun X, Lawson D. Speech processors for auditory prostheses: combined use of DRNL filters and virtual channels. *Seventh Quarterly Progress Report*, NIH project N01-DC-2-1002. Bethesda, MD: Neural Prosthesis Program, National Institutes of Health; 2003.

45. Wilson BS, Schatzer R, Lopez-Poveda EA, Sun X, Lawson DT, Wolford RD. Two new directions in speech processor design for cochlear implants. *Ear Hear*. 2005;26: 73S–81S.

46. Buechner A, Brendel M, Krüeger B, Frohne-Büchner C, Nogueira W, Edler B, Lenarz T. Current steering and results from novel speech coding strategies. *Otol Neurotol*. 2008;29:203–207.

47. Litvak LM, Krubsack DA, Overstreet EH. Method and system to convey the within-channel fine structure with a cochlear implant. US Patent 7317945; 2008.

48. Nogueira W, Litvak L, Edler B, Ostermann J, Buechner A. Signal processing strategies for cochlear implants using current steering. *EURASIP J Adv Signal Processing*. 2009;2009:1–20.

49. Brendel M, Buechner A, Krueger B, Frohne-Buechner C, Lenarz T. Evaluation of the Harmony sound processor in combination with the speech coding strategy HiRes 120. *Otol Neurotol*. 2008;29:199–202.

50. Donaldson GS, Dawson PK, Borden LZ. Within-subjects comparison of the HiRes and Fidelity120 speech processing strategies: speech perception and its relation to place-pitch sensitivity. *Ear Hear*. 2011;32: 238–250.

51. Drennan WR, Won JH, Nie K, Jameyson E, Rubinstein JT. Sensitivity of psychophysical measures to signal processor modifications in cochlear implant users. *Hear Res*. 2010;262:1–8.

52. Berenstein CK, Mens LH, Mulder JJ, Vanpoucke FJ. Current steering and current focusing in cochlear implants: comparison of monopolar, tripolar, and virtual channel electrode configurations. *Ear Hear*. 2008;29:250–260.

53. Firszt JB, Koch DB, Downing M, Litvak L. Current steering creates additional pitch percepts in adult cochlear implant recipients. *Otol Neurotol*. 2007;28:629–636.

54. McDermott HJ, McKay CM. Pitch ranking with non-simultaneous dual electrode electrical stimulation of the cochlea. *J Acoust Soc Am*. 1994;96:155–162.

55. Kwon BJ, van den Honert C. Dual-electrode pitch discrimination with sequential interleaved stimulation by cochlear implant users. *J Acoust Soc Am*. 2006;120:EL1–EL6.

56. Smith ZM, Delgutte B, Oxenham AJ. Chimaeric sounds reveal dichotomies in auditory perception. *Nature*. 2002;416:87–90.

57. Zeng FG, Nie K, Stickney GS, et al. Speech recognition with amplitude and frequency modulations. *Proc Natl Acad Sci U S A*. 2005;102:2293–2298.

58. Xu L, Pfingst BE. Relative importance of temporal envelope and fine structure in

lexical-tone perception. *J Acoust Soc Am.* 2003;114:3024–3027.

59. Arnoldner C, Riss D, Brunner M, Baumgartner WD, Hamzavi JS. Speech and music perception with the new fine structure speech coding strategy: preliminary results. *Acta Otolaryngol.* 2007;127:1298–1303.

60. Krenmayr A, Visser D, Schatzer R, Zierhofer C. The effects of fine structure stimulation on pitch perception with cochlear implants. *Cochlear Implants Int.* 2011;12:S70–S72.

61. Zeng FG. Temporal pitch in electric hearing. *Hear Res.* 2002;174:101–106.

62. Wilson BS, Lawson DT, Finley CC, Zerbi M. Speech processors for auditory prostheses: randomized update orders; slow rate CIS implementations; channel number manipulations; evaluation of other promising processing strategies; performance of CIS and CA processors in noise; and use and possible development of new test materials. *Tenth Quarterly Progress Report*, NIH project N01-DC-9-2401. Bethesda, MD: Neural Prosthesis Program, National Institutes of Health; 1991.

63. Riss D, Arnoldner C, Reiss S, Baumgartner WD, Hamzavi JS. 1-year results using the Opus speech processor with the fine structure speech coding strategy. *Acta Otolaryngol.* 2009;129:988–991.

64. Riss D, Hamzavi JS, Katzinger M, Baumgartner WD, Kaider A, Gstoettner W, Arnoldner C. Effects of fine structure and extended low frequencies in pediatric cochlear implant recipients. *Int J Pediatr Otorhinolaryngol.* 2011;75:573–578.

65. Vermeire K, Punte AK, Van de Heyning P. Better speech recognition in noise with the fine structure processing coding strategy. *ORL J Otorhinolaryngol Relat Spec.* 2010;72:305–311.

66. Riss D, Arnoldner C, Baumgartner WD, Kaider A, Hamzavi JS. A new fine structure speech coding strategy: speech perception at a reduced number of channels. *Otol Neurotol.* 2008;29:784–788.

67. Magnusson L. Comparison of the fine structure processing (FSP) strategy and the CIS strategy used in the MED-EL cochlear implant system: speech intelligibility and music sound quality. *Int J Audiol.* 2011; 50:279–287.

68. Brill S, Möltner A, Harnisch W, Müller J, Hagen R. *Temporal fine structure coding in low frequency channels: Speech and prosody understanding, pitch and music perception, and subjective benefit evaluated in a prospective randomized study.* Presented at the 2007 Conference on Implantable Auditory Prostheses, Lake Tahoe, CA, USA, July 15–20, 2007. (Abstract 1E on p. 24 in the conference proceedings.)

69. Schatzer R, Krenmayr A, Au DK, Kals M, Zierhofer C. Temporal fine structure in cochlear implants: preliminary speech perception results in Cantonese-speaking implant users. *Acta Otolaryngol.* 2010; 130:1031–1039.

70. Helms J, Müller J, Schön F, Moser L, Arnold W, et al. Evaluation of performance with the COMBI40 cochlear implant in adults: a multicentric clinical study. *ORL J Otorhinolaryngol Relat Spec.* 1997;59:23–35.

71. Krueger B, Joseph G, Rost U, Strauss-Schier A, Lenarz T, Buechner A. Performance groups in adult cochlear implant users: speech perception results from 1984 until today. *Otol Neurotol.* 2008;29:509–512.

72. Niparko JK, Tobey EA, Thal DJ, Eisenberg LS, Wang NY, et al. Spoken language development in children following cochlear implantation. *JAMA.* 2010;303:1498–1506.

73. Holt RF, Svirsky MA. An exploratory look at pediatric cochlear implantation: is earliest always best? *Ear Hear.* 2008;29:492–511.

74. Dorman MF, Gifford RH. Combining acoustic and electric stimulation in the service of speech recognition. *Int J Audiol.* 2010;49:912–919.

75. Wilson BS, Dorman MF. Cochlear implants: a remarkable past and a brilliant future. *Hear Res.* 2008;242:3–21.

76. Spahr AJ, Dorman MF. Performance of subjects fit with the Advanced Bionics CII and Nucleus 3G cochlear implant devices. *Arch Otolaryngol Head Neck Surg.* 2004; 130:624–628.

77. Wilson BS, Lopez-Poveda EA, Schatzer R. Use of auditory models in developing coding strategies for cochlear implants. In: Meddis R, Lopez-Poveda EA, Popper A, Fay RR, eds. *Computational Models of the Auditory System*. New York, NY: Springer-Verlag; 2010:237–260.

78. Wilson BS, Dorman MF, Woldorff MG, Tucci DL. Cochlear implants: matching the prosthesis to the brain and facilitating desired plastic changes in brain function. *Prog Brain Res*. 2011;194:117–129.

79. Oxenham AJ, Bernstein JG, Penagos H. Correct tonotopic representation is necessary for complex pitch perception. *Proc Natl Acad Sci U S A*. 2004;101:1421–1425.

80. Wilson BS, Dorman MF. Cochlear implants: current designs and future possibilities. *J Rehabil Res Dev*. 2008;45:695–730.

Chapter 5

Cochlear Implant Candidate Selection

RENÉ H. GIFFORD

INTRODUCTION

Determining cochlear implant candidacy is not necessarily a straightforward process. Cochlear implant criteria have rapidly evolved since the Food and Drug Administration (FDA) first approved multichannel cochlear implants for adults and children in 1985 and 1990, respectively. Candidacy criteria vary with patient age, etiology of hearing loss, type of insurance coverage, and even across the different implant manufacturers. Further clouding the question of candidacy is the presence of overlapping indications with cochlear implants, hearing aids, bone-anchored auditory prostheses, middle ear implants, and shorter electrode cochlear implants for hearing preservation (ie, Nucleus Hybrid and MED-EL electric and acoustic stimulation, EAS). Thus, one could imagine the confusion surrounding the selection of appropriate cochlear implant candidates—even among the most knowledgeable members of a cochlear implant team.

Conversely, clinicians who do not frequently work with cochlear implants may not even be aware of how many patients can potentially benefit from this technology.

There are a number of aspects requiring consideration in the process of cochlear implant candidate selection. Many are related to the audiologic evaluation including audiometric and speech recognition testing. Others are related to speech and language development, primarily for pediatric candidates. There are also medical, radiologic, and psychological issues requiring consideration. This chapter discusses the process of cochlear implant candidate selection including aspects to be considered from the perspective of the audiologist, speech-language pathologist, social worker, and/or psychologist as well as the medical/surgical team. This chapter further describes the elements of cochlear implant candidate selection for adults and children with hearing loss as it stands today and discusses those elements that, as a field, we may want to consider in the evaluation process.

AUDIOLOGIC EVALUATION

ASSESSMENT OF HEARING STATUS

Virtually all cochlear implant evaluations will begin in the Audiology clinic. By the time an adult patient is referred for a cochlear implant evaluation, they have likely been followed for a number of years by an audiologist for hearing aid fittings and follow-up. These patients have also likely been seen by an otolaryngologist to gain medical clearance for hearing aids. Thus, by the time an adult patient arrives for a cochlear implant evaluation, he or she is typically aware that hearing aids are not providing adequate benefit for successful communication and is ready to take the next step. From a professional perspective, this generally is a different experience from that commonly faced by the rehabilitative audiologist recommending hearing aids—where denial and hesitation are more often the norm.

For pediatric patients, the cochlear implant evaluation is ordinarily preceded by numerous appointments in the diagnostic Audiology clinic for behavioral hearing testing as well as objective estimates of auditory function. Thus, the cochlear implant evaluation does not typically involve the diagnosis of a severe-to-profound hearing loss as children almost always present to the evaluation with a confirmed diagnosis and hearing aid experience. Thus, the family arrives at the appointment with knowledge and at least partial acceptance of the diagnosis. This helps facilitate discussion about cochlear implants generally without the presence of a raw emotional component that is known to accompany new diagnoses.

Despite the fact that most patients, both adult and pediatric, will present to the cochlear implant evaluation with prior audiograms, it is recommended that comprehensive audiometric testing be completed. For pediatric patients, this is an obvious opportunity to gain additional ear specific information, particularly for frequencies, as the prior audiograms may have been lacking as well as immittance and, minimally, ear specific speech awareness thresholds. For adult patients, comprehensive audiologic testing is recommended as a part of the implant evaluation including air-conduction thresholds for octave frequencies 125 through 8000 Hz as well as bone conduction, immittance, and standard speech audiometry (ie, ear specific speech reception thresholds and word recognition). Obtaining thresholds at 125 Hz is particularly important given that the professions of otology and audiology are becoming increasingly cognizant of minimally traumatic surgical techniques and low-frequency hearing preservation following cochlear implantation.[1-4] Thus, having this baseline information is critical if we are to investigate the presence of residual acoustic hearing in the implanted ear following surgery.

Otoacoustic emissions (OAEs) can also provide valuable information obtained during the cochlear implant evaluation, particularly for pediatric patients. Although most newborn hearing screening programs utilize OAEs as a first-pass screening tool,[5-7] not all children will have had this completed. Virtually every cochlear implant audiologist has at least one story about a patient presenting for an evaluation who is diagnosed with auditory neuropathy spectrum disorder (ANSD) *after* the cochlear implant evaluation. Although ANSD does not preclude a patient from cochlear implantation,[8-12] it is important to have an accurate diagnosis in place as well so as to explore all possible rehabilitative options prior to pursuing surgical intervention.

Most adult patients presenting for a cochlear implant evaluation will have been wearing hearing aids for a number of years. In fact, limited benefit from "appropriately fitted hearing aids" is listed as a requirement for determination of candidacy by all three cochlear implant manufacturers (Cochlear Americas package insert, Advanced Bionics package insert; MED-EL package insert). Thus, even if an adult had present OAEs at lower frequencies in the past, the use of amplification has been shown to be associated with secondary loss of OAEs per long-term use.[13] Hence, the use of OAEs in the adult cochlear implant evaluation is generally not included in most clinical protocols.

COCHLEAR IMPLANT CRITERIA: AUDIOMETRIC THRESHOLDS

Cochlear implant criteria, with respect to audiometric thresholds, differ across implant manufacturers. For pediatric candidacy, there is an additional element of age-specific audiometric criteria. For children aged 12 to 24 months, the current criteria specify bilateral profound sensorineural hearing loss (Cochlear Americas package insert, Advanced Bionics package insert, MED-EL package insert). This is not to imply that children with less severe hearing losses would not benefit from cochlear implantation. Rather, the historical concern was that establishing behavioral thresholds or minimal response levels in the youngest children was more difficult than for older children, and hence the criteria were more stringent for the youngest candidates. This concern may not be as valid today given the audiologic

checks and balances that are at our disposal for both behavioral and physiologic measures of auditory function. In fact, this is also an argument for lowering the official FDA approved age for cochlear implantation from 12 months to slightly younger, perhaps in the 6- to 9-month range.[14,15] Research has demonstrated higher levels of word and language acquisition[16–18] and speech perception[19] for children implanted early—even for those implanted under 12 months of age compared to those in the 2nd year of life. The reality is that if a child under 2 years of age with less severe hearing loss or under 12 months and not making auditory progress with full-time use of appropriately-fitted hearing aids and recommended intervention, that child would meet "candidacy" for cochlear implantation based upon professional clinical judgment.

For children over 2 years of age, the audiometric criteria are slightly more lenient including bilateral severe-to-profound sensorineural hearing loss, allowing for slightly more residual acoustic hearing for candidacy qualification. Again, however, if a child has moderate-to-profound sensorineural hearing loss and is not making auditory progress with well-fitted hearing aids and intervention, the cochlear implant team has the professional clinical judgment to determine candidacy on a case-by-case basis.

Adult audiometric criteria also differ across the manufacturers as well as across insurance carriers. Advanced Bionics and MED-EL specify bilateral severe-to-profound sensorineural hearing loss for adult implant candidacy. On the other hand, both Cochlear Americas and Medicare[20] specify bilateral moderate to profound sensorineural hearing loss, recognizing that individuals with sloping hearing losses will not always obtain benefit from amplification allowing for successful communication.

SPEECH RECOGNITION TESTING

RECORDED MATERIALS

A central component of all adult implant evaluations and pediatric cochlear implant evaluations for older children involves the behavioral assessment of speech recognition abilities. Many individuals with hearing loss report that in order to "hear," they rely heavily on visual cues such as lip reading and more global nonverbal communication. Thus, in order to gain an understanding of an individual's auditory-based speech recognition abilities, speech stimuli are presented without visual cues.

The most important aspect surrounding the administration of speech recognition testing involves the use of recorded speech materials. Using recorded materials for speech recognition assessment has been advocated since 1946 when the Father of Audiology, Dr. Raymond Carhart, suggested that the use of a phonograph recording would increase the test stability across conditions.[21] Unfortunately, however, over two-thirds of audiologists report that they routinely use monitored live voice (MLV) for administration of speech recognition materials,[22,23] although it is unclear whether that estimate included audiologists involved in determining cochlear implant candidacy. Roeser and Clark[24] examined word recognition performance obtained with recorded materials as compared to MLV for 32 ears. They reported that word recognition scores for MLV and recorded stimuli were significantly different for 23 of the 32 ears (or 72% of the population) with the difference between the two scores being as high as 80 percentage points. Thus these data confirm the critical need for the elimination of monitored live voice presentation particularly for the assessment of cochlear implant candidacy.* Currently, Cochlear Americas, MED-EL, and Medicare specify the use of recorded stimuli for the implant evaluation. Given the prevalence of recorded materials available on both compact disc as well as digitized for transmission from the output of the computer sound card directly to the audiometer makes for simple and inexpensive use as well as presentation.

PRESENTATION LEVEL

A second important aspect of speech recognition testing for cochlear implant evaluations involves the presentation level of the recorded speech stimuli. For years the accepted presentation level for the stimulus was 70 dB SPL as this was thought to be necessary in order to provide audibility for individuals with severe-to-profound hearing loss. The problem with using a presentation level of 70 dB SPL is that it is not representative of average conversational level speech. Rather, in a study funded by the Environmental Protection Agency, Pearsons and colleagues[25] reported that average conversational speech was 60 dB SPL and that 70 dB SPL was: (1) representative of raised level or loud speech and (2) not sustainable from a talker's perspective

---

*Some speech materials used for pediatric testing currently do not have recorded versions. These include Glendonald Auditory Screening Procedure (GASP) words and sentences[96] and ESP low verbal pattern perception.[39] These materials, however, are not indicated for use in the determination of implant candidacy and thus do not influence whether or not a child qualifies for cochlear implantation.

for an extended period of time. Later, a number of studies have evaluated speech perception performance for both preimplant[26] and postimplant recipients[27,28] at multiple presentation levels including 50, 60, and 70 dB SPL. They found that postoperative performance for both 60 and 70 dB SPL levels were essentially identical[27,28] but that *preoperative* performance was significantly poorer for 60 dB SPL as compared to 70 dB SPL.[26] Thus, using 70 dB SPL as the presentation level for determining implant candidacy puts the individual at a disadvantage as it: (1) is not representative of average conversational levels in the real world, (2) has the potential to artificially inflate one's speech recognition performance, and (3) can potentially disqualify an individual from candidacy who could derive significant benefit from cochlear implantation. Both Cochlear Americas[29] and Advanced Bionics[30] have recently completed clinical trials which have incorporated a 60-dB-SPL level (A weighting) for presentation of speech stimuli. Thus, best practices recommendations have included the use of recorded speech materials presented at 60 dB A[†] for assessment of speech recognition performance for pre- as well as postimplant testing.

SPEECH RECOGNITION TEST MATERIALS FOR DETERMINING CANDIDACY: ADULTS

A variety of speech recognition materials are available and could be used in the assessment of cochlear implant candidacy including monosyllabic words, sentences, and sentences in noise. With respect to adult cochlear implant candidacy, the minimum speech test battery (MSTB) was originally developed in 1996 when representatives from the American Academy of Otolaryngology-Head and Neck Surgery, the American Academy of Audiology, and an experienced group of clinicians/scientists from the cochlear implant manufacturers met to determine the MSTB recommended for audiologic cochlear implant candidacy and for longitudinal assessment of postoperative performance.[31] The MSTB committee recommended that patient speech recognition performance should be assessed with both monosyllabic words (consonant nucleus consonant, CNC, words[32]; and the Hearing in Noise Test (HINT) sentences[33] presented in quiet and in a fixed-level noise background. Although the MSTB committee did not specify a criterion performance level for determining implant candidacy, they recommended that "at each preoperative and postoperative evaluation, one 50-word CNC list and two 10-sentence HINT lists should be presented in quiet." The committee also recommended that the HINT sentences be presented in fixed-level noise at +10, +5, or even 0 dB signal-to-noise ratio (SNR) as necessary to avoid ceiling effects.[31] Despite these recommendations, current adult cochlear implant candidacy in the United States, with respect to speech recognition performance, has traditionally been based *solely* on sentence recognition performance in a quiet background. Generally, the HINT

[†]The use of A weighting for sound level meter measurements is recommended due to the fact that linear weighting, which is implied in an SPL reference unless otherwise specified, provides noisier recordings due to flat frequency response through the lower frequency region. In contrast, the A-weighted frequency response rolls off for lower frequencies having reached 20 dB of attenuation (relative to pass-band) at 100 Hz.

sentences had been presented in quiet and used for qualification purposes. Cochlear Americas and Medicare, however, do not specify a sentence metric but rather refer to open-set sentence recognition materials for determining candidacy.

Recently a committee of audiologist clinician/scientists convened to discuss the assessment of speech perception for cochlear implant recipients.[34] Based on clinical survey data and literature review, the committee recommended a speech perception test battery for assessing both pre- and postimplant performance. The recommended test battery was estimated to take approximately 30 to 45 minutes to administer, which is an important consideration given the busy clinical environment. The recommended battery included CNC words,[32] AzBio sentences,[35,36] and AzBio sentences presented in multitalker babble using a +5 dB SNR ratio or one list pair of the Bamford-Kowal-Bench-Sentence-in-noise (BKB-SIN) test.[37,38] The recommended use of the AzBio sentences over the seemingly ubiquitous HINT sentences stemmed from the finding that the HINT sentences suffer from ceiling effects for post- and even some preimplant individuals.[36] In fact, the cochlear implant manufacturers in the United States have now moved to include the AzBio sentences in a new battery of tests that will serve as the standard for evaluation of pre- and postimplant assessments of speech recognition. The implant companies have recommended a test battery including AzBio sentences, BKB-SIN sentences in noise, and CNC monosyllabic words. The use of words, sentences in quiet, and sentences in noise provides information on the individual's performance in a variety of listening conditions as well as verification of subject performance via cross-checking across the dif-

ferent speech recognition materials and the known inter-relationship of individual performance on those measures.[34,36] In fact, the most recent MSTB manual released in July 2011 specifies the use of CNC monosyllables, AzBio sentences in quiet (and possibly in noise), as well as the Bamford-Kowal-Bench, speech in noise (BKB-SIN) metric.

As with the other previously discussed aspects of implant candidacy, each manufacturer outlines a slightly different set of indications found in the FDA-approved Physician's Package Insert labeling for each device. At the time of chapter preparation, Advanced Bionics specified HINT sentence recognition up to 50% in the best aided condition. Cochlear Americas specified sentence recognition up to 50% correct in the ear to be implanted and up to 60% in the best aided condition (Cochlear Americas package insert). MED-EL listed HINT sentence recognition up to 40% correct in the best aided condition. Last, Medicare criteria were also outlined independently to include sentence recognition performance up to 40% correct in the best aided condition.

SPEECH RECOGNITION TEST MATERIALS: OLDER CHILDREN

Current implant candidacy criteria for older children are generally based on either mono- or multisyllabic word recognition depending on which is most developmentally appropriate for the child being evaluated. The tests that are listed by the cochlear implant manufacturers in their FDA labeling are as follows (presented in order of developmentally appropriate progression): Early Speech Perception (ESP) test,[39] Multisyllabic lexical Neighborhood Test (MLNT[40]), the Lexical Neighborhood Test (LNT[40]), the Phonetically Balanced Kindergarten (PBK[41]) word recognition test, and HINT sentences for children (HINT-C[42]).

The older child for whom these metrics are considered developmentally appropriate is required to exhibit considerably lower performance than even that listed for adult FDA implant labeling. Word recognition candidacy criteria for the older child ranges from 12 to 30% correct in the best aided condition across the three manufacturers. Advanced Bionics further lists performance up to 30% correct for HINT-C sentences, when developmentally appropriate for children over 4 years, although the same company lists up to 50% HINT sentence recognition performance for adult candidates. The need for the expansion of pediatric cochlear implant criteria has been and remains a hot topic, as an ever increasing amount of research emerges supporting a relatively narrow critical period for cochlear implantation for the development of listening and spoken language[16–18,17,39,43,44] and auditory pathway maturation.[45–51] Thus, the combined fields of otology, audiology, and speech-language pathology are right to question the most stringent candidacy criteria for the youngest of auditory language learners.

EVALUATION OF AUDITORY SKILLS AND PROGRESS IN INFANTS AND YOUNGER CHILDREN: BIRTH TO 3 YEARS

Determining a child's auditory skills and progress with hearing aids prior to determining implant candidacy is not as easy as studying the audiogram. It is well known that similar audiograms do not necessarily yield similar levels of benefit from amplification across a range of hearing loss severities and configurations. Given that speech recognition performance cannot be completed for infants and many toddlers, it is critical that the candidacy evaluation process include assessment of auditory skills, development, and progress with hearing aids. From the perspective of the audiologist, these skills will most likely be assessed via parental history and administration of validated questionnaires that are designed to gauge a child's auditory-based responsiveness to sounds in their environment.

One of the most common questionnaires used for children from birth to 3 years is the Infant-Toddler version of the Meaningful Auditory Integration Scale (IT-MAIS).[52] All three cochlear implant companies make reference to the MAIS[53] and/or IT-MAIS for use in determining lack of auditory progress with amplification. For the youngest of children, the 10-item IT-MAIS is frequently used due to the widespread familiarity of the metric as well as the ease and time required of administration (approximately 10 minutes). The IT-MAIS is designed to be administered in a structured parental interview format and thus requires that the clinician interpret open-ended responses and assign a numerical score ranging from 0 (never) to 4 (always).

The Auditory Skills Checklist (ASC[54]) was developed in response to the increasing number of children being implanted under 12 months of age. The ASC is a 35-item questionnaire that assesses detection, discrimination, identification and comprehension. Similar to the IT-MAIS, the ASC is designed to be administered in a parental interview style as well as via clinician observation for which the parent/administrator assigns a rating ranging from 0 to 2 as follows: 0, child does have the skill; 1, child has demonstrated emerging skill development; 2, child consistently demonstrates skill. The ASC can be administered along with the IT-MAIS as it is expected that the ASC can be used over a longer period of time (for children implanted up to 3 years of age) and will provide a detailed assessment over smaller increments of auditory skill development.

Other parental questionnaires designed to assess spontaneous and prompted responsiveness to sound for infants and toddlers have surfaced and are gaining popularity amongst clinicians. The LittlEars Auditory Questionnaire[55,56] is comprised of 35 yes/no questions designed to gauge a child's auditory-based responses to different sounds and environments. The questions are organized hierarchically with a progression of difficulty so that the parent can stop answering questions following six consecutive "no" answers. It is designed for use in children up to 24 months of age for normal hearing or 24 months following implantation, although a child would be expected to reach ceiling levels prior to that test point. Administration of the LittlEars takes very little time because it does not require parental interview and does not take up time during the actual appointment.

Another questionnaire that offers valuable information in the candidacy process, although designed primarily for use following implantation, is the Functioning after Pediatric Cochlear Implantation (FAPCI) questionnaire.[57] The 23-item FAPCI is considered appropriate for children aged approximately 2 to 5 years and

does not require parental interview for administration. Using the FAPCI during the candidacy process provides clinicians and families with a baseline against which future growth in auditory skills can be gauged.

The Functional Auditory Performance Indicators (FAPI[58]) assesses seven categories of auditory development including sound awareness, meaningful sounds, auditory feedback, sound localization, discrimination, short-term auditory memory, and linguistic auditory processing. The clinician assigns a score for each category as emerging (0 to 35%), in process (36 to 79%), or acquired (80 to 100%). The FAPI can be used in children as young as a few months of age and can continue to be used until "acquired" scores are obtained for all categories.

The Early Listening Function (ELF[59]) questionnaire is also appropriate for children from birth to 3 years. It is different from the others in that it is designed to assess a child's responsiveness to certain sounds from multiple distances both in quiet and noise. It is consists of 12 listening *situations* where the parent and clinician will observe the child and record the distance at which the child responds to the auditory stimulus.

Individual clinics will determine which auditory questionnaires best meet the needs of their patient population and their families. Being more important than the actual questionnaires used is that the clinicians within a given program be consistent across all patients. The cochlear implant team should closely monitor the auditory progress of children during the hearing aid trial period being careful to analyze the child's complete auditory profile and not fall into the trap of failing to see "beyond the audiogram."

EVALUATION OF AUDITORY SKILLS AND PROGRESS IN PRESCHOOL TO SCHOOL-AGE CHILDREN

As with infant and toddlers, assessment of auditory skills and development for older children cannot always be well predicted by the audiogram. Although behavioral assessment of auditory skills should always be attempted for preschool and school-aged children, due to a number of factors, behavioral assessment may not be possible or only very limited information may be gleaned. For this reason, there are several auditory skill questionnaires designed for use with preschool and school-aged children.

The Meaningful Auditory Integration Scale (MAIS[53]) is a 10-item parental interview style questionnaire designed for assessing auditory skills including spontaneous responses to sounds for children aged 3 to 5 years. All three cochlear implant manufacturers make reference to this questionnaire for determining auditory progress, or lack thereof, with appropriately fitted amplification.

The Parents' Evaluation of Aural/oral Performance of Children or the PEACH is a 13-item questionnaire that was designed for parental estimation of their child's functional aural and oral abilities in everyday life.[60] It is considered appropriate for administration to children aged 3 to 7 years. The parents are asked to reflect on their child's listening behavior over the previous week and requires that an answer ranging from 0 (never or 0%) to 4 (always or 75 to 100%) be assigned to questions relating to listening in both quiet and noisy situations.

The 23-item FAPCI questionnaire[57] can be administered to parents of children aged 2 to 5 years. As stated previously, although the FAPCI was originally intended to track postoperative progress, using it during the candidacy process provides clinicians and families with a baseline against which future growth in auditory skills can be gauged.

As with the questionnaires discussed for the younger children, individual clinics will determine the appropriateness of the different instruments and appropriateness for their patient population. What is most important is consistency across clinicians and patients within a cochlear implant program.

TESTING CONDITIONS

The testing conditions for determining cochlear implant candidacy are not widely agreed upon amongst clinicians. All three manufacturers use the term "best aided condition" when referring to speech recognition performance for both adults and children. Medicare criteria also specify the "best aided condition" as the performance to be considered for determining implant candidacy. Only one of the manufacturers, Cochlear Americas, specifically states different performance criteria for the ear to be implanted as compared to the best aided listening condition, allowing for binaural summation and/or asymmetry between the ears. The problem is that different clinicians can interpret the term "best aided condition" differently. In the case of asymmetric hearing loss and/or speech recognition performance across the ears, the best aided condition may be a gross overestimation of performance as compared to performance for the proposed ear to be implanted. The most recent MSTB as well as Fabry and colleagues[60] recommend individual ear testing for postoperative assessment of performance. Thus, it would follow that we should be assessing individual ear performance preoperatively, as well. As the implant manufacturers propose new candidacy indications for FDA approval, it is very likely that more emphasis will be placed on assessing the ear to be implanted as well as a best aided condition.

SUBJECTIVE EVALUATION OF ADULT PREIMPLANT PERFORMANCE

Evidence-based practice is gaining increasingly more attention in clinical patient care as insurance companies require proof of treatment efficacy for coverage purposes. Evidence-based practice in audiology has largely been associated with hearing aid fittings; however, evidence-based practice has an active role in the preimplant evaluation and postoperative fitting and assessment of patients with cochlear implants, as well. Objective measures of postoperative speech perception performance and subjective assessments of perceived performance and/or benefit may not be in good agreement with one another.[62] One likely explanation is that the laboratory-like conditions assessed in the audiometric test booth may not truly reflect real-world listening conditions. Furthermore, subjective assessment instruments can also serve to validate the efficacy of a particular treatment option, such as cochlear implantation. Although we recognize the efficacy of cochlear implantation with respect to restoration of hearing and speech recognition, we do

not routinely assess the effect of cochlear implants on a recipient's social or emotional welfare or the more global effect on one's quality of life. On another level, the use of subjective measures during the *preoperative* assessment can provide an element of information that is not necessarily contained within the objective scores of speech recognition.

There are a number of instruments used to assess subjective benefit, performance and/or quality of life following cochlear implantation. Although the 24-item Abbreviated Profile of Hearing Aid Benefit[63] was designed to gauge degree of benefit following hearing aid fittings, due to the ease of administration and the relative brevity of the questionnaire, it is often used in cochlear implant programs. The APHAB self-assessment scale evaluates listening difficulties experienced in four areas: ease of communication, background noise, reverberation, and aversiveness of sound. Thus, the difference in listening difficulties found pre- and post-implant provides an index of the benefit associated with cochlear implantation.

The Client-Oriented Scale of Improvement (COSI[64]) is a clinical assessment instrument developed by National Acoustic Laboratories for evaluating individually-determined outcomes following amplification. The COSI can be easily adapted for use with cochlear implant recipients as the patient can identify listening situations in which he/she would like improved with cochlear implants. Although the COSI is a great tool for use with patients, it is limited in its across-patient comparison due to the individual nature of the instrument.

The Nijmegen Cochlear Implant Questionnaire (NCIQ[65]) is a 60-item, quality-of-life instrument designed for use with adult cochlear implant recipients. The NCIQ assesses six domains including basic sound perception (eg, environmental sounds), advanced sound perception (eg, modulation of one's own voice, speech intelligibility), speech perception, self-esteem, activity, and social interactions. The NCIQ was designed for administration both pre- and postimplant.

The 25-item Cochlear Implant Function Index (CIFI[66]) is a self-assessment instrument that was designed and validated for use with adult cochlear implant recipients. The CIFI evaluates an individual's reliance on visual cues, use of the telephone, communication at work as well as hearing in noise, in groups, and in large room settings. As with the other instruments, the CIFI is recommended for administration both pre- and postimplant.

More generic quality of life assessment instruments are also available and are widely used in cochlear implant research, although they may also be useful in the clinical environment. Health-related, quality of life questionnaires can assign a numerical value to duration of life as modified by the impairments (eg, hearing loss), functional states, perceptions, and social opportunities that can be influenced by disease, injury, treatment, or policy.[67] The Health Utilities Index (HUI®) Mark III[68] is a multidimensional instrument that assesses individual abilities on attributes including vision, hearing, speech, ambulation, dexterity, emotion, cognition, and pain. There are multiple questionnaire formats available including self-assessment, clinician-administered, and even proxy-assessment versions. Although these were designed with a clinical research focus, one could reasonably incorporate such an instrument into clinical protocol for cochlear implant candidate selection and assessment of health-related changes following cochlear implantation.

SPEECH AND LANGUAGE EVALUATION: PEDIATRIC CANDIDACY

The speech-language pathologist plays a critical role in the cochlear implant candidate selection process for infants and children. Often, a child presenting for cochlear implant evaluation will have little or no language when considering either manual or spoken communication abilities. The evaluation of speech, and more importantly, language should be scheduled to coincide with an audiology appointment so that the hearing aid settings are first verified prior to the assessment using either probe microphone measurements or test box verification using either patient-specific or average age corrected real ear to coupler difference (RECD) corrections.

When commencing a "hearing aid trial" for infants who are thought to meet cochlear implant candidacy based on the severity of the hearing loss, it is critical to also schedule a speech-language evaluation to determine baseline language skills against which future development can be gauged. The specific metrics used by the speech-language pathologist will be dependent on both the chronologic age as well as the "hearing" age of the child. During the hearing aid trial period, it is expected that the child make *at least* month-for-month auditory progress and well as speech and language developmental progress with amplification in order to be deriving appropriate benefit from hearing aids. What that means is that if a child has been fitted with hearing aids for 3 months, they should make *at least* 3 months of progress in auditory skills and speech-language development. If this is not the case for a child making full-time use of amplification and appropriate intervention, then cochlear implantation should be considered.

It is expected that a child receive at least two speech-language evaluations during the candidacy selection process during the hearing aid trial. Furthermore, it is critical that children receive appropriate intervention including regular visits from a member of the early intervention team, speech-language therapy, as well as active parental involvement to supplement therapy with proper modeling of spoken language development. The cochlear implant team can glean considerable information from parental compliance of not only full-time use of amplification, but also to the recommended therapy schedule during the candidacy selection process. It sets an important precedent for what will be expected following cochlear implant surgery as intensive intervention and therapy will be required if the child is to make full use of the audibility provided by the new, electrical signal.

THE ROLE OF THE SOCIAL WORKER AND/ OR PSYCHOLOGIST IN THE DETERMINATION OF COCHLEAR IMPLANT CANDIDACY

The role of the social worker and/or psychologist in the determination of cochlear implant candidacy can be pivotal for both adult and pediatric recipients. Psychological evaluations are generally not routinely scheduled for all adult cochlear implant evaluations as was the common practice when cochlear implants were first introduced clinically; however, scheduling a visit with a psychologist and/or social worker in select adult cases can provide valuable information for not only the cochlear implant team, but also for the patient and his or her family. For example, adult patients who were prelingually deafened as well as individuals who have had sudden onset profound hearing loss are obvious populations that could benefit from a preoperative psychological evaluation and/or appointment with a social worker specially trained to work with hearing-impaired individuals. The goal of the cochlear implant team is to evaluate each patient individually and recommend psychological and/or social worker attention for adult candidates on a case-by-case basis, as needed.

The role of the social worker and/ or psychologist in the determination of pediatric cochlear implant candidacy is perhaps of greater importance than that for adult patients. A psychological evaluation, particularly a developmental psychological evaluation, may be ordered by the cochlear implant team in the event that concerns are raised regarding the overall cognitive and mental functioning of the child. Other areas where a psychologist and/or social worker can provide invaluable assistance is for families struggling with the diagnosis and implications of having a child who will be dependent on the cochlear implant technology for hearing and communication. Other areas within the scope of the psychologist and/or social worker in determining implant candidacy include evaluation of family dynamics and level of dedication to the recommended postoperative therapy schedule. Such guidance can be sought after and/or recommended by the cochlear implant team pre- and post-implant, as needed.

MEDICAL/SURGICAL ISSUES

The cochlear implant surgeon, typically an otologist or neurotologist, provides a discernable critical role in the determination of implant candidacy. The otologist's role in cochlear implantation is discussed at length in Chapters 7–10. Surgeons complete a thorough preoperative evaluation in addition to being responsible for the implant surgical procedure and postoperative otologic medical care. The otologist and his or her medical team ensures that all cochlear implant candidates are up to date on their immunizations prior to cochlear implantation. The immunization schedule is provided in the Appendix.

The otologist will also review the patient's current medication list and devise a plan for the management of anticoagulant medications prior to the scheduled cochlear implant surgery. The otologist will also order a preanesthetic medical evaluation or preoperative evaluation to ensure that the candidate is able to undergo surgery and the associated anesthetic risk. The preoperative evaluation includes assessment of vital signs and general medical evaluation to identify the presence of health problems that may affect peri- and/or postanesthetic care. Furthermore, the otologist typically will refer pediatric patients to ophthalmology as well as medical genetics. Approximately 40% of children with sensorineural hearing loss have other medical and/or developmental comorbidities including cognitive, visual, motor, behavioral, and learning.[69–72] Thus, the otologist will also refer to additional medical specialties such as Neurology, Physical Medicine and Rehabilitation, and Developmental Pediatrics, as needed.

Otologists also routinely order imagining studies including CT and/or MRI to determine cochlear patency as well as to rule out cochlear or other temporal bone anomalies that could impact the surgical insertion of the device. Cochlear and temporal bone anomalies, however, are not necessarily contraindicated for cochlear implantation although it is critical that the surgical team be aware of such issues. High-resolution CT is typically ordered for all patients having met audiologic criteria for cochlear implantation. MRI, on the other hand, is generally ordered for adult patients exhibiting audiometric asymmetry as well as for pediatric patients who have either exhibited no behavioral hearing via audiometric testing and/or who are suspect for cochlear nerve deficiency. For further information on radiologic imaging studies as pertaining to cochlear implant candidacy, see Chapter 6.

BIMODAL HEARING AND BILATERAL COCHLEAR IMPLANTATION

Up to this point, this chapter has focused on the determination of whether a patient meets cochlear implant candidacy or not. Although this is an important consideration, there are many other concerns to be factored with respect to candidacy. When multichannel cochlear implants were first FDA approved in 1985, patients were required to have bilateral profound sensorineural hearing loss and little to no speech recognition abilities. Furthermore, these patients would receive a single cochlear implant and thus have hearing restored unilaterally. Implant criteria have evolved significantly since that time and even more so over the past several years.

Individuals with increasing amounts of residual acoustic hearing and higher levels of preoperative speech recognition are receiving cochlear implants and deriving significant communicative benefit.[73–77]

Most patients being considered for cochlear implant candidacy will retain "bilateral" hearing in the sense that they will either hear bimodally, with one cochlear implant and aided acoustic hearing in the nonimplanted ear, or will hear with two cochlear implants. At the time of chapter preparation, bilateral cochlear implantation was considered standard of care treatment for individuals with bilateral severe-to-profound sensorineural hearing loss for the largest of private health insurance companies in the United States such as Aetna, Blue Cross Blue Shield, Cigna, Great West, Health Partners, Kaiser California, Medica, Priority Health, and TRICARE (although this list is in no way exhaustive). Furthermore, the William House Cochlear Implant Study Group[78] and Papsin and colleagues[79] have both recognized bilateral cochlear implantation as accepted medical practice and stated that it should be considered standard of care treatment for severe-to-profound sensorineural hearing loss.

One of the most frequently asked questions from patients and clinicians alike deals with whether or not a particular patient should get one or two cochlear implants. Providing a thorough literature review on this topic could fill the pages of an entire book. The short answer is that there are no definitive data that define the audiometric thresholds, configuration of hearing loss, or levels of speech perception performance that can serve as a preoperative indicator to determine whether an individual should pursue one versus two implants. For children acquiring spoken language *through*

the use of cochlear implants, there are an increasing number of reports indicating that bilateral cochlear implantation, at a young age, yields higher levels of speech perception,[80,81] rapid language acquisition achieving age-appropriate norms at younger ages,[82] binaural summation,[83–86] equivalent head shadow across ears,[84,85] binaural squelch,[84,87] and improved localization abilities.[80,88–91]

DIRECTIONS FOR THE FUTURE

It is estimated that 28.0 to 34.3 million people in the United States, or roughly 10% of the population, report significant hearing difficulty.[92,93] The NIDCD further estimates that up to 750,000 Americans have severe-to-profound sensorineural hearing loss.[93] As of 2008, Wilson and Dorman[94] reported that the cumulative number of implanted devices worldwide exceeded 120,000. Wilson and Dorman[95] further reported that approximately 37% of the worldwide cochlear implant recipients were located in the United States. With roughly 44,400 cochlear implant recipients in the United States as of 2008, that number represented just under 6% of the approximate 750,000 severe to profound, hearing-impaired population. Thus, it is reasonable to assume that we have only scratched the surface in offering this technology to those individuals who could potentially derive benefit. It is unclear why so many cochlear implant "candidates" are not being identified. Potential reasons include lack of knowledge on the part of the hearing aid consumer, or on the part of the dispenser (whether it be an audiologist or hearing aid dealer), use of inappropriate preimplant assessment materials, overall lack of public awareness, or some combination of these as well as other possible factors. Thus, the future will likely see significant increases in the number of adult and pediatric cochlear implant recipients.

Other directions for the future may consider physiologic and/or behavioral estimates of listening effort, listening fatigue, or stress as associated to listening. Many patients report that although they are able to "get by" with their current hearing aids, they are completely exhausted by the end of the workday. Evaluating such variables may one day prove useful in the qualification of initial cochlear implant candidacy as well as for determining when a bimodal listener should pursue a second cochlear implant.

CONCLUSION

The opening of this chapter stated that determining cochlear implant candidacy is not a straightforward process. The determination of cochlear implant candidacy is truly a *process* that is accomplished via the collective teamwork of a multidisciplinary group of professionals. Many patients and their families are astonished at the intricacies involved in a cochlear implant evaluation. Given the expansion of cochlear implant criteria for both adults and children and increased incidence of hearing preservation with cochlear implantation, the cochlear implant selection process will continue to evolve.

Cochlear implants have been labeled as the most successful and effective implantable prosthesis in terms of restoring function to its recipients.[96] Cochlear implants have been shown to literally change the course of a child's life and re-store hearing and communication abilities to adults with acquired deafness. Furthermore, it is important to recognize that candidacy criteria have dramatically evolved over the past several decades and that cochlear implants are no longer only for individuals with profound sensorineural deafness. A number of studies have demonstrated the efficacy of cochlear implants for individuals falling outside current candidacy indications with respect to both audiometric thresholds and speech perception performance.[64–68] Despite the efficacy of cochlear implantation and associated aural habilitation and/or rehabilitation in the treatment of severe-to-profound sensorineural hearing loss, it is of critical importance that candidacy be carefully determined to ensure that the least invasive treatment option be determined for all patients. The multidisciplinary cochlear implant team offers patients the highest level of care and information needed to progress through the candidacy selection process.

REFERENCES

1. Gstoettner WK van de Heyning P, O'Connor AF, et al. Electric acoustic stimulation of the auditory system: results of a multicentre investigation. *Acta Otolaryngol.* 2008;128:968–975.
2. Skarzynski H, Lorens A, Piotrowska A, Anderson I. Partial deafness cochlear implantation provides benefit to a new population of individuals with hearing loss. *Acta Otolaryngol.* 2006;126:934–940.
3. Gantz BJ, Hansen MR, Turner CW, Oleson JJ, Reiss LA, Parkinson AJ. Hybrid 10 clinical trial: preliminary results. *Audiol Neurotol.* 2009;14 (suppl 1):32–38.
4. Carlson MC, Driscoll CLW, Gifford RH, et al. Implications of minimizing trauma dur-

ing conventional length cochlear implantation. *Otol Neurotol.* 2011;32(6):962–968.

5. American Academy of Pediatrics (AAP) Joint Committee on Infant Hearing (JCIH). Year 2007 position statement: principles and guidelines for early hearing detection and intervention programs. *Pediatrics.* 2007;120(4):898–921.

6. White KR, Vohr BR, Meyer S, et al. A multisite study to examine the efficacy of the otoacoustic emission/automated auditory brainstem response newborn hearing screening protocol: research design and results of the study. *Am J Audiol.* 2005; 14:S186–S199.

7. Gravel JS, White KR, Johnson JL, et al. A multisite study to examine the efficacy of the otoacoustic emission/automated auditory brainstem response newborn hearing screening protocol: recommendations for policy, practice, and research. *Am J Audiol.* 2005;14(2):S217–S228.

8. Shallop JK, Peterson A, Facer GW, Fabry LB, Driscoll CLW. Cochlear implants in five cases of auditory neuropathy: postoperative findings and progress. *Laryngoscope.* 2001;111:555–562.

9. Peterson A, Shallop J, Driscoll C, et al. Outcomes of cochlear implantation in children with auditory neuropathy. *J Am Acad Audiol.* 2003;14:188–201.

10. Rance G, Barker EJ. Speech perception in children with auditory neuropathy/dyssynchrony managed with either hearing aids or cochlear implants. *Otol Neurotol.* 2008;29:179–182.

11. Teagle HFB, Rousch PA, Woodard JS, et al. Cochlear implantation in children with auditory neuropathy spectrum disorder. *Ear Hear.* 2010;31:325–335.

12. Breneman A, Gifford RH, DeJong MD. Cochlear implantation in children with auditory neuropathy spectrum disorder: long-term outcomes. *J Am Acad Audiol.* In press.

13. Deltenre P, Mansbach AL, Bozet C, Christiaens F, Barthelemy P, Paulissen D, et al. Auditory neuropathy with preserved cochlear microphonics and secondary loss of otoacoustic emissions. *Audiology.* 1999; 38(4):187–195.

14. Cosetti M, Roland JT Jr. Cochlear implantation in the very young child: issues unique to the under-1 population. *Trends Amplif.* 2010;14(1):46–57.

15. Kim LS, Jeong SW, Lee YM, Kim JS. Cochlear implantation in children. *Auris Nasus Larynx.* 2010;37(1):6–17.

16. Bergeson TR, Houston DM, Miyamoto RT. Effects of congenital hearing loss and cochlear implantation on audiovisual speech perception in infants and children. *Restor Neurol Neurosci.* 2010;28:157–165.

17. Houston DM, Miyamoto RT. Effects of early auditory experience on word learning and speech perception in deaf children with cochlear implants: implications for sensitive periods of language development. *Otol Neurotol.* 2010;31:1248–1253.

18. Niparko JK, Tobey EA, Thal DJ, et al. Spoken language development in children following cochlear implantation. CDaCI Investigative Team. *JAMA.* 2010 Apr 21; 303(15):1498–1506.

19. Tajudeen BA, Waltzman SB, Jethanamest D, Svirsky MA. Speech perception in congenitally deaf children receiving cochlear implants in the first year of life. *Otol Neurotol.* 2010 Oct;31(8):1254–1260.

20. Centers for Medicare and Medicaid Services (CMS). CMS Manual System, Pub 100–103, Medicare National Coverage Determination, Subject: Cochlear Implantation Transmittal 42. Baltimore, MD: Department of Health & Human Services, Center for Medicare and Medicaid Services; 2005.

21. Carhart R. Monitored live-voice as a test of auditory acuity. *J Acoust Soc Am.* 1946; 17:339–349.

22. Martin FN, Champlin C, Chambers JA. Seventh survey of audiometric practices in the United States. *J Am Acad Audiol.* 1998; 9(2):95–104.

23. Medwetsky L, Sanderson D, Young D. A national survey of audiology clinical practices, Part 1. *Hear Rev.* 1999;6 (11):24–32.

24. Roeser R, Clark J. Live voice speech recognition audiometry—stop the madness. *Audiology Today.* 2008;20:32–33.
25. Pearsons KS, Bennett RL, Fidell S. *Speech Levels in Various Noise Environments* (Report No. EPA-600/1-77-025). Washington, DC: U.S. Environmental Protection Agency; 1977.
26. Alkaf FM, Firszt JB. Speech recognition in quiet and noise in borderline cochlear implant candidates. *J Amer Acad Audiol.* 2007;18(10):872–882.
27. Firszt JB, Holden LK, Skinner MW, et al. Recognition of speech presented at soft to loud levels by adult cochlear implant recipients of three cochlear implant systems. *Ear Hear.* 2004;25(4):375–387.
28. Skinner MW, Holden LK, Holden TA, Demorest ME, Fourakis MS. Speech recognition at simulated soft, conversational, and raised-to-loud vocal efforts by adults with cochlear implants. *J Acoust Soc Am.* 1997;101(6):3766–3782.
29. Balkany T, Hodges A, Menapace C, et al. Nucleus Freedom North American clinical trial. *Otolaryngol Head Neck Surg.* 2007; 136:757–762.
30. NCT01066780 ClearVoice Sound-processing Strategy for AB HiRes 120 Cochlear Implant Users. 2010; Advanced Bionics, United States: Food and Drug Administration Clinical Trial.
31. Nilsson MJ, McCaw VM, Soli S. *Minimum Speech Test Battery for Adult Cochlear Implant Users: User Manual.* Los Angeles, CA: House Ear Institute; 1996.
32. Peterson GE, Lehiste I. Revised CNC lists for auditory tests. *J Speech Hear Disorders.* 1962;27:62–72.
33. Nilsson M, Soli S, Sullivan J. Development of the Hearing-in-Noise test for the measurement of speech reception thresholds in quiet and in noise. *J Acoust Soc Am.* 1994;95:1085–1099.
34. Fabry D, Firszt JB, Gifford RH, Holden LK, Koch D. Evaluating speech perception benefit in adult cochlear implant recipients. *Audiology Today.* 2009;21:37–42.
35. Spahr AJ, Dorman MF. Effects of minimum stimulation settings for the Med El Tempo+ speech processor on speech understanding. *Ear Hear.* 2005;26(4 suppl):2S–6S.
36. Gifford R, Shallop JK, Peterson AM. Speech recognition materials and ceiling effects: considerations for cochlear implant programs. *Audiol Neurotol.* 2008;13:193–205.
37. Killion M, Niquette, P, Revit L, Skinner M. Quick SIN and BKB-SIN, two new speech-in-noise tests permitting SNR-50 estimates in 1 to 2 min (A). *J Acoust Soc Am.* 2001; 109(5):2502–2512.
38. Etymotic Research, Inc. BKB-SIN Test. Speech-in-Noise Test Version 1.03, 2005. http://www.etymotic.com
39. Moog JS, Geers A. *Early Speech Perception Test for Profoundly Hearing-Impaired Children.* St. Louis, MO: Central Institute for the Deaf; 1990.
40. Kirk KI, Pisoni DB, Osberger MJ. Lexical effects on spoken word recognition by pediatric cochlear implant users. *Ear Hear.* 1995;16:470–481.
41. Haskins H. *A Phonetically Balanced Test of Speech Discrimination for Children.* Unpublished dissertation, Chicago, IL: Northwestern University; 1949.
42. Gelnett D, Sumida A, Nilsson M, Soli SD. *Development of the Hearing-in-Noise Test for Children (HINT-C).* Paper presented at the annual meeting of the American Academy of Audiology. Dallas, TX; 1995.
43. Habib MG, Waltzman SB, Tajudeen B, Svirsky MA. Speech production intelligibility of early implanted pediatric cochlear implant users. *Int J Pediatri Otorhinolaryngol.* 2010 Aug;74(8):855–859.
44. Hayes H, Geers AE, Treiman R, Moog JS. Receptive vocabulary development in deaf children with cochlear implants: achievement in an intensive auditory-oral educational setting. *Ear Hear.* 2009 Feb:30(1):128–135.
45. Gilley PM, Sharma A, Dorman MF. Cortical reorganization in children with cochlear implants. *Brain Res.* 2008;1239:56–65.

46. Kral A, Tillein J, Heid S, Klinke R, Hartmann R. Cochlear implants: cortical plasticity in congenital deprivation. *Prog Brain Res*. 2009;157:283–313.

47. Kral A, Eggermont J. What's to lose and what's to learn: development under auditory deprivation, cochlear implants and limits of cortical plasticity. *Brain Res Rev*. 2007 Nov;56(1):259–269.

48. Ponton CW, Eggermont JJ, Don M, et al. Maturation of the mismatch negativity: effects of profound deafness and cochlear implant use. *Audiol Neurootol*. 2000 May–Aug;5(3–4):167–185.

49. Sharma A, Nash AA, Dorman M. Cortical development, plasticity and re-organization in children with cochlear implants. *J Commun Disord*. 2009 Jul–Aug;42(4):272–279.

50. Sharma A, Dorman MF. Central auditory development in children with cochlear implants: clinical implications. *Adv Otorhinolaryngol*. 2006;64:66–88.

51. Gordon KA, Wong DD, Valero J, Jewell SF, Yoo P, Papsin BC. Use it or lose it? Lessons learned from the developing brains of children who are deaf and use cochlear implants to hear. *Brain Topogr*. 2011 Apr 11. [Epub ahead of print].

52. Zimmerman-Phillips S, Robbins AM, Osberger MJ. Assessing cochlear implant benefit in very young children. *Ann Otol Rhinol Laryngol Suppl*. 2000;185, 42–43.

53. Robbins AM, Renshaw JJ, Berry SW. Evaluating meaningful auditory integration in profoundly hearing-impaired children. *Am J Otology*. 1991;12 (suppl):144–150.

54. Meinzen-Derr J, Wiley S, Creighton J, Choo D. Auditory Skills Checklist: clinical tool for monitoring functional auditory skill development in young children with cochlear implants. *Ann Otol Rhinol Laryngol*. 2007;116(11):812–818.

55. Weichbold V, Tsiakpini L, Coninx F, D'Haese P. Development of a parent questionnaire for assessment of auditory behaviour of infants up to two years of age. *Laryngorhinootologie*. 2005;84(5):328–334.

56. Coninx F, Weichbold V, Tsiakpini L, et al. Validation of the LittlEARS((R)) Auditory Questionnaire in children with normal hearing. *Int J Pediatr Otorhinolaryngol*. 2009;73(12):1761–1768.

57. Lin FR, Ceh K, Bervinchak D, Riley A, Miech R, Niparko JK. Development of a communicative performance scale for pediatric cochlear implantation. *Ear Hear*. 2007;28(5):703–712.

58. Stredler-Brown A, DeConde Johnson C. *Functional Auditory Performance Indicators: An Integrated Approach to Auditory Development* [Online]. Denver: Colorado Department of Education, Special EducationServices Unit; 2003. http://www.cde.state.co.us/cdesped/SpecificDisability-Hearing.html

59. Anderson KL. *Early Listening Function (ELF): Discovery Tool for Parents and Caregivers of Infants and Toddlers*. http://www.hear2learn.com/Inventories/ELF_Questionnaire.pdf

60. Ching TY, Hill M. The Parents' Evaluation of Aural/Oral Performance of Children (PEACH) scale: normative data. *J Am Acad Audiol*. 2007;18(3):220–235.

61. Fabry D, Firszt JB, Gifford RH, Holden L, Koch D. Evaluating speech perception benefit in adults with cochlear implants. *Audiology Today*. 2009;21:36–43.

62. Wackym PA, Runge-Samuelson CL, Firszt JB, Alkaf FM, Burg LS. More challenging speech-perception tasks demonstrate binaural benefit in bilateral cochlear implant users. *Ear Hear*. 2007;28:80S–85S.

63. Cox RM, Alexander GC. The abbreviated profile of hearing aid benefit. *Ear Hear*. 1995;16:176–186.

64. Dillon H, James A, Ginis J. The Client Oriented Scale of Improvement (COSI) and its relationship to several other measures of benefit and satisfaction provided by hearing aids. *J Am Acad Audiol*. 1997;8:27–43.

65. Hinderink JB KP, Broek PVD. Development and application of a health-related quality-of-life instrument for adults with cochlear implants: the Nijmegen Cochlear

Implant Questionnaire. *Otolaryngol Head Neck Surg.* 2000;123:756–765.

66. Coelho DH, Hammerschlag PE, Bat-Chava Y, Kohan D. Psychometric validity of the Cochlear Implant Function Index (CIFI): a quality of life assessment tool for adult cochlear implant users. *Cochlear Implants Int.* 2009;10(2):70–83.

67. Patrick DL, Erickson P. *Health Status and Health Policy: Quality of Life in Health Care Evaluation and Resource Allocation.* New York, NY: Oxford University Press; 1993.

68. Furlong WJ, Feeny DH, Torrance GW, Barr RD. The Health Utilities Index (HUI) system for assessing health-related quality of life in clinical studies. *Ann Med.* 2001; 33:375–384.

69. Fortnum HM, Summerfield AQ, Marshall DH, Davis AC, Bamford JM. Prevalence of permanent childhood hearing impairment in the United Kingdom and implications for universal neonatal hearing screening: questionnaire based ascertainment study. *Br Med J.* 2001 Sep 8;323(7312):536–540.

70. Gallaudet Research Institute. *Regional and National Summary Report of Data from the 2008 Annual Survey of Deaf and Hard of Hearing Children and Youth.* Washington, DC: Gallaudet University; 2008.

71. Roberts C, Hindley P. Practitioner review: The assessment and treatment of deaf children with psychiatric disorders. *J Child Psychol Psychiatry.* 1999;40(2):151–167.

72. Van Naarden K, Decouflé P, Caldwell K. Prevalence and characteristics of children with serious hearing impairment in metropolitan Atlanta, 1991–1993. *Pediatrics.* 1999 Mar;103(3):570–575.

73. Cullen RD, Higgins C, Buss E, Clark M, Pillsbury HC III, Buchman CA. Cochlear implantation in patients with substantial residual hearing. *Laryngoscope.* 2004;114: 2218–2223.

74. Novak MA BJ, Koch DB. Standard cochlear implantation of adults with residual low-frequency hearing: implications for combined electro-acoustic stimulation. *Otol Neurotol.* 2007;28(5):609–614.

75. Gifford RH, Dorman MF, McKarns SA, Spahr A. Combined electric and contralateral acoustic hearing: word and sentence recognition with bimodal hearing. *J Speech Lang Hear Res.* 2007;50(4):835–843.

76. Gifford RH, Dorman MF, Shallop JK, Sydlowski S. Evidence for the expansion of adult cochlear implant candidacy. *Ear Hear.* 2010;31(2):186–194.

77. Adunka OF, Buss E, Clark M, Pillsbury H, Buchman C. Effect of preoperative residual hearing on speech perception after cochlear implantation. *Laryngoscope.* 2004; 118:2044–2049.

78. Balkany T, Hodges A, Telischi F, et al. William House Cochlear Implant Study Group: position statement on bilateral cochlear implantation. *Otol Neurotol.* 2008; 29(2):107–108.

79. Papsin BC, Gordon KA. Bilateral cochlear implants should be the standard for children with bilateral sensorineural deafness. *Curr Opin Otolaryngol Head Neck Surg.* 2008;16:69–74.

80. Lovett RE, Kitterick PT, Hewitt CE, Summerfield AQ. Bilateral or unilateral cochlear implantation for deaf children: an observational study. *Arch Dis Child.* 2010; 95:107–112.

81. Wolfe J, Baker S, Caraway T, et al. 1-year postactivation results for sequentially implanted bilateral cochlear implant users. *Otol Neurotol.* 2007;28:589–596.

82. Wie OB. Language development in children after receiving bilateral cochlear implants between 5 and 18 months. *Int J Pediatr Otorhinolaryngol.* 2010;74(11): 1258–1266.

83. Dorman MF, Yost WA, Wilson BS, Gifford RH. Speech perception and sound localization by adults with bilateral cochlear implants semin hear. *Semin Hear.* 2011; 32:73–89.

84. Buss E, Pillsbury HC, Buchman CA, et al. Multicenter U.S. bilateral MED-EL cochlear implantation study: speech perception over the first year of use. *Ear Hear.* 2008; 29(1):20–32.

85. Litovsky R, Parkinson A, Arcaroli J, Sammeth C. Simultaneous bilateral cochlear implantation in adults: a multicenter clinical study. *Ear Hear.* 2006;27(6):714–731.

86. Koch DB, Soli S, Downing M, Osberger MJ. Simultaneous bilateral cochlear implantation: prospective study in adults. *Cochlear Implants Int.* 2010;11(2):84–99.

87. Eapen RJ, Buss E, Adunka MC, Pillsbury HC 3rd, Buchman CA. Hearing-in-noise benefits after bilateral simultaneous cochlear implantation continue to improve 4 years after implantation. *Otol Neurotol.* 2009 Feb;30(2):153–159.

88. Beijin JW, Snik AF, Mylanus EA. Sound localization ability of young children with bilateral cochlear implants. *Otol Neurotol.* 2007;8:479–485.

89. Grieco-Calub TM, Litovsky RY. Sound localization skills in children who use bilateral cochlear implants and in children with normal acoustic hearing. *Ear Hear.* 2010;31(5):645–656.

90. Godar SP, Litovsky RY. Experience with bilateral cochlear implants improves sound localization acuity in children. *Otol Neurotol.* 2010;31:1287–1292.

91. Van Deun L, van Wieringer A, Scherf F, et al. Earlier intervention leads to better sound localization in children with bilateral cochlear implants. *Audiol Neurotol.* 2010;15:7–17.

92. Kochkin S. MarkeTrak VIII: consumer satisfaction with hearing aids is slowly increasing. *Hear J.* 2010;63(1):19–32.

93. NIDCD. Cochlear Implants. 2005; NIH Publication No. 00–4798.

94. Wilson BS, Dorman MF. Cochlear implants: a remarkable past and a brilliant future. *Hear Res.* 2008 Aug;242(1–2):3–21.

95. Wilson BS, Dorman MF. Cochlear implants: current designs and future possibilities. *J Rehabil Res Dev.* 2008;45:695–730.

96. Erber NP. *Auditory Training.* Washington, DC: Alexander Graham Bell Association for the Deaf; 1982.

Chapter 6

Imaging of Cochlear Implantation

SUYASH MOHAN, ELLEN G. HOEFFNER, AND LAURIE A. LOEVNER

INTRODUCTION

A cochlear implant (CI) is an electronic device used to rehabilitate patients with profound (>90 dB) and severe (between 70 and 90 dB) sensorineural hearing loss (SNHL) who are refractory to conventional hearing augmentation. It is partly worn externally and partly implanted in the ear and provides a direct stimulation of the spiral ganglion cells of the cochlear nerve by bypassing the destroyed hair cells. Imaging plays an important part in the workup of cochlear implant candidates, and an understanding of imaging evaluation procedures is essential. It is also imperative to be familiar with the growing number of imaging options (particularly magnetic resonance imaging pulse sequences) to optimize evaluation of cochlear implant candidates. In this chapter, we discuss and illustrate what head and neck surgeons need to know before cochlear implantation, findings that contraindicate implantation and those that could significantly alter surgical technique, radiologic assessment of correct positioning, and potential complications.

Cochlear implants were first developed in France in 1957 by Djourno and Eyriès,[1] who described how to stimulate the cochlear nerve by electric currents. In fact, auditory excitation was already demonstrated by Volta at the end of the 18th century. At the beginning, development of cochlear devices was limited by the size of electronic components and by the weight of batteries. House developed the concept of a single-channel electrode stimulation.[2] More recently, Merzenich[3] developed cochlear stimulation by a multichannel electrode array, which is currently employed.

HEARING AUGMENTATION DEVICES

Normal hearing requires that all elements of the auditory pathway have intact structure and function. Sound vibrations cause movement of the tympanic membrane and the middle ear ossicles, creating fluid waves in the cochlea that stimulate the inner hair cells. The hair cells transduce these movements into electrical signals that are transmitted by the cochlear nerves to the spiral ganglia and the auditory nerve. The various causes of SNHL disrupt the structure, function, or both of one or more components of the inner ear. There are three devices available for hearing augmentation: a hearing aid, a cochlear implant, and an auditory brainstem implant (ABI).

HEARING AID

A hearing aid functions as an amplifier by magnifying received acoustic signals. Once magnified, the acoustic signal travels along the auditory pathway normally. If potential augmentable hearing is present, a conventional hearing aid is the initial device of choice. The greatest limitation of a hearing aid is not technologic; rather, it relates to the number of surviving functional cochlear hair cells. If only a small percentage of the cochlear hair cells are viable, their stimulation by amplification of the sound signal cannot completely compensate for the hearing loss caused by the nonfunctional hair cells.

COCHLEAR IMPLANT

Implants provide a direct stimulation of the residual spiral ganglion cells of the cochlear nerve by bypassing the destroyed hair cells. A cochlear implant differs from a hearing aid in that the auditory signal–sound wave received by the device is processed (not just amplified) and converted into an electrical impulse.[4] Cochlear implants are intended for patients with severe to profound SNHL. Sound and speech are captured by a microphone worn behind the ear and sent to a speech processor, which may be incorporated with the microphone behind the ear or worn remotely. The speech processor digitally encodes the speech with use of various encoding strategies, depending on the manufacturer and model of the implant. It then sends the encoded signal to a transmitter. The transmitter is located behind the ear and overlies the implanted stimulator, being held in place by a magnet attached to the implanted stimulator. The transmitter then sends the signal transcutaneously to the implanted stimulator, which in turn directly stimulates the spiral ganglion cells and axons of the cochlea by means of an electrode array implanted in the basal turn. This process bypasses the severely degenerated hair cells in the organ of Corti. The impulse then travels normally along the remainder of the auditory pathway.

The components of a cochlear implant device include:

a) Externally worn components: a speech processor placed in a pocket receiving speech stimuli, and an ear-level microphone, placed behind the ear and worn like a hearing aid. The microphone is connected to the transmitter.

b) Internally implanted components: a transmitter or receiver/stimulator coil, firmly fixed beneath the retroauricular soft tissues within a well drilled-out area of the temporal squama. This transmitter has a transducer coil coupled across the skin by a magnet disk with a receiver coil.

c) An electrode array inserted into the scala tympani of the basal turn via the round window for a distance of 20 to 24 mm.

Different models with a variable number of electrodes exist for adult and children. All are now multichannel intracochlear array devices. Three main systems are in use worldwide—the Nucleus device (Nucleus 22/24 Cochlear Corp, USA), the Ineraid, and the Clarion device (Advanced Bionic Corp, USA). Digisonic (MXM) is used in Europe.

AUDITORY BRAINSTEM IMPLANT (ABI)

An ABI is similar to a cochlear implant in the way it receives and processes sound. It differs from a cochlear implant in that an electrical impulse is sent directly to the cochlear nuclei in the brainstem, bypassing the organ of Corti and the cochlear nerve.

COCHLEAR IMPLANT CANDIDATES

CLINICAL EVALUATION

The goal of clinical and imaging evaluation is to select those patients who will benefit the most from implantation. Cochlear implant candidates should usually be over 12 months of age, have bilateral profound or severe hearing loss, receive no enough benefit from external hearing aid with less than 30% of intelligibility, and have a high motivation for rehabilitation.[5] The rate of success of implantation is higher in acquired deafened patients than in prelingually deafened patients. In prelingually deafened patients, the best results are obtained in children operated as early as possible as the development and volume of the cochlear nerve depends on auditory stimulation. Adults who lose normal hearing do very well following implantation because they have a lifetime of auditory memory to call upon when the auditory system is stimulated.

A detailed review of hearing history is the first step in evaluating a potential cochlear implant candidate. Some common questions that are asked include: When did hearing loss begin? Has hearing loss been gradual, or have there been sudden drops or fluctuations? Did both ears progress together? When did the patient begin wearing hearing aids? Is there a family history of hearing loss? Has there been excessive noise exposure or ototoxic medication? Patients then undergo a series of hearing tests and must demonstrate certain levels of hearing loss to qualify for a cochlear implant. A com-plete neurotologic and head and neck examination is also performed. Particular attention is paid to evidence of subtle otologic malformations and syndromic features. Most commonly, the examination findings are normal. Laboratory testing varies considerably depending on the clinical picture. A patient with rapidly progressive bilateral fluctuating hearing loss will undergo a battery of tests to assess for autoimmune or inflammatory disorders. An elderly patient with an extensive history of noise exposure doesn't necessarily need to undergo any tests other than imaging. Most patients who receive implants have hearing loss due to genetic factors (familial hearing loss, syndromic and nonsyndromic deafness), noise exposure, or infectious and inflammatory diseases. The expected degree of success will depend on the clinical situation.

IMAGING EVALUATION

COMPUTED TOMOGRAPHY

CT has been the predominant imaging modality for evaluation of the temporal bone and has previously been the primary modality for evaluation of cochlear implant candidates. However, with the advent of high-resolution MR imaging of the temporal bone, the role of CT in workup is continually being reevaluated.[6] Nevertheless, useful and unique information can still be obtained with CT, particularly in pediatric implant candidates.[7,8] CT technique generally consists of thin-collimation (≤1 mm) scanning performed contiguously or with a 0.5- to 1-mm overlap. Raw data can be retrospectively processed with a sharp bone algorithm. Scanning time is substantially reduced in helical CT, offering an advantage in nonsedated pediatric patients. Image reformation allows coronal imaging in adult patients who are unable to attain adequate neck hyperextension for direct coronal imaging (Fig 6–1). Helical CT can be performed at submillimeter (0.5-mm) increments with a 0.5-mm overlap.[9]

MR IMAGING

Recent advances in MR imaging technology have added to the importance of this modality in the evaluation of cochlear implant candidates. There are a number of coil and pulse sequence options available for imaging of the temporal bone. Each option has advantages and disadvantages, depending on the manufacturer of the imaging system.

A standard birdcage head coil is the standard multipurpose coil used for head imaging. It is very versatile, providing an acceptable signal-to-noise (S/N) ratio and homogeneity throughout the superficial and deep imaging volume. With its "sweet spot," a surface coil provides a considerably better S/N ratio than does a birdcage coil.

The depth of penetration of a surface coil depends on the diameter of the coil, and deeper structures are not as well seen as with the birdcage coil. The recent development of hybrid phased-array coils and integrated phased-array imaging systems has allowed simultaneous data acquisition with custom-designed surface coils and the vendor head coil.[10] The improved superficial S/N ratio of the surface coils (although it can be slightly less than that attainable with surface-coil-only imaging) allows higher-resolution cochlear imaging while maintaining the improved S/N ratio of the head coil for deeper structures.

Imaging of the temporal bone for potential cochlear implantation is best performed with T2-weighted sequences, which provide optimal contrast between nerves and cerebrospinal fluid (CSF) and between the membranous and bony labyrinth. Two-dimensional rapid acquisition with refocused echoes sequences (2D fast spin-echo or turbo spin-echo imaging) provides the desired contrast, but resolution is limited to approximately 1 to 2 mm per section. The intrinsic contiguous-section feature and superior S/N ratio of three-dimensional (3D) sequences permit improved resolution with an achievable section thickness of 1 mm or less, resulting in better visualization and evaluation of the IAC and inner ear. The 3D fast-recovery fast spin-echo pulse sequence[11,12] makes use of a negative 90° pulse at the end of the echo train, so that bright fluid signal intensity can be achieved with a repetition time of 2 seconds or less. Draw-

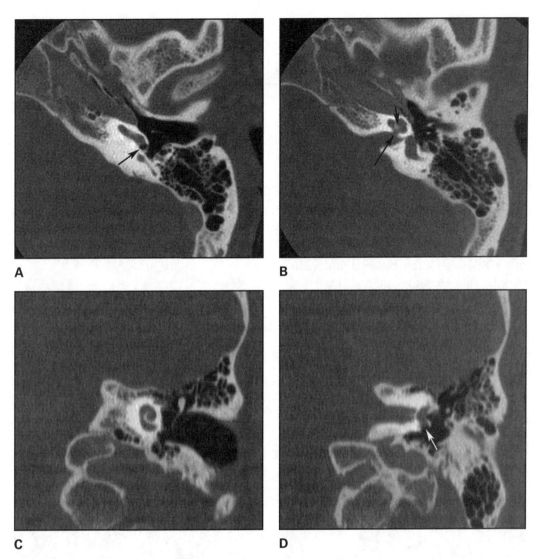

Figure 6–1. *Direct axial images obtained with 0.625-mm slice thickness at a 0.312-interval.* **A.** *Image through the basal turn of the cochlea and round window niche (arrow).* **B.** *Direct axial CT superior to (A) at level of modiolus (short arrow) and cochlear nerve canal (long arrow). Coronal reformatted images 0.625-mm thickness and 0.312-spacing.* **C.** *The cochlea is well seen on coronal reformatted image.* **D.** *Slightly posterior to (C) the round window niche (arrow) is seen on a coronal reformatted image.*

backs include blurring from T2 decay during the echo train and generally lower S/N unit acquisition time compared with gradient-echo methods. CISS[13] is a 3D gradient-echo pulse sequence that allows reduced sensitivity to susceptibility changes and flow while retaining the bright fluid signal intensity achievable with true fast imaging with steady-state precession (FISP). On General Electric (Milwaukee, Wisc) scanner, CISS is called "*f*ast *i*maging *e*mploying *st*eady-state *a*cquisition with phase *cycling*," or FIESTAC.) Three-dimensional true-FISP[14] is a gradient-echo pulse sequence in which the net gradient areas are zero during any repetition time interval. Advantages of true-FISP include excellent signal to noise efficiency. Drawbacks include banding artifacts in the presence of susceptibility changes. Reducing the repetition time can minimize these artifacts, as does using the phase cycling of CISS. The implementation of 3D true-FISP on General Electric scanner is called 3D FIESTA. No matter which pulse sequence is chosen, the thinner sections of a 3D data set allow optimal multiplanar reformatting. Better image resolution of the nerves can be achieved with oblique sagittal imaging perpendicular to the plane of the IAC (Fig 6–2). The cochlea can be further evaluated by generating MIP images. The process is the same as that used in MR angiography, except the inner ear is targeted in the reformatting process.

Advantages of MRI over CT are to distinguish between cochlear fibrosis and ossification and to diagnose cochlear nerve agenesis. Moreover, MRI may depict unsuspected acoustic nerve or central acoustic pathway anomalies including acoustic nerve tumours (Tables 6–1 and 6–2).

The main disadvantages of MRI are its additive cost as MRI does not replace CT. Good quality MR images in deaf patients are more difficult to obtain, as difficulties of communication may lead to movement artefacts. Moreover, sedation is needed in children.

FUNCTIONAL MRI

Recently developed, fMRI is a new noninvasive technique to test cerebral function. It is based on the concept that blood has oxygenation-sensitive paramagnetic characteristics. It can test cerebral auditory

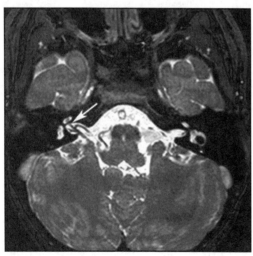
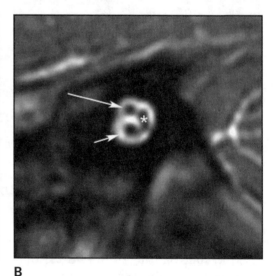

A   B

Figure 6–2. A. *Axial 3D TSE T2-weighted image shows the cochlear nerve (arrow) within the internal auditory canal (IAC).* ***B.*** *The 4 cranial nerves within the IAC are well seen on this oblique sagittal reformatted image, with the facial (long arrow) and cochlear (short arrow) nerves anteriorly and the superior and inferior vestibular nerves posteriorly (*).*

Table 6–1. Key Points for Preoperative Imaging Studies for Cochlear Implantation

Contraindications for cochlear implantation	• Absent cochlear nerve: diameter of IAM (mid-part) <3 mm increases the risk of a congenital absence or of severe hypoplasia of the acoustic nerve • Absent cochlea • Absent modiolus: diameter <3 mm in CT, or a modiolar surface <4 mm^2 in MR are at risk of absence of cochlear nerve
Alter surgical technique or modify implant device	• Cochlear ossification (partial or total; length in basal turn) • Hyperostosis of the round window niche • Persistent membranous labyrinth inflammation • Inner ear at risk of "Gusher": endolymphatic sac dilatation; abnormal cochlear segmentation, deficient modiolus, semicircular canal, or vestibular dilatation • Stenosis of the basal turn: otosclerosis foci • Paget disease • Lobstein disease
Increasing surgical risk	• Hypoplastic mastoid process • Inflammed middle ear • Dehiscent or aberrant facial nerve • Mastoid emissary vein • Deep sigmoid sinus • Exposed jugular bulb • Aberrant carotid artery • Persistent stapedial artery

Table 6–2. Role of Preoperative MRI

- To identify cochlear fluid fibrosis
- To identify active fibrosis
- To depict cochlear nerve agenesis and cochlear anomalies
- To detect an occult acoustic nerve tumour
- To detect brainstem anomalies (infarct, trauma, congenital)

pathway and, therefore, may add criteria in predicting who are good candidates for cochlear implantation. The response to auditory stimuli is obtained on the superior temporal gyrus and predominates on the left side in a right-handed group.[15]

CONTRAINDICATIONS FOR COCHLEAR IMPLANTATION

The absolute requirements for cochlear implantation are the presence of a cochlea (either normal or malformed) and of a cochlear nerve. Cochlear aplasia is readily apparent at computed tomography (CT) or MR imaging (Fig 6–3). Absence of the cochlear nerve is best seen on oblique sagittal MR images obtained through the internal auditory canal (IAC) (Fig 6–4). Normally, the cochlear nerve lays on the inferior part of the internal auditory meatus, measures approximately 0.4 mm and is larger than the facial nerve, which is taken as reference. The embryologic development of the inner ear is complex.[16,17] The independent development

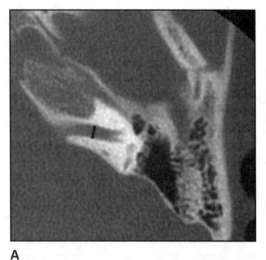

A

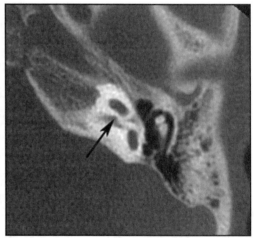

B

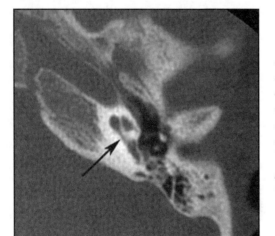

C

Figure 6–3. *Axial CT images in a 6 year old boy with CHARGE syndrome.* ***A.*** *The internal auditory canal (IAC) in narrow (black line) measuring 2.4 mm in diameter.* ***B.*** *Slightly inferior image demonstrates absence of the bony cochlear nerve canal (arrow), a finding suggestive of an absent cochlear nerve.* ***C.*** *Despite presumed absence of the cochlear nerve, a dysplastic cochlea is present (arrow).*

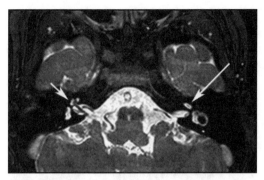

A

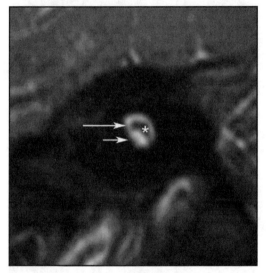

B

Figure 6–4. *3-year-old with profound left hearing loss.* ***A.*** *Axial 3D TSE T2-weighted image demonstrates an absent cochlear nerve and cochlear nerve canal on the left (long arrow), compared to normal structures on the right (short arrow).* ***B.*** *Oblique sagittal reformatted image shows absence of the cochlear nerve (short arrow) in the anterior inferior quadrant of the internal auditory canal (IAC). A normal facial nerve is seen in the anterior superior quadrant of the IAC (long arrow) and normal vestibular nerves in the posterior IAC (*).*

of the organ of Corti and cochlear nerve explains how a normal-appearing (or nearly so) cochlea does not ensure the presence of a normal cochlear nerve.

Cochlear dysplasias (ie, Mondini dysplasias) do not contraindicate cochlear implantation (Fig 6–5). Although no correlative studies have been performed, cochlear implantation is expected to provide some clinical benefit regardless of the degree of dysplasia.

OTHER IMPORTANT IMAGING FINDINGS THAT CAN IMPACT SURGERY

In addition to cochlea–cochlear nerve aplasia and dysplasia as discussed above, other imaging findings can also impact surgery.

OTOMASTOIDITIS

Acute otitis media is treated prior to implantation to avoid potential labyrinthitis or meningitis. Isolated mastoid air cell opacification from chronic mastoiditis may not require treatment prior to implantation. If signs and symptoms of inflammation are present, a canal wall-up mastoidectomy may be performed prior to implantation. Dense mastoid sclerosis can potentially complicate the creation of the implant well reservoir and limit exposure to the middle ear. If the changes are asymmetric, the aerated side may be chosen for implantation.

LABYRINTHITIS

SNHL can result from meningitis, with subsequent labyrinthine fibrosis and eventual ossification. Cochlear ossification with luminal obstruction is not a contraindication for implantation but is important to

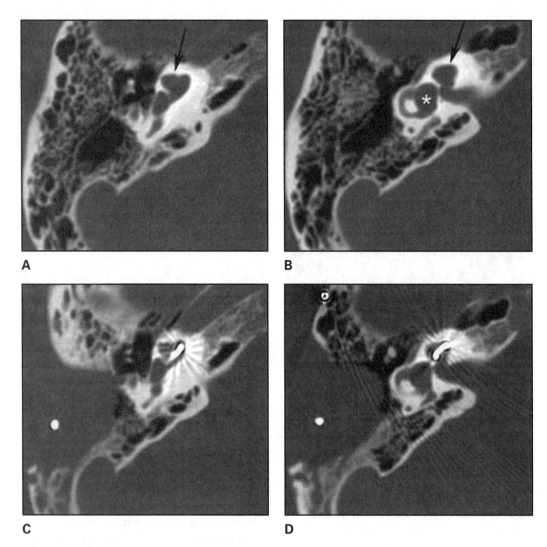

Figure 6–5. *A* and *B. Axial CT images show an empty, cystic cochlea with absent modiolus* (arrows) *consistent with incomplete partition type I (IP-I). A dilated vestibule, also part of IP-I, is seen (*).* *C* and *D. Axial CT images at similar levels following cochlear implantation show the electrode coiled in the dysplastic cochlea.*

identify preoperatively. Cochlear ossification makes the cochleostomy more challenging and often results in choosing an implant with a shorter electrode array. MR imaging is superior to CT in assessing the presence or absence of fibrosis within the cochlea (Fig 6–6).

FACIAL NERVE DEHISCENCE AND OTOSCLEROSIS

Facial nerve compromise or paralysis resulting from cochlear implantation is rare. Recognizing facial nerve dehiscence

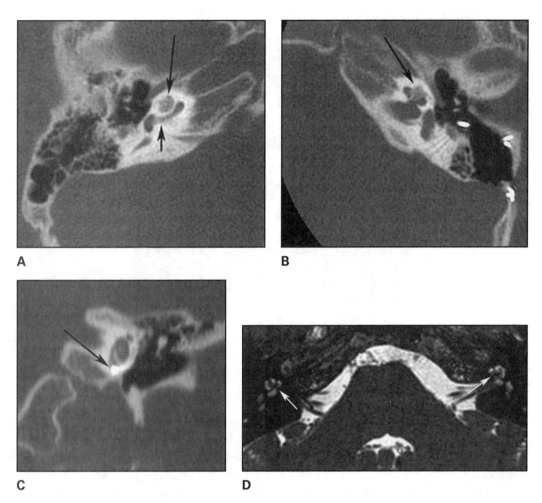

A

B

C

D

Figure 6–6. A. *Ossification completely obliterates the middle and apical turns (long arrow) of the right cochlea and partially obliterates the basal turn (short arrow) on axial CT image, compatible with labyrinthitis ossificans in a 7-year-old with postmeningitic deafness.* ***B.*** *Similar findings are seen in the middle and apical turns of the left cochlea (arrow).* ***C.*** *Coronal reconstructed image demonstrates cochlear implant electrode could only be partially inserted into the basal turn of the cochlea (arrow) related to ossification encountered at the time of surgery.* ***D.*** *Axial 3D TSE T2-weighted image shows foci of low signal (arrows) in the basal turn or each cochlea compatible with fibrosis or ossification in a 20-year-old with postmeningitic deafness.*

or an atypical course preoperatively can help prevent this complication. Facial nerve dehiscence is readily apparent at CT (Fig 6–7).

Retrofenestral otosclerosis is not a contraindication for cochlear implantation. However, facial nerve stimulation following transplantation is more common in patients with otosclerosis and is likely related to conduction of current through otospongiotic bone.[18] This problem is usually corrected by programming out the electrodes causing the stimulation. Sagittal T2-weighted MR images are essential

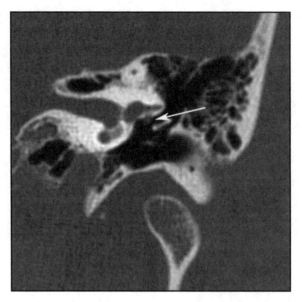

Figure 6–7. *Direct coronal CT image shows absence of bony covering surrounding the tympanic segment of the facial nerve (arrow), compatible with dehiscence.*

in evaluating toddlers or older pediatric patients with hearing loss and facial nerve paralysis. Although rare, an absent facial nerve can be differentiated from an absent cochlear nerve and would not prevent implantation on the affected side.

ENLARGED ENDOLYMPHATIC DUCT AND SAC

Meningitis following implantation is very rare and is likely caused by a CSF leak. Preoperative imaging can be used to identify patients in whom a potential intraoperative CSF leak ("gusher") may be encountered. For example, in SNHL associated with an enlarged endolymphatic duct and sac, the dilated sac is seen at MR imaging, whereas CT readily depicts the enlarged vestibular aqueduct (Fig 6–8).

The relationship of an enlarged cochlear duct to the CSF perilymph gusher phenomenon is less certain.[19] The risk of a CSF gusher is also significantly increased in the presence of a bulbous, dilated distal IAC, often associated with absence of the bone partition that separates the distal canal and the base of the cochlea.[20–22] The potential for a gusher to occur during cochleostomy does not preclude implantation. It is important to identify the anomaly preoperatively because the leak is readily treated with packing of the fascia and soft tissue around the electrode array at cochleostomy.

VASCULAR CONDITIONS

Abnormal middle ear vascular anatomy could potentially complicate mastoidectomy and cochleostomy. Anomalies such

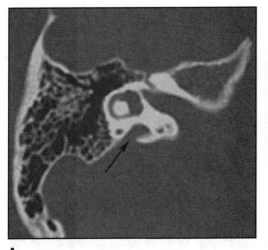

A

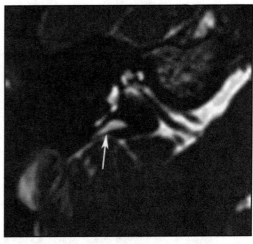

B

C

Figure 6–8. A. *Axial CT image through right temporal bone demonstrates enlarged vestibular aqueduct (arrow).* ***B.*** *Axial 3D TSE T2-weighted image through right temporal bone shows the enlarged endolymphatic duct (arrow).* ***C.*** *Image slightly inferior to B shows enlarged endolymphatic sac (arrow).*

as a high-riding jugular bulb and an aberrant carotid artery are often apparent clinically and are easily confirmed with MR imaging or CT (Fig 6–9).

OTHER IMAGING FINDINGS

Various unusual and unsuspected causes of sensorineural loss may be encountered during imaging evaluation. Implantation should not be performed on the ipsilateral side in a patient with a brainstem infarct involving the cochlear nuclei that leads to unilateral SNHL. Demyelinating processes, such as multiple sclerosis, can cause SNHL if the plaque involves the cochlear nucleus. Hemosiderosis from previous subarachnoid hemorrhage can cause cranial neuropathies including SNHL. Although such hemosiderosis is not a contraindication for cochlear implantation, the degree of hearing recovery in this setting remains unknown.

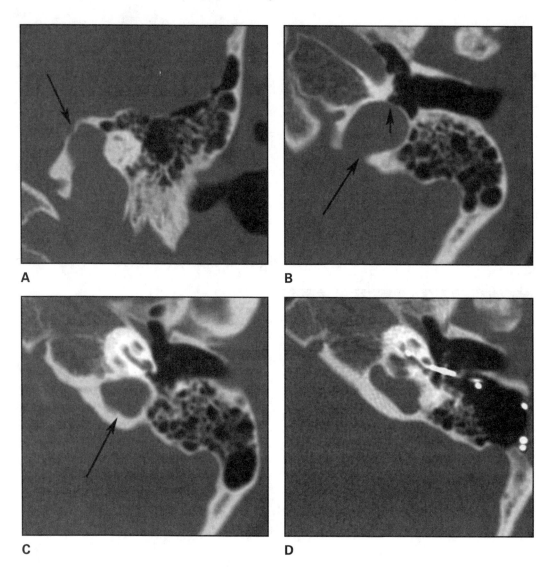

Figure 6–9. A. *Coronal and (**B, C**) axial CT images demonstrate a high riding jugular bulb (long arrows) with a focal area of dehiscence on a precochlear implant CT.* **D.** *Patient underwent cochlear implant surgery without complication.*

SURGICAL TECHNIQUE

The surgical procedure usually performed for cochlear implantation is a canal wall-up mastoidectomy. The facial recess cells are opened into the middle ear cavity, thereby, allowing surgical access to the round window. The electrode is advanced into the basal turn of cochlea either directly through the round window or via a cochleostomy. The electrode is advanced into scala tympani for approximately one and a half turns or for a distance of 20 to 24 mm (Fig 6–10). Patients functioning with more than 15 active electrodes per-

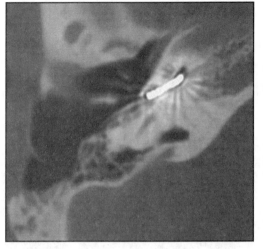

A

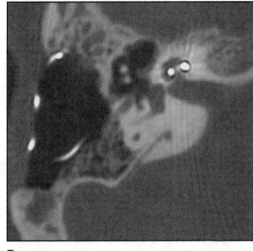

B

C

Figure 6–10. *Axial CT images show the normal appearance of a cochlear implant coiled for one and a half turns in the cochlea.*

form better on auditory tests than patients with fewer active electrodes.[23] The entire procedure usually takes about 2 hours and is often performed on an outpatient basis. Most clinicians currently favor placing the implant in the better hearing ear. Experience has yielded improved results, likely reflecting more surviving neural elements available for implant stimulation. There are always exceptions, particularly in patients who are extremely anxious about "saving" their better hearing ear.

SURGICAL COMPLICATIONS

Complications from implantation of newer model cochlear implants occur in less than 1% of adults and children.[5] Many such complications are related to the scalp flap (infection, necrosis, thickening) (Fig 6–11). Tinnitus and vertigo may occur but usually resolve spontaneously. Facial nerve stimulation can rarely

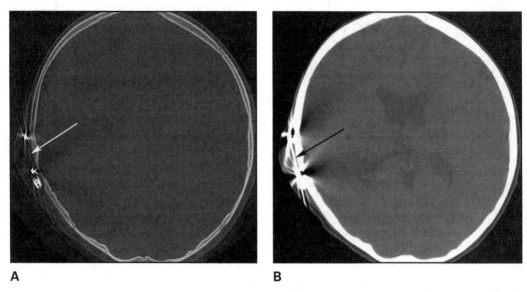

A   B

Figure 6–11. *Axial head CT images show nonspecific soft tissue swelling (arrows) overlies the receiver-stimulator component of the cochlear implant, which at surgery was a liquefied hematoma.*

occur following an aggressive cochleostomy and electrode extrusion through the cochlear wall.

POSTSURGICAL FOLLOW-UP

ELECTRODE POSITION

Postoperative radiographic documentation may be necessary to underline the position of the implanted electrode and to assess the implant's function. Audiometric testings detect better than radiographic evaluation failure of a cochlear implant. Radiographic evaluation may ensure intracochlear position, detect electrode kinking, and serve as a reference. Plain x-ray films (profile and modified Stenvers's views) suffice to depict the pathway of the electrode array (Fig 6–12).[24] To appre-

ciate surgical insertion depth, a vertical line called VL1 parallel to the superior semicircular canal is drawn. A second horizontal line passing by the basal turn and perpendicular to VL1 is drawn. Section of these two lines point to the level of the round window niche, the slots of the electrode array should not be lateral to this point. Spiral HRCT may help to depict the location of electrode array due to its capacity of multiplanar reconstructions.

CAUSES OF IMPLANT FAILURE

A common cause of device failure is extrusion or malpositioning of the electrode, which can lead to mechanical malfunction. It is important for the radiologists to recognize this important aspect of device failure. Comparison of follow-up radio-

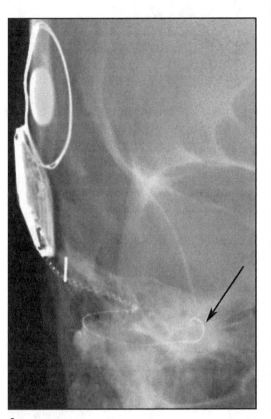 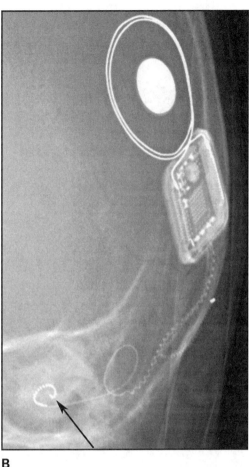

A   B

Figure 6–12. **A.** *Frontal skull x-ray shows electrode from cochlear implant coiled in the cochlea (*arrow*).* **B.** *Frontal skull x-ray shows a kink in the electrode coiled in the cochlea (*arrow*) in a normally functioning cochlear implant.*

graphs or postimplant CT with prior post-operative studies can allow detection of retraction or of change in the position of the electrode (Fig 6–13). In patients with malpositioned electrode another attempt can be made by correctly reimplanting the electrode. Possible sites of electrode malpositioning include electrode coiled into the middle ear cavity or mastoid bowl, incomplete or incorrect insertion of the electrode in the cochlea, electrode malpositioned into the cochlear aqueduct, petrous carotid canal, or eustachian tube, and electrode abutting the labyrinthine part of the facial nerve.

MRI SAFETY IN COCHLEAR IMPLANTATION

MRI has been contraindicated in patients with cochlear implants as ferromagnetic

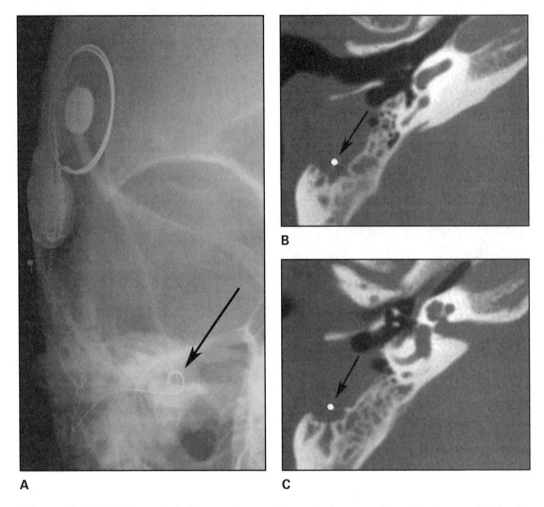

A

B

C

Figure 6–13. A. *Frontal skull x-ray shows electrode from cochlear implant coiled in the cochlea (arrow).* ***B*** *and* ***C.*** *4 years later, axial CT images show extrusion of the electrode with the tip in the mastoid region (arrows) rather than the cochlea.*

materials in the implant, and the magnet used to "anchor" the transmitter transcutaneously to the implanted receiver-stimulator, were both incompatible with the MRI environment with concerns regarding torque, force, demagnetization, artifacts, induced voltages, and heating. However, preliminary experiments with MED-EL Combi 40+ cochlear implants in cadavers and patients using a 0.2 T unit have shown some promising results.[25,26]

Companies have begun to manufacture MRI compatible implants without ferromagnetic materials and with magnets that can be surgically removed prior to imaging. The microphone, speech processor, and transmitter are also removed before the patient is placed in the imager. The implant (minus the magnet) does result in local artifact, but the remainder of the examination is unaffected. Binding of CI with mold material and gauze has recently been attempted before MRI and it is shown that patients can safely undergo 1.5 T MRI after CI, if the device is tightly bound before scanning. No CI malfunction, displacement, or magnet displacement was observed, with minimal risks, compared with the risk and inconvenience of removing the magnet before the study.[27] It remains imperative to exhaustively review the case prior to imaging a patient with a cochlear implant. The exact type of implant must be verified with the surgical history and the MRI compatibility of the implant must be ascertained.

FUTURE IMAGING OF IMPLANT CANDIDATES

Future imaging of implant candidates may include routine virtual endoscopy of the IAC and cochlea, although the utility of this procedure will need to be determined. Objective measurements of cochlear nerve diameter may prove to be of prognostic value in determining the potential benefit of a cochlear implant.[28]

CONCLUSIONS

In conclusion, cochlear implants are now a well-accepted treatment in patients with profound and severe SNHL. It is a safe surgical procedure with good results in terms of overall hearing improvement. Imaging studies are a part of the candidate evaluation, pre- and postsurgical assessment and device failure. Both CT and MR should be used as they delineate in different manners cochlear and middle ear anatomy, and look for labyrinthine ossification and malformations. Imaging studies may orient and modify surgical strategy. Functional MRI is a new way for testing candidates of cochlear implantation. Radiologists will assume a larger role in evaluating these patients as the number of procedures escalates. An understanding of imaging evaluation procedures and relevant findings is essential.

REFERENCES

1. Djourno A, Eyries C. Prothèse auditive par excitation à distance du nerf sensoriel à l'aide d'un bobinage inclus à demeure. *Presse Med.* 1957;35:1417–1423.
2. House WF, Urban J. Long-term result of electrode implantation and electronic stimulation of the cochlea in man. *Ann Otol Rhinol Laryngol.* 1973;82:504–518.
3. Merzenich MM, Michelson RR, Petit LC, et al. Cochlear prosthesis: further considerations clinical observations preliminary results of physiological studies. *Laryngoscope.* 1973;83:1116–1122.
4. Lo W. Imaging of cochlear and auditory brain stem implantation. *Am J Neuroradiol.* 1998;19:1147–1154.
5. Cochlear implants in adults and children. NIH Consensus Conference, *J Am Med.* 1995;274:1955–1961.
6. Ellul S, Shelton C, Davidson H, Harnsberger H. Preoperative cochlear implant imaging: is magnetic resonance imaging enough? *Am J Otol.* 2000;21:528–533.
7. Alexander A, Caldemeyer K, Rigby P. Clinical and surgical application of reformatted high-resolution CT of the temporal bone. In: Tanenbaum L, ed. *CT in Neuroimaging Revisited.* Philadelphia, PA: Saunders; 1998:631–650.
8. Fishman A, Holliday R. Principles of cochlear implant imaging. In: Waltzman SB, Cohen NL, eds. *Cochlear Implants.* New York, NY: Thieme; 2000:79–115.

9. Caldemeyer K, Sandrasegaran K, Shinaver C, Mathews V, Smith R, Kopecky K. Temporal bone: comparison of isotropic helical CT and conventional direct axial and coronal CT. *Am J Roentgenol.* 1999;172:1675–1682.

10. Kocharian A, Lane J, Bernstein M, et al. Hybrid phased array for improved internal auditory canal imaging at 3.0-T MR. *J Magn Reson Imaging.* 2002;16:300–304.

11. Oshio K, Williamson CS, Winalski S, Miyamoto S, Kosugi S, Suzuki K. Fast recovery RARE for knee imaging [Abstr]. In: *Proceedings of the Sixth Meeting of the International Society for Magnetic Resonance in Medicine.* Berkeley, CA: International Society for Magnetic Resonance in Medicine; 1998.

12. Schmalbrock P. Comparison of three-dimensional fast spin echo and gradient echo sequences for high-resolution temporal bone imaging. *J Magn Reson Imaging.* 2000;12:814–825.

13. Casselman JW, Kuhweide R, Deimling M, Ampe W, Dehaene I, Meeus L. Constructive interference in the steady-state-3DFT MR imaging of the inner ear and cerebellopontine angle. *Am J Neuroradiol.* 1993; 14:47–57.

14. Duerk JL, Lewin JS, Wendt M, Petersilge C. Remember true FISP? a high SNR, near 1-second imaging method for T2-like contrast in interventional MRI at .2 T. *J Magn Reson Imaging.* 1998;8:203–208.

15. Millen SJ, Haughton VM, Yetkin Z. Functional magnetic resonance imaging of the central auditory pathway following speech and puretone stimulus. *Laryngoscope.* 1995;105:1305–1309.

16. Van De Water T. Tissue interactions and cell differentiation: neurone-sensory cell interaction during otic development. *Development.* 1988;103 (suppl):185–193.

17. Van De Water T, Frenz D, Giraldez F, et al. Growth factors and development of the statoacoustic system. In: Romand R, ed. *Development of Auditory and Vestibular Systems 2.* New York, NY: Elsevier; 1992: 1–32.

18. Kelsall D, Shallop JK, Brammeier TG, Prenger EC. Facial nerve stimulation after Nucleus 22-channel cochlear implantation. *Am J Otol.* 1997;18:336–341.

19. Jackler RK, Hwang PH. Enlargement of the cochlear aqueduct: fact or fiction? *Otolaryngol Head Neck Surg.* 1993;109:14–25.

20. Reardon W, Bellman S, Phelps P, Pembrey M, Luxon L. Neuro-otological function in X-linked hearing loss: a multipedigree assessment and correlation with other clinical parameters. *Acta Otolaryngol.* 1993;113:706–714.

21. Piussan C, Hanauer A, Dahl N, et al. X-linked progressive mixed deafness: a new microdeletion that involves a more proximal region in Xq21. *Am J Hum Genet.* 1995;56:224–230.

22. Curtin H, Vignaud J, Bar D. Anomaly of the facial canal in a Mondini malformation with recurrent meningitis. *Radiology.* 1982;144:335–341.

23. Proops DW, Stoddart RL, Donaldson I. Medical, surgical and audiological complications of the first 100 adult cochlear implant patients in Birmingham. *J Laryngol Otol.* 1999;24(suppl):14–17.

24. Marsh MA, Jin Xu, Blamey PJ, et al. Radiologic evaluation of multichannel intracochlear implant insertion depth. *Am J Otol.* 1993;14(4):366–391.

25. Smith WMM, Banks PA, Prost KL, Firszt RW, Jill B. *Effect of MR imaging on internal magnetic strength in patients with Med-El cochlear implants.* Presented at 36th annual meeting ASHNR 2002 Cleveland, Ohio, 11–15 September, 2002.

26. Witte RJ, Lane JI, Driscoll CL, et al. Pediatric and adult cochlear implantation. *Radiographics.* 2003;23(5):1185–1200.

27. Crane BT, Gottschalk B, Kraut M, Aygun N, Niparko JK. Magnetic resonance imaging at 1.5 T after cochlear implantation. *Otol Neurotol.* 2010;31(8):1215–1220.

28. Glastonbury C, Davidson H, Harnsberger H, Butler J, Kertesz T, Shelton C. Imaging findings of cochlear nerve deficiency. *Am J Neuroradiol.* 2002;23:635–643.

Chapter 7

Surgical Technique for Cochlear Implants in Adults

JASON BRANT, D. C. BIGELOW, AND MICHAEL J. RUCKENSTEIN

INTRODUCTION

Just as the technology of the cochlear implant has evolved over the past 3 decades, so too has the implantation surgery. Implantation with preservation of residual hearing is now possible, and many surgeons are now availing themselves of more minimal techniques. This chapter details the main surgical techniques employed to date.

INDICATIONS

At present, cochlear implants are indicated for postlingually deafened adults and prelingually and postlingually deafened children as follows.

ADULTS

➤ Severe-to-profound bilateral sensorineural hearing loss (Pure-tone average ≥70 dB

➤ 50% sentence recognition or poorer (eg, HINT, AzBio) in ear to be implanted (aided results) (FDA Criteria)
➤ 60% sentence recognition or poorer (eg, HINT, AzBio) in opposite ear and binaurally (aided) (FDA Criteria)
➤ 40% sentence recognition or poorer (eg, HINT, AzBio) in ear to be implanted (aided results) (Medicare Criteria)

CHILDREN (25 MONTHS–17 YEARS)

➤ Severe-to-profound sensorineural hearing loss in both ears
➤ Up to 30% score on MLNT (Multisyllabic Lexical Neighborhood Test)/LNT
➤ No progress in auditory skill development with hearing aids and intervention

INFANTS (12–24 MONTHS)

➤ Profound sensorineural hearing loss in both ears
➤ No progress in auditory skill development with hearing aids and intervention

➤ High motivation and appropriate expectations from family

A more detailed analysis of indications for cochlear implantation is provided in Chapter 5.

CONTRAINDICATIONS

➤ Congenital or acquired absence of the VIIIth cranial nerve
➤ Congenital absence of the labyrinth (Michel's Aplasia)
➤ Adult patient (20 years old and older) with congenital/prelingual deafness who has never acquired speech
➤ Cognitive impairment that would prevent adequate rehabilitation (eg, acquired dementia)
➤ Lack of adequate support or motivation so as to ensure attendance at activation and programming sessions

TECHNIQUE

CLASSICAL TECHNIQUE

Although minor alterations have been made, the basic procedure of a mastoidectomy with posterior tympanotomy for access to the round window and promontory has remained relatively unchanged since it was first described.[1]

The side of the scalp is shaved, prepped, and draped. The position of the implant is marked, lying at an angle of 45° to 60° with respect to the temporal line. The incision line is designed and marked to make sure the receiver lies approximately 1.5 cm posterior to the incision (Fig 7–1). An extended postauricular skin incision is made and a skin flap is raised in the plane of the temporalis fascia. This provides a relatively avascular plane, and is most easily identified superiorly. It is carried inferiorly being careful to remain

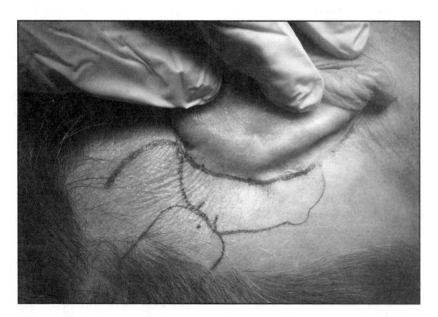

Figure 7–1. *The positions of the receiver and processor are marked using the provided templates. The incision is marked to ensure that the receiver lies posterior to the incision line.*

superior to the lambdoid suture. This ensures that large branches of the occipital artery and vein are avoided. While designing the skin flap over the receiver unit it should be noted that this provides a barrier to the transmission of energy from the external hardware. Current models require the skin flap to be no more than 10- to 12-mm thick. This must be balanced against a skin flap that is too thin. Exposure of hair follicles during the thinning process predisposes to infection, skin breakdown, and eventual extrusion of the implanted device.

An anteriorly based pericranial flap is elevated (Fig 7–2). The incision begins just superior to the external auditory meatus and is carried posteriorly along the temporal lines for 2 to 3 cm to create a flap that will cover the anterior portion of the implant. The incision is then carried inferiorly to the level of the occipital crest, and anterior-inferiorly to the mastoid tip. The last portion of the incision should remain superior to the attachment of the sternocleidomastoid muscle. The flap is then elevated and reflected anteriorly exposing the mastoid cortex.

A subperiosteal pocket is then elevated in a posterior-superior direction that will hold the implanted receiver (Fig 7–3). A bony seat (well) and superior and inferior tie-down holes are then drilled into the parietal bone underlying the pocket (Fig 7–4). This recess acts to immobilize the device, protect it from trauma, and create a more aesthetically pleasing final result. Complications of this method are rare but serious, including CSF leak, subdural hematoma, epidural hematoma, lateral sinus thrombosis, and cerebral infarction.[2,3]

After the cortex is exposed a complete mastoidectomy is performed. Technique differs slightly from chronic ear surgery in that complete saucerization is not performed. Small superior, posterior, and inferior overhangs are left to help

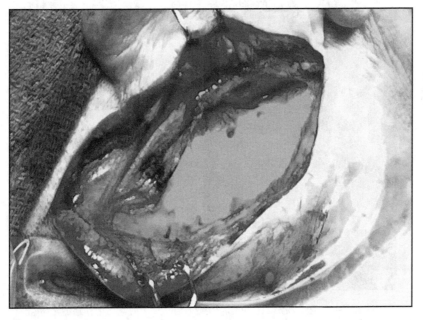

Figure 7–2. *An anteriorly based pericranial flap is raised to the level of the external auditory meatus.*

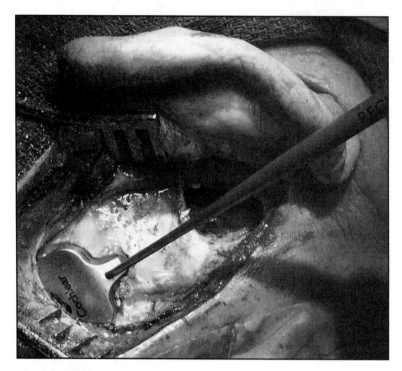

Figure 7–3. *A subpericranial pocket is made and the position of the processor marked using the provided template.*

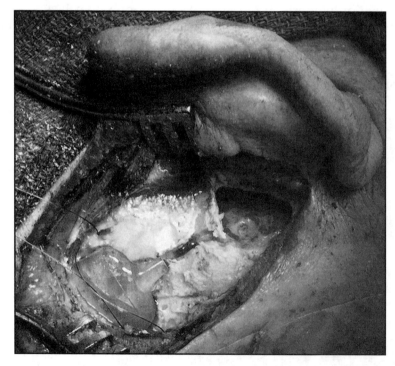

Figure 7–4. *The bony well for the receiver and electrode is drilled together with tie-down holes to secure the implant.*

control the electrode. It also is not necessary to completely expose sigmoid and mastoid tip air cells. A widely opened facial recess achieves access to the promontory and round window. Care should be taken to preserve a layer of bone over the facial nerve; however, the anterior-medial portion of the fallopian canal is occasionally removed just below the pyramidal process to adequately expose the round window. The posterior external auditory canal wall should be maximally thinned in order to provide a site-path for cochleostomy and electrode insertion. Care should be taken to not penetrate the canal wall, and often the chorda tympani nerve can be preserved.

At this point, the round window membrane can be visualized approximately 1 to 1.5 mm inferior to the stapedius tendon, and the round window overhang should be removed if present to positively identify the membrane. If the round window is used as the route for insertion of the electrode, then the drilling portion of the procedure is complete. Alternatively, a cochleostomy may be drilled in the promontory 1 mm anterior and inferior to the round window membrane. The surface of the promontory is carefully removed until the fibrous layer of the endosteum of the scala tympani is revealed. The bony edges are smoothed and the endosteum is elevated circumferentially from the bone.[4] Care should be taken to prevent the introduction of bone dust or blood into the cochlea. The depth of the bone can be approximated by noting that the endosteum is contiguous to the round window. The size of the cochleostomy varies by manufacturer and ranges from 1.0 to 1.4 mm.

Before insertion of the electrode the receiver pocket is irrigated with antibiotic containing saline. The receiver is inserted and secured using a single nonabsorbable suture looped through the superior and inferiorly drilled holes. Some surgeons prefer placing four 3-mm titanium reconstruction screws around the receiver and then looping the suture around the screws to secure the implant in place.

Immediately prior to electrode insertion, the endosteum is incised with a fine needle. Depending on the electrode, insertion techniques differ. Advanced Bionics electrodes are delivered with a custom insertion tool. Cochlear Nucleus electrodes are currently inserted using an "advance off-stylet" technique that allows the precurved electrode to curl tightly around the modiolus. The MED-EL electrode is inserted, somewhat ironically, with insertion tools manufactured for the Nucleus implant, and is designed to sit along the lateral wall of the cochlea. The cochleostomy is then covered with pericranium, temporalis fascia, or muscle. Incomplete or inadequate closure of the cochleostomy can theoretically predispose to meningitis.

The wound is then closed in layers after meticulous irrigation. A light mastoid dressing is kept in place overnight and removed the morning after surgery. Adult patients generally can be discharged the same day of surgery.

MODIFICATIONS TO THE CLASSIC TECHNIQUE

As surgery for cochlear implants has evolved, a trend toward a more "minimal approach" has been advocated by a number of authorities. Such modifications to the surgery technique, theoretically, can decrease flap complications, surgical time, head shave, pain, and hematoma/seroma formation. Other modifications, in particular to the cochleostomy, have been motivated by the desire to preserve residual hearing using so-called "soft surgery" techniques.

Incision

Flap-related complications including dehiscence, infection, and necrosis have been the most commonly reported surgical complications of cochlear implantation.[5-8] A wide variety of modifications to the incision and flap were proposed although few gained wide appeal. The trend in all surgery is smaller incisions with less tissue dissection and this holds true with cochlear implantation. Currently, a 3- to 4-cm incision located 1 cm posterior to the retroauricular crease is in common use (Fig 7–5). It provides adequate exposure for implantation, requires little to no hair removal, heals rapidly, and allows for initial device activation at about 2 weeks postoperation. This incision has been used by one the authors (MJR) in over 100 consecutive surgeries without significant complications including no cases of wound dehiscence and flap necrosis.

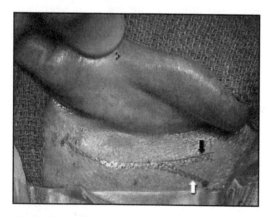

Figure 7–5. *A smaller incision of 3 to 4 cm is a viable alternative to the incision pictured in Figure 7–1. The superior arch of the incision may either follow the postauricular crease (black arrow) or a small posterior limb may be incised (white arrow).*

Device Fixation

Secure fixation of the receiver unit is critical to the long-term success of implantation. Electrode fatigue and shearing can result from improperly secured implants.[9] Traditionally, a well is drilled in the bony cortex into which the receiver is recessed and monocortical holes are drilled surrounding the implant through which nonresorbable suture (eg, 2-0 Prolene) is placed to tie down the receiver (see Fig 7–4). A channel is drilled through the bone leading from the receiver well to the mastoid cavity into which the electrode is placed.

Although these techniques certainly ensure that the receiver and electrode remain stable, several factors have led many surgeons to question their necessity, particularly in adult patients. In patients who undergo revision or explantation surgery, the implant, particularly the receiver, is always found encased in a thick fibrous capsule. The capsule binds the receiver in place, making it immovable. Another important consideration is the change in electrode design that has occurred. Both MED-EL and Nucleus receivers currently are housed in thin, low-profile Silastic housings. Undoubtedly, Advanced Bionics will pursue similar modifications to their electrode. These low profile designs mitigate the need to recess the receiver into bone to prevent excess tension on the flap and unsightly bulges on the side of the skull.

A number of alternative fixation techniques have been described that can be successfully coupled to a minimal incision. One such technique, described by Balkany and his colleagues, involves the creation of a tight pericranial pocket into which the receiver is placed (Fig 7–6).[11] Once the receiver is in position, a suture is placed through the anterior portion of

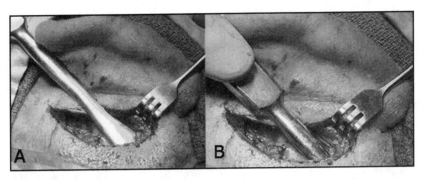

Figure 7–6. *A "Balkany pocket" is elevated. This tight periosteal pocket is designed to approximate the width (A) and the height (B) of the receiver.*

the pericranium to further prevent displacement of the receiver. Similar techniques have been used by a number of surgeons, allowing for successful placement of the receiver without incurring potential complications associated with drilling on the dura including CSF leak, epidural, or subdural hematomas.[11]

Cochleostomy Versus Round Window Insertion

Two major factors have refocused surgeons' attention on the cochleostomy site. With the exception of the data presented in one recent study, the weight of the current evidence indicates that the auditory performance is directly correlated with the amount of the electrode that resides within the scala tympani.[12–15] Recent efforts have also focused on the preserving residual hearing in the implanted ear ("soft surgery"). Thus, the current consensus is that the cochleostomy should be performed to facilitate the placement of the electrode into the scala tympani and minimize insertion trauma.

Round window insertion has regained considerable popularity (Figs 7–7 and 7–8). Using the round window as a gateway

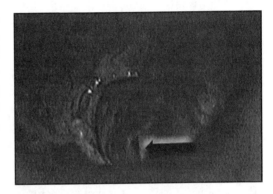

Figure 7–7. *A small slit is made in the round window membrane using a fine pick.*

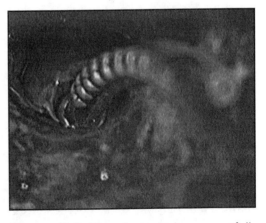

Figure 7–8. *The electrode is successfully and completely inserted into the cochlea through the round window.*

to the cochlea has several advantages.[16] It offers an unambiguous landmark that leads directly into the scala tympani. Other than a small amount of bony overhang that must be removed to visualize the round window membrane, there is no drilling on the cochlea, thus eliminating potential acoustic and physical trauma to the cochlea and its associated structures. Other authorities favor drilling a small cochleostomy inferior to the round window membrane.[17,18] Although more time consuming and potentially somewhat more traumatic, the feeling is that by avoiding the most basal "hook" region of the cochlea, more favorable and less traumatic insertion vectors can be achieved using the cochleostomy.[17–19] Clearly, the surgeon should be familiar and comfortable with both techniques. That said, we have found that we can insert electrodes through the round window membrane in 90% of cases using electrodes manufactured by MED-EL, Cochlear, and Advanced Bionics.[20] When the round window insertion was not possible, it typically resulted from the mastoid segment of the facial nerve lying directly lateral the round window, obscuring more than 50% of the niche.

SPECIAL CONSIDERATIONS

Abnormalities in the cochlea itself, or in the surrounding anatomy, require special considerations at the time of surgery.

The Malformed or Dysplastic Cochlea

The surgical management of patients with malformed or dysplastic cochleae (eg, Mondini, common cavity malformations) is covered extensively in Chapter 8 of this book.

Cochlear Ossification (Labyrinthitis Ossificans)

Ossification of the cochlear lumen can occur in a variety of conditions, most commonly in cases of otosclerosis and subsequent to pneumococcal meningitis.[21] Other disorders that cause cochlear ossification include autoimmune inner ear disease, sickle cell disease, trauma, and chronic otitis media. Fortunately, in the majority of cases, the ossification is restricted to the most basal region in the area of the round window.[21] The ossification can extend along to the basal turn and becomes more problematic when it involves the ascending portion of the basal turn. Complete ossification of the basal turn presents a particular challenge to the surgeon.

Most cases of ossification occur at the round window and in the adjacent area of the basal turn of the cochlea. This can be addressed through the facial recess using a 1-mm diamond or cutting bur angled to extend the opening of the basal turn anteriorly until a lumen is encountered. A standard electrode insertion can then be performed.

If the ossification extends further down the basal turn, the drilling can continue anteriorly until a lumen is encountered.[22] It is critical that the dissection not exceed 8 mm in length as extension beyond the cochlea can result in violation of the carotid artery. It is a good a good idea to place a mark on the bur at the 8-mm point to remind the surgeon when the critical depth is approaching. Encountering any bleeding during the drilling usually indicates that the surgeon is uncovering the vasa vasorum of the carotid and that the dissection should be halted. If a lumen is encountered during this portion of the dissection then the electrode should be inserted at this point using the position of the round window to guide the depth of electrode insertion.

Failure of the surgeon to open into the scala tympani by drilling out the horizontal portion of the basal turn of the cochlea necessitates an attempt to perform a scala vestibuli insertion.[22] The original cochleostomy is extended superiorly and anteriorly to open the scala vestibuli. If this maneuver results in the opening into a patent scala vestibuli lumen, then the electrode can be inserted into the scala vestibuli and a good result can be anticipated.

If the techniques described above do not result in the opening of a patent cochlear lumen, then a more extensive dissection is required.[23–25] Several anatomic landmarks must gain the surgeon's attention in order for this dissection to be safe and successful. The carotid artery runs anterior to the basal turn of the cochlea. The tympanic segment of the facial nerve runs superior to the basal turn. The labyrinthine segment of the facial nerve lies just posterior to the superior portion of the basal turn. Drilling out the basal turn of the cochlea can be achieved using one of two approaches. A radical mastoidectomy can be performed with closure of the eustachian tube orifice and the ear canal.[23,24] This affords broad exposure to the middle ear space. An alternate approach is to maintain the canal wall and use a combined approach through the facial recess and through the ear canal after a broad tympanomeatal flap is elevated (Fig 7–9).[25]

Once exposure is achieved, the position of the carotid artery is identified. The eustachian tube orifice is a highly reliable landmark to begin this dissection as the carotid artery lies directly medial the orifice. The dissection can then be

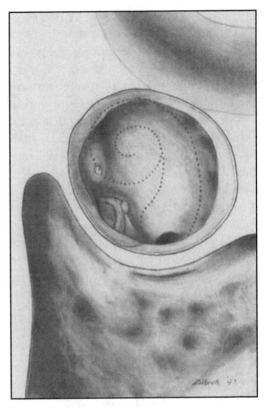

Figure 7–9. *Transcanal view of the middle ear with the malleus and incus removed and the superiorly based tympanomeatal flap elevated. Note the relationship of the basal turn of the cochlea with the round window, carotid canal, processus cochleariformis, and oval window. From Balkany et al,[25] used with permission.*

carried inferiorly using a 2- to 3-mm diamond bur to identify the carotid artery within the middle ear. The incudostapedial joint is separated and the malleus and incus removed after the tensor tympani is cut. The dissection is carried along the ascending portion of the basal turn until about the level of the cochleariform process, at which point it is taken posteriorly, with care to stay inferior to the tympanic segment of the facial nerve. The dissection is terminated anterior and slightly inferior to the oval window. This dissection creates a trough into which the electrode can be placed. Retaining the round window overhang and placing the electrode through this small tunnel around the round window facilitates retention of the electrode in the trough. If a canal wall-down approach is performed, then soft tissue such as fat can be placed into the middle ear/mastoid defect lateral to the electrode to further anchor it in place. A small variation of this approach is to begin the dissection anterior to the oval window to see if a lumen is present in this portion of the basal turn. If a lumen is opened, then a spilt electrode can be placed, with one limb going into the horizontal drill out of the basal turn, and the second limb going through the more apical cochleostomy.

Chronic Otitis Media With or Without Cholesteatoma

Due to the risk of infection involving the device and compromising the soft tissue flaps, there can be no active infection of the middle ear and mastoid at the time of surgery. That said, once infection has been controlled, there should be no impediments to pursue implantation.

In patient with chronic otitis media without cholesteatoma, a dry perforation may be repaired at the time of cochlear implant surgery or it can be repaired, with the cochlear implant surgery staged for 3 to 6 months after the tympanoplasty. If the ear is actively draining, then the ear must be treated medically, and if necessary with a tympanomastoidectomy, to ensure an infection free surgical site at the time of implantation.

If cholesteatoma is present, then depending on the extent of the lesion, a tympanomastoidectomy and cochlear implantation can be performed as a pri-mary surgery. Alternatively, a staged procedure can be performed to eradicate the cholesteatoma and a cochlear implantation can be performed at a later date. If a canal wall-down mastoidectomy is either required at the time of the surgery or has been performed in the past, then it most prudent to perform radical mastoidectomy to eradicate all disease, obstruct the eustachian tube, and close the ear canal. The authors favor soft tissue obliteration of the dead space, typically with fat placed in the cavity lateral to the implant.

SURGICAL COMPLICATIONS

DIZZINESS, VERTIGO, AND IMBALANCE

Postoperative vertigo and imbalance are the most common complaints associated with the surgery.[26–32] If vertigo occurs, it will be in the immediate postoperative period and will resolve over the course of 24 to 48 hours. A residual sense of imbalance may persist for 1 to 2 weeks. This occurs in less than 10% of cases. Vestibular rehabilitation physical therapy is helpful in hastening the recovery from these symptoms. Vestibular suppressants should be avoided after the initial vertigo has resolved.

ALTERED TASTE

Dysgeusia from damage to the chorda tympani nerve occurs in less than 5% of cases.[26–30] At times, when the facial recess is particularly narrow, the chorda tympani nerve must be deliberately sacrificed to obtain adequate visualization. The only real management for this complication is avoidance, with particular care to avoid damaging the chorda tympani when opening the facial recess.

WOUND COMPLICATIONS

Wound infections and dehiscence were a particular issue in the initial days of cochlear implants surgery. Modifications to the incision and flap construction, as detailed above, and the advent of minimal incisions, have resulted in a significant drop in the incidence of wound complications.[26-30,32]

Infection of the wound in the immediate postoperative period is managed with parenteral or oral antibiotics. Small areas of dehiscence can usually be managed with temporary discontinuation of the use of the processor and local wound care. More significant areas of dehiscence, particularly in the area overlying the receiver, require explantation of the device and closure of the defect with a local flap. Reimplantation can occur once the wound has completely healed. Cutting the electrode off receiver and leaving in place facilitates reimplantation.

CNS COMPLICATIONS

MENINGITIS

A sharp rise in the incidence of post-implantation meningitis from 2000 to 2002 prompted an international panel to address the causes and suggest solutions. The cases of meningitis were more commonly, but not uniquely, associated with an Advanced Bionics electrode implanted with a Silastic positioner.[31,33] It was noted that most cases occurred within one year

of implantation, and were more common in children less than 5 years of age. There were several risk factors that predisposed to meningitis including a higher rate of spontaneous meningitis in profoundly deaf patients, impaired immune status, history of meningitis, and the presence of other neurologic prosthesis (eg, VP shunts). Otologic risk factors include otitis media that can spread through the scala tympani in implanted patients, and inner ear malformations (eg, Mondini dysplasias) that are more likely to have CSF fistulas. Surgical risk factors include bacterial colonization due to surgical trauma, lack of soft tissue packing at the cochleostomy site, and the use of accessory implants for positioning. Recommendations to avoid meningitis include patient education before surgery, strict reporting of all cases to the manufacturer for continued monitoring, urgent and appropriate treatment of OM postimplant, vaccination against *S. pneumoniae* and *H. influenzae*, packing of the cochleostomy with soft tissue, and use of less traumatic electrode arrays.

If a patient does develop meningitis postoperatively it must be treated aggressively as it can be fatal. Organisms cultured from the CSF of patients include (in descending frequency) *Streptococcus pneumoniae*, *Streptococcus viridans*, *Haemophilus influenzae*, and *Escherichia coli*. Although vaccination reduces the risk, there are reports of patients being infected with both *H. influenzae* and *S. pneumoniae* following appropriate vaccination. Empiric treatment does not differ from that of non-otogenic meningitis if the tympanic membrane is intact and includes IV vancomycin and ceftriaxone. In cases of TM perforation or ventilation tubes *Pseudomonas* must be considered and meropenem or cefepime should be substituted for ceftrixone. Due to local variability in susceptibilities an infectious disease expert should be consulted.[15]

In patients with meningismus and an implant, CT should be obtained to assess for fluid in the middle ear, soft tissue masses, and osteolytic areas around the cochlea. A middle ear and mastoid exploration should be conducted with complete removal of inflammatory tissue including bone to the level of the sigmoid sinus or dura if needed. The site of chochleostomy should be inspected. If purulent drainage is seen from the cochleostomy site the electrodes may have to be removed and a labyrinthectomy performed. If there is evidence of bony destruction on the CT a total middle ear obliteration with a vascularized flap should be performed. If there is a perilymph fistula but no clear purulence antibiotic solution can be injected into the middle ear, the mastoid left to drain, and parenteral antibiotics given until symptoms resolve. In this case function of the implant may be preserved.[15]

CSF LEAK

CSF leak can occur from the inner ear if there is an abnormal communication with the CSF, as seen in cases of inner ear dysplasias.[29-32] This is managed with packing of the cochleostomy and middle ear space. CSF leak may also occur from inadvertent violation of the dura when drilling the mastoidectomy or when creating the well. In either case, the leak should be repaired immediately.

RARE INTRACRANIAL COMPLICATIONS

Other rare intracranial complications include cerebral infarction, epidural hema- toma, temporal lobe infarction with lateral sinus thrombosis, and epidural hema- toma.[31] The risk of these complications decreases with decreased drilling in the calvarium for device fixation.

FACIAL PARALYSIS

The most common approach to the round window and promontory is through the facial recess which puts the facial nerve at risk for damage during posterior tympanotomy.

Fortunately, facial paralysis is a rare complication that occurs in less than 1% of cases.[28,29] Damage to the nerve occurs in its descending (mastoid) segment and postoperative paralysis warrants a decom- pression of this region with repair if the nerve is transected.

REFERENCES

1. Clark GM, Pyman BC, Bailey QR. The sur- gery for multiple-electrode cochlear im- plantations. *J Laryngol Otol.* 1979;93(03): 215–223.

2. Balkany TJ, Whitley M, Shapira Y, et al. The temporalis pocket technique for cochlear implantation: an anatomic and clinical study. *Otol Neurotol.* 2009;30(7):903–907.

3. Gosepath J, Maurer J, Mann WJ. Epidural hematoma after cochlear implantation in a 2.5-year-old boy. *Otol Neurotol.* 2005; 26(2):202–204.

4. Cohen N. Cochlear implant soft surgery: Fact or fantasy? *Otolaryngol Head Neck Surg.* 1997;117(3):214–216.

5. Cohen NL, Hoffman RA. Complications of cochlear implant surgery in adults and children. *Ann Otol Rhinol Laryngol.* 1991; 100(9 pt 1):708–711.

6. Cohen NL, Hoffman RA. Surgical compli- cations of multichannel cochlear implants

in North America. *Adv Otorhinolaryngol.* 1993;48:70–74.

7. Hoffman RA, Cohen NL. Complications of cochlear implant surgery. *Ann Otol Rhinol Laryngol Suppl.* 1995;166:420–422.

8. Telian SA, El-Kashlan HK, Arts HA. Minimizing wound complications in cochlear implant surgery. *Am J Otol.* 1999;20(3): 331–334.

9. Otto RA, Lane AP, Carrasco VN. A new technique for securing cochlear implants. *Otolaryngol Head Neck Surg.* 1999;120(6): 897–898.

10. Davis BM, Labadie RF, McMenomey SO, Haynes DS. Cochlear implant fixation using polypropylene mesh and titanium screws. *Laryngoscope.* 2004;114(12):2116–2118.

11. Balkany TJ, Whitley M, Shapira Y, et al. The temporalis pocket technique for cochlear implantation: an anatomic and clinical study. *Otol Neurotol.* 2009;30(7):903–907.

12. Aschendorff A, Kromeier J, Klenzner T, Laszig R. Quality control after insertion of the nucleus contour and contour advance electrode in adults. *Ear Hear.* 2007;28(2 suppl):75S–79S.

13. Finley CC, Holden TA, Holden LK, et al. Role of electrode placement as a contributor to variability in cochlear implant outcomes. *Otol Neurotol.* 2008;29(7):920–928.

14. Skinner MW, Holden TA, Whiting BR, et al. In vivo estimates of the position of advanced bionics electrode arrays in the human cochlea. *Ann Otol Rhinol Laryngol* (suppl). 2007;197:2–24.

15. Wanna, GB, Noble JH, McRackan TR, et al. Assessment of electrode placement and audiological outcomes in bilateral cochlear implantation. *Otol Neurotol.* 2011;32(3):428–432.

16. Roland PS, Wright CG, Isaacson B. Cochlear implant electrode insertion: the round window revisited. *Laryngoscope.* 2007;117(8): 1397–1402.

17. Adunka OF & Buchman CA. Scala tympani cochleostomy I: results of a survey. *Laryngoscope.* 2007;117(12):2187–2194.

18. Adunka OF, Radeloff A, Gstoettner WK, Pillsbury HC, Buchman CA. Scala tympani cochleostomy II: topography and histology. *Laryngoscope.* 2007;117(12):2195–2200.

19. Souter MA, Briggs RJ, Wright CG, Roland PS. Round window insertion of precurved perimodiolar electrode arrays: how successful is it? *Otol Neurotol.* 2011; 32(1):58–63.

20. Ruckenstein MJ, Bigelow DC, Montes M., Rotz J. *The round window, is it the cochleostomy of choice?* 11th International Conference on Cochlear Implants and other Auditory Implantable Technologies. Stockholm, Sweden; 2011, July.

21. Green JD Jr, Marion MS, Hinojosa R. Labyrinthitis ossificans: histopathologic consideration for cochlear implantation. *Otolaryngol Head Neck Surg.* 1991;104(3): 320–326.

22. Balkany T, Gantz BJ, Steenerson RL, Cohen NL. Systematic approach to electrode insertion in the ossified cochlea. *Otolaryngol Head Neck Surg.* 1996;114(1):4–11.

23. Telian SA, Zimmerman-Phillips S, Kileny PR. Successful revision of failed cochlear implants in severe labyrinthitis ossificans. *American J Otol.* 1996;17(1):53–60.

24. Gantz BJ, McCabe BF, Tyler RS. Use of multichannel cochlear implants in obstructed and obliterated cochleas. *Otolaryngol Head Neck Surg.* 1988;98(1):72–81.

25. Balkany T, Bird PA, Hodges AV, Luntz M, Telischi FF, Buchman C. Surgical technique for implantation of the totally ossified cochlea. *Laryngoscope.* 1998;108(7): 988–992.

26. Collins MM, Hawthorne MH, el-Hmd K. Cochlear implantation in a district general hospital: problems and complications in the first five years. *J Laryngol Otol.* 1997; 111(4):325–332.

27. Proops DW, Stoddart RL, Donaldson I. Medical, surgical and audiological complications of the first 100 adult cochlear implant patients in Birmingham. *J Laryngol Otol* (suppl). 1999;24:14–17.

28. Green KMJ, Bhatt YM, Saeed SR, Ramsden RT. Complications following adult cochlear implantation: experience in Manchester. *J Laryngol Otol.* 2004;118(6):417–420.

29. Dutt SN, Ray J, Hadjihannas E, et al. Medical and surgical complications of the second 100 adult cochlear implant patients in Birmingham. *J Laryngol Otol.* 2005; 119(10):759–764.

30. Arnoldner C, Baumgartner W-D, Gstoettner W, Hamzavi J. Surgical considerations in cochlear implantation in children and adults: a review of 342 cases in Vienna. *Acta Otolaryngol.* 2005;125(3):228–234.

31. Dodson KM, Maiberger PG, Sismanis A. Intracranial complications of cochlear implantation. *Otol Neurotol.* 2007;28(4): 459–462.

32. Migirov L, Dagan E, Kronenberg J. Surgical and medical complications in different cochlear implant devices. *Acta Otolaryngol.* 2009;129(7):741–744.

33. Lalwani A, Cohen N. Longitudinal risk of meningitis after cochlear implantation associated with the use of the positioner. *Otol Neurotol.* 2011;32:1082–1085.

Chapter 8

Cochlear Implants: Surgical Techniques, Special Considerations—Pediatric and Malformed Cochleae

LUV JAVIA

INTRODUCTION

The widespread institution of universal newborn hearing screening has led to the early identification of profound sensorineural hearing loss in infants and children. Moreover, advances in diagnostic testing have led to increased reliability in the diagnosis of sensorineural hearing loss in younger infants. With increased experience and elucidation of its benefits in younger patients, pediatric cochlear implantation has become a widely available treatment option for many children with profound sensorineural hearing loss. Outcomes from pediatric cochlear implantation have shown that surgery in children can be performed safely and with positive effects on auditory system development and language skills. Anatomic and developmental considerations specific to pediatric implant recipients need to be taken into consideration and influence surgical techniques derived from adult cochlear implantation. Moreover, as cochlear implant candidacy has been expanded to children with certain cochleovestibular anomalies, it is imperative that cochlear implant surgeons be familiar with germane surgical issues, challenges and potential complications inherent to these patients.

COCHLEAR IMPLANTATION OF PEDIATRIC COCHLEAE

GENERAL CONSIDERATIONS

Cochlear implantation involves the manipulation of delicate otologic structures and implant hardware necessitating meticulous technique and unique considerations.

This is more so the case with pediatric patients in whom, although inner ear structures including the cochlea are adult size, other anatomic differences need specific mention. Pediatric soft tissues are often thinner than adults and require a delicate touch to prevent seromas, hematomas, and other postoperative complications. Moreover, the mastoid cavity itself is smaller in younger children and may have bone marrow, the latter of which can result in bleeding and difficulty with visualization if not properly managed.

Careful surgical planning starts with the incision. Shaving of hair should be kept to a minimum to prevent postoperative infectious complications; often in younger children shaving can be avoided altogether. The incision should take into consideration adequate exposure for drilling the mastoidectomy and adequate soft tissue coverage of the implanted receiver-stimulator unit. The standard approach involves a 4- to 5-cm postauricular incision that should be set posteriorly enough from the anterior border of the mastoid tip and postauricular crease to preserve vascular supply from branches of the postauricular artery (Fig 8–1). Some have advocated for small incision techniques, which is discussed later.

Unnecessary manipulation of soft tissues, very large flaps with significant dead space, posterior bony canal wall

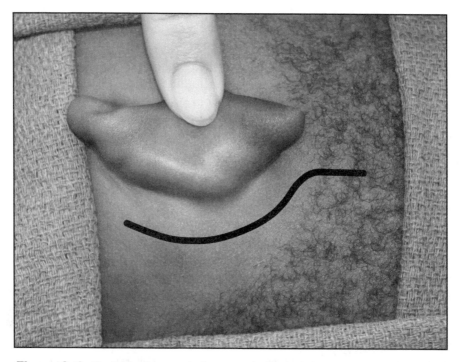

Figure 8–1. *Traditional extended retroauricular incision technique. The heavy black line shows the position of a 4- to 5-cm extended retroauricular incision. Careful attention is paid to minimizing the amount of hair that needs to be shaved. Moreover, the incision is placed 10 mm posterior to the retroauricular crease; preservation of the branches of the postauricular artery helps to prevent postoperative infectious complications and flap breakdown.*

fenestration especially if not recognized and repaired during the initial operation, extreme thinning of the posterior bony canal wall, and inadequately treated signs of infection may contribute to surgical complications that may be prevented. In a large series examining complications encountered in pediatric cochlear implantation, Bhatia et al[1] report that excessive thinning of the posterior canal wall may have led to atrophy of the posterior canal wall and the development of a retraction pocket and cholesteatoma in one case. This is particularly an issue in the pediatric population as concomitant eustachian tube dysfunction and middle ear disease often seen in children can complicate postoperative care. Côté et al[2] report that the high rate of middle ear pathology, such as acute otitis media, eustachian tube dysfunction, and retraction pockets, may explain why three cases of cable erosion and extrusion in the external auditory canal (EAC) associated with a cholesteatoma were observed. Reports of cholesteatoma in implanted children range from 0.27 to 0.89%. Accidental posterior external canal wall fenestration should be meticulously reconstructed and an overly thinned wall should be strengthened with bone pate to prevent future cholesteatoma formation or electrode erosion. Furthermore, management of an ipsilateral cholesteatoma in an ear with a cochlear implant is complex and should be individualized. Cartilage graft tympanoplasty may need to be performed to prevent retraction pocket progression or to prevent extrusion of an electrode array when it comes into contact with a tympanic membrane.[3]

Acute otitis media and otitis media with effusion is not infrequently encountered in a pediatric cochlear implant population and should be treated appro-priately with antibiotics and potentially placement of ventilation tubes to prevent infectious complications such as implant infection and meningitis. Studies have not demonstrated any increased incidence of acute otitis media in implanted children, and treatment of acute otitis media and otitis media with effusion with ventilation tubes in implanted children has not been associated with increased complications.[4]

There is evidence that the presence of chronic health conditions may increase the risk of complications. Hopfenspirger et al[4] report that 5 of the 12 (42%) children with chronic health conditions developed infectious complications postoperatively. Their practice includes covering fresh implant wounds with an occlusive dressing for two weeks after cochlear implantation in children with tracheostomies due to concerns of infectious soiling. They advocate for closer monitoring and an extended course of postoperative antibiotic prophylaxis in children with chronic health conditions.

PLACEMENT AND FIXATION OF THE RECEIVER-STIMULATOR

The careful placement of the receiver-stimulator is an important surgical consideration as complications related to device migration are reported to be approximately 5%.[5] Moreover, the developing motor coordination skills and increased head-to-body ratio of infants and young children place them at increased risk for blunt trauma injury to the head.[6] The receiver-stimulator should not be placed too close to the postauricular crease such that it may rub against the ear level processor resulting in skin breakdown, discomfort, and potentially infection or extrusion. Functional disconnect can result from the receiver-stimulator being positioned not only too close to the post-auricular crease and ear level processor, but also from an excessively posterior placement increasing interactions with a car seat or headrest.

A variety of receiver-stimulator fixation techniques have been reported in the literature. The classic fixation method involves creating a bony well and using nonabsorbable sutures through monocortical or bicortical holes drilled in the calvarium surrounding the receiver-stimulator. As the pediatric calvarium can be as thin as 1 mm in areas and dural exposure is usually seen when drilling the well for the receiver-stimulator, meticulous technique is required to prevent injury. A central bony island can be created to protect the underlying dura and prevent broad dural exposure. Complications including dural injuries, cerebrospinal fluid leaks, and intracranial complications have been reported. Intracranial complications include epidural hematoma, cerebral infarction, laceration of the superficial branch of the middle meningeal artery, and subdural hematoma.[7] These risks, although rare, have prompted the development of myriad other fixation techniques using a variety of alloplastic materials such as titanium plates, resorbable plates, polypropylene mesh, Gore-Tex sheets, and titanium anchor screws with nonabsorbable sutures.[6] More recent fixation methods have relied less on alloplastic materials and more on the inherent anatomy of the calvarium. Obviating the need for plates, screws, meshes, or other alloplastic materials also avoids additional costs.

Adunka et al[8] describe a straightforward technique in which the receiver-stimulator is fixed using a bony well for the device and suture fixation through the native cranial periosteum, avoiding transcortical holes, screws, and foreign materials other than sutures which can also be employed with minimal access surgical techniques. After elevation of a periosteal pocket and creation of a well with a central bony island, the receiver-stimulator is placed into the pocket/well and the posterior periosteum overlying the seated receiver-stimulator is then sutured to itself (3-0 Vicryl) using either a simple or mattress configuration to tighten the periosteal pocket snugly over the device. This technique avoids transcortical suture or screw placement that can result in cerebrospinal fluid leaks, dural injury, or intracranial hematomas. This approach relies on the natural periosteal attachments to the calvarial bone surrounding the receiver-stimulator and does still require the creation of a bony well. This technique was found to require fewer tools and be less time consuming than the standard calvarial suture method; moreover, there were no complications involving device migration, extrusion, or intracranial injury.[6]

Balkany et al[9] describe another technique for placement of the receiver stimulator that obviates the bony well and relies on the natural calvarial anatomy. They describe a t-pocket technique in which a subpericranial pocket is created without drilling a bony well which is limited anteriorly by a condensation of temporalis facsia and pericranium at the temporal-parietal suture, and posteroinferiorly by a dense pericranial attachment at the lambdoid suture. The aperture of the pocket is anterior-inferior at the squamous suture, between the temporal-parietal and lambdoid sutures. Due to the size of the pediatric skull and a more vertical orientation of the lambdoid and temporal-parietal sutures, young children may be best implanted in a more vertical position than older patients. The vertical orientation avoids an occipital magnet location and areas of greater calvarial curvature in very young children. The authors advise against its use in revision cases where the soft-tissue envelope can be less secure. They report no cases of migration or intracranial complications in 107 pediatric patients with a mean duration of follow-up of 16.4 months.

At our institution, we employ two other techniques for receiver-stimulator fixation. Both techniques use a resorbable plating system and start with the creation of a tight pocket without drilling a bony well down to the dura. Instead, the receiver-stimulator is placed into the pocket and a resorbable plate is fashioned such that the shoulder and fantail of the implant are secured down to the calvarium with two resorbable screws (Fig 8–2). In the second method, a tight pocket is similarly fashioned, and the pericranium is tacked down to the calvarium with a resorbable screw and washer made from one resorbable hole of a plate (Fig 8–3). The pericraniopexy is performed by placing two screws with washers, one on either side of the fantail and anterior to the shoulder of the receiver-stimulator. Advantages of these techniques include speed of technique, secure fixation of the implant, and avoidance of dural exposure as no bony well is made.

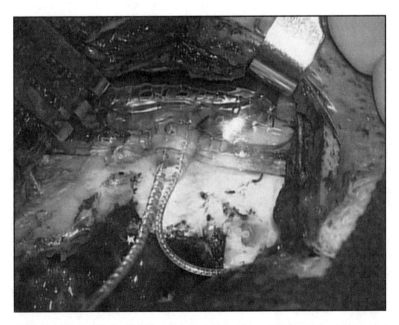

Figure 8–2. Plate fixation technique. Resorbable plate is heated and conformed to the shoulder and fantail region of the receiver-stimulator template. The receiver-stimulator is placed into a tight pericranial pocket and then fixed to the calvarium with the resorbable plate. A bony well is not drilled. Two resorbable screws are used to secure the resorbable plate (Synthes, Inc; West Chester, PA). Courtesy of John Germiller, MD.

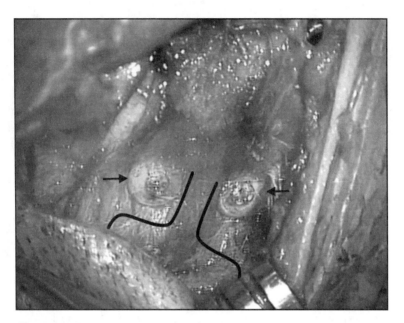

Figure 8–3. *Pericraniopexy fixation technique. The receiver-stimulator is placed into a tight pericranial pocket and then the pericranium at the mouth of the pocket is fixed to the calvarium with a resorbable screw and washer (arrows). The pericranium is secured with a screw and washer on either side of the fantail, just in front of the shoulder of the receiver-stimulator. The washer is fashioned by cutting one hole off a resorbable plate (Synthes, Inc; West Chester, PA). Courtesy of John Germiller, MD.*

Due to the increased frequency of minor head trauma and thinner soft tissue envelope encountered in the pediatric population as compared to adults, Davids et al[10] believe that good fixation is especially important. Based on personal experience, they advocate that a tie-down procedure ideally should be performed in all pediatric cases, even those with thick cortical bone. The authors believe this to be a key factor in their low rates of soft tissue complications (1.51%).

SMALL INCISION TECHNIQUE

Traditional implant surgery employs a 4- to 5-cm retroauricular incision (see Fig 8–1); however, recent reports have proposed a smaller incision technique (Fig 8–4).[11] James et al report using a 25-mm long incision placed just anterior to the posterior-superior edge of the ear level template.[12] Despite the incision being 25 mm, the soft tissue and skin are able to stretch to accommodate the large width of the receiver-stimulator. This placement of the incision is usually just anterior to the hairline and thus avoids incisions through the scalp, which have potential for cosmetic issues such as a hairless scar. Overzealous retraction should be avoided to prevent postoperative wound edema. Potential advantages of this technique are reduced edema, dead space, and vascular compromise that may have an effect on postoperative infection rates. Additionally, the lack of edema and decrease in pain may

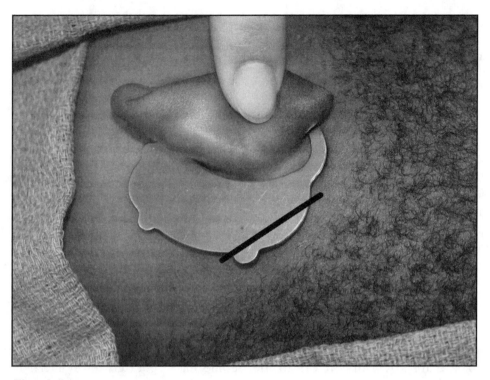

Figure 8–4. *Small incision technique. A 25-mm incision (heavy black line) is located slightly overlapping the posterior-superior portion of the ear level processor template. Hair does not usually need to be shaved.*

allow for earlier mapping and device activation.[10]

The implant angle has evolved from a retroverted to an anteverted orientation to optimize the cosmetic and functional characteristics of the behind the ear processor as well as to maintain a low wound complication rate. A survey conducted of patient/parent satisfaction reveals that the fact that patients have been consistently satisfied over time suggests that the cosmetic, functional and wound implications are minimal.[13]

SUPRAMEATAL APPROACH IN CHILDREN

Classically, cochlear implantation has been completed by performing a mastoidec-tomy and posterior tympanotomy, or facial recess approach. However, a new approach was proposed by Kronenberg called the suprameatal approach (SMA) involving exposure of the middle ear through the external auditory canal and insertion of the electrode into the cochlea via a suprameatal tunnel instead of the mastoid cavity.[14] Proponents of the SMA argue that risk of injury to the facial nerve and chorda tympani nerve are avoided, the latter of which is important more recently as patients are increasingly receiving bilateral cochlear implants. The SMA technique has been used in infants as young as 10 to 12 months.[15]

Briefly, the middle ear is entered via an endaural tympanotomy after completing a retroauricular incision of about 2 to 3 cm. Next, a suprameatal tunnel is drilled superoposterior to the spine of Henle toward the posterior part of the aditus ad antrum, carefully avoiding injury to the middle fossa dura during drilling of the suprameatal tunnel. When the body of the incus is visualized drilling is stopped; the horizontal semicircular canal is visualized as well. The antrum is connected to the recessus epitympanicus via a groove drilled lateral to the body of the incus. A second incision of 2 to 3 cm is made temporoparietally to drill the bony well and place the receiver-stimulator. A subperiosteal tunnel is created between the two incisions and the electode is passed through this and the suprameatal tunnel into the middle ear. The electrode is then inserted through a cochleostomy placed anteroinferior to the oval window in the promontory.[16]

There are a few drawbacks to the SMA. Due to the transmeatal line of sight of the cochleostomy, the surgeon gets a perpendicular view of the inferior cochlea, hindering the view of the electrode array tip along the course of the basal turn after insertion. Therefore, proponents of this practice advocate for using fluoroscopy intraoperatively to confirm electrode positioning both before and after stylet removal. As compared to the classic approach, the SMA technique has an increased risk for electrode array kinking due to the difficult 30° more superior insertion. Moreover, there is a relatively steep angle of insertion of the electrode that increases the risk of rotating the electrode in an upward direction as a consequence of touching the outer wall of the scala tympani as the electrode is advanced. This ruptures the basal membrane and the integrity of the scala media, resulting in loss of all preexisting residual hearing. This approach is also more difficult in patients with a low-lying tegmen/

dura; consequently the incus may need to be removed when creating the suprameatal tunnel.[16,17]

Proponents believe that there are several advantages of the SMA technique including a better exposure of the electrode due to direct middle ear access. Interestingly, it is necessary to remove bone from the posterosuperior wall of the external ear canal to obtain a wider view of the middle ear contents to facilitate electrode maneuverability. Moreover, due to avoidance of a mastoidectomy and facial recess approach, operative time may be decreased compared to the classical approach performed by inexperienced or moderately experienced ear surgeons. The facial nerve is protected in the SMA technique by the body of the incus; likewise, the chorda tympani nerve is spared. Some have reported fewer facial nerve paralysis and postoperative infections of the mastoid with the SMA technique.[16,17]

COCHLEAR IMPLANTATION IN CHILDREN YOUNGER THAN ONE YEAR OF AGE

The United States Food and Drug Administration has approved cochlear implants for children with bilateral profound sensorineural hearing loss down to one year of age except in the case of meningitis when there are concerns of intracochlear scarring and ossification. Additionally, children fitted with implants at an early age have been shown to improve their expressive and receptive language skills. Auditory performance scores rapidly normalize in children implanted before the age of 2 years, whereas such a result was rarely achieved in those implanted after the age of 4 years. Moreover, the earlier the cochlear implantation before 2 years of age, the closer the onset of babbling, and subsequent auditory performance at a chronological age comparable to normal-hearing infants.[18] In this context, children younger than one have received cochlear implants with the youngest one being performed at an age of 4 months.[19] But even prior to implantation, two considerations need to be adequately addressed: audiologic certainty of the diagnosis of profound sensorineural hearing loss and the parental acceptance of such a diagnosis and treatment course. The challenge of diagnosing profound sensorineural hearing loss in children younger than one has some implant surgeons cautioning against implantation in this population.

Cochlear implantation in children younger than 1 year has several unique concerns. The delicate skin and subcutaneous tissues demand the utmost care and attention to prevent wound complications. Moreover, as the skull is very thin, extreme care should be taken preoperatively when creating bone markings transcutaneously with a needle and methylene blue, as the skull integrity can be breached causing dural injury. If this were to happen, the dura should be inspected and evidence for bleeding sought. Due to the relatively poorly developed mastoid tip, infants can have a laterally positioned stylomastoid foramen and superficial facial nerve that can lie just under the skin. The skin incision should not be extended as inferiorly and special care should be taken when lifting periosteum off the mastoid in this region to avoid injuring a superficial facial nerve. Implantation has been accomplished through both traditional extended postauricular and small incision techniques.

James et al compared the mastoid characteristics on preoperative CT temporal bone scans between infants and chil-dren between 13 months and 3.5 years of age and reported that the mastoid marrow content on CT scan was significantly greater in this age group ($p < 0.001$), but pneumatization was always adequate for safe identification of surgical landmarks.[20] They found that there was an increase in pneumatization of the mastoid bone and reduction in marrow content that occurs with age. Pneumatization increases to approximately 60% by 2 years of age, when very little marrow remains at the level of the round window on CT scans. Thus, although the overall mastoid space may be decreased in infants, this is not typically restrictive and instead the implant surgeon must be ready to deal with bleeding that can be encountered with marrow, particularly when drilling a facial recess. Expeditious but safe drilling employing bone wax, a diamond burr reverse drilling technique, thrombin soaked Gelfoam, and/or coagulation of emissary veins can help control hemorrhage.[20,21] Pneumatization of the mastoid antrum is usually present, facilitating the identification of the incus and horizontal semicircular canal; however, three patients have been described with virtually no pneumatization. As the cochlea is adult sized, it is not surprising that full insertion of the electrode did not generally seem to be an issue in reports.

Hemostasis while performing cochlear implantation in infants is of the utmost importance to prevent hypovolemia and cardiovascular collapse. Hypovolemic effects can be anticipated from blood loss over 10% of the total blood volume. This equates to an approximate loss of 80 mL blood in an average 10 kg 12-month-old. The margin of safety is even lower in a 6-month-old with a weight of 8 kg where hypovolemic effects can be seen at a loss of 65 mL.[20] All groups reporting on cochlear implantation in infants prominently highlight the importance of having a pediatric anesthesiologist who is more familiar with the unique physiologic characteristics present in this age group. The impact of concurrent medical factors such as cardiovascular disease, preterm birth, and low birth weight needs to be examined during candidacy considerations.

Issues of skull growth and electrode migration are also a consideration in this very young population as pediatric head circumference undergoes tremendous change in the first year of life, especially compared to growth occurring after one year of age. Interestingly, this risk is low and thus band fixation of the electrode to the buttress is not advocated.[18,21] Moreover, careful attention should be given when positioning the receiver-stimulator as the calvarium can be more curved; a coil position of above the apex of the pinna can help prevent interactions dislodging the coil when the infant is in a car seat or stroller.[20] Due to the calvarial growth and potential trauma incurred during the process of learning how to walk in this population, fixation is advised to prevent long-term complications.

Several groups have reported that cochlear implantation is safe in this age group, with complications comparable to surgery in older children and adults. Rare complications reported include flap breakdown requiring device reimplantation, intraoperative cerebrospinal fluid leak, device failure, hematoma, and minor wound trauma/cellulitis.[15,18–22]

Audiologic outcome data is limited at this time. The average CAP function of age for three age groups of children (including one infant group) indicated that the highest score was achieved in all three groups, but at more delayed intervals in the older age groups. Thus if one considers only the highest score of the CAP testing as the target, very early implantation does not seem justified. However, the rate of receptive language growth as assessed with PPVT-R provides distinctive evidence that only the children implanted as infants have scores overlapping the line of normal-hearing children, with the distinction between children implanted younger than 11 months and older than 11 months remaining statistically significant even after 9 years of cochlear implant use. TROG outcomes clearly indicate that only children from the infant implant age group (74%) were in the 76 to 100 percentile at 5 years follow-up. At 9 years follow-up, 100% of children in the infant group, 45% in the second group (12 to 23 months), and 20% in the third group (24 to 36 months) were in the 76 to 100 percentile. Based on their data, Colleti et al[19] comment that infants implanted between 4 and 11 months can be expected to exhibit levels of spoken language competence that are on a par with hearing age-mates much before they enter the (Italian) primary school, whereas children fitted with cochlear implants after 12 months of age may experience some difficulties catching up with hearing age-mates. Further experience and research will give us more information on complications and audiologic outcomes in the infant implant age group.

HEARING PRESERVATION PEDIATRIC COCHLEAR IMPLANTATION

Data primarily from adult patients suggest that preservation of residual hearing in cochlear implant recipients can result in increased hearing performance in noisy listening environments, improved music perception and appreciation, and increased realism of sounds and voices. The mechanism of injury and loss of residual hearing during cochlear implantation is thought to be primarily related to the acoustic trauma of drilling a cochleostomy and mechanical trauma of electrode insertion resulting in fractures of the osseous spiral lamina, disruption of the basilar membrane, or tearing of the endosteum of the scala tympani. Other causes include disturbances of cochlear fluid homeostasis, bacterial infection, osteoneogenesis, or cochlear fibrosis from a foreign body reaction to electrode components, bone dust, or blood.[23]

Several surgical techniques have been described that aim to improve residual hearing after cochlear implantation. These are aimed at introducing the electrode into the basal turn of the cochlea while preserving function in the apical regions. Soft surgery techniques that are aimed at minimal disruption of intracochlear structures include using a smaller bur to make the cochleostomy, delineating the endosteum of the scala tympani prior to entering in a controlled fashion with dissectors, avoiding suctioning of perilymph fluid, gentle electrode introduction, and the use of lubricants such as hyaluronate.[24] Additional surgical modifications include a shorter insertion depth, off-stylet technique, changes in the angle of insertion, and modiolar-hugging electrode arrays. The significance of the various factors on audiologic outcomes is still being elucidated and is a source of some debate.

Brown et al[23] examined attempts at hearing preservation in pediatric cochlear implant recipients employing a full insertion, standard electrode array. The advantage of using a full-length electrode array instead of a shorter, basal region array is that future progression of low-frequency hearing loss can be better remedied as more apical electrodes can be activated over time. This may be especially important in children as the progression of hearing loss is at a greater rate than in adults. Also, apical electrodes can initially be inactivated and thus be used in an electroacoustical stimulation strategy. Brown et al were able to achieve complete residual hearing preservation (change in low frequency PTA ≤10 dB) in 14 of 31 (45.2%) of patients and partial hearing preservation (change in low frequency PTA between 0 and 40 dB) in 28 of 31 (90.3%) of patients.

Others have examined partial insertion techniques via a round window insertion to a shortened depth and report 9 out of 9 children with preservation of at least some residual hearing, with 8 of the 9 viable candidates for electroacoustical stimulation employing both a hearing aid and cochlear implant in one ear.[25] Gantz et al[26] have implanted a Nucleus Hybrid S12 array that is 10 mm in length instead of the standard 24 mm of the Nucleus Freedom and employs 10 contacts instead of 22. They performed bilateral cochlear implants in children with one ear receiving the Nucleus Hybrid S12 array and the other a standard Nucleus Freedom array and reported speech recognition performance that seemed to be similarly high in both ears. Proponents of using a shorter electrode in children believe that the standard length electrode may cause too much intracochlear damage to the scala media, organ of Corti, and support cells; damage which may prevent the use of future, potential therapies grounded in molecular or genetic regeneration.

Clearly, much more research needs to be done to elucidate whether hearing preservation techniques can be reliably reproduced and organized as a strategy, and whether this translates into a practical, acoustic performance advantage for pediatric patients.

BILATERAL PEDIATRIC COCHLEAR IMPLANTATION

Bilateral cochlear implantation has been performed in pediatric patients as it is thought to provide increased resolution of sound localization and increased performance in difficult or noisy environments. This can be performed sequentially in which implants are performed at two separate surgeries, or they can be done simultaneously with both implants placed at one surgical visit. Simultaneous implantation can increase the anesthetic time and blood loss at one surgical procedure, an important consideration in infant implant recipients where there is a narrower margin of safety with blood loss and anesthetic time. Sequential surgeries require two anesthetic exposures. Ramsden et al[27] examined their first 50 consecutive simultaneous cochlear implantations and compared them to historical sequential implantations. They found that the group of children receiving simultaneous bilateral cochlear implants showed no difference in complications, length of hospital stay, or use of analgesia and antiemetics compared with children receiving single implants. Interestingly, the simultaneously implanted children had a reduced cumulative surgical time.

An advantage of bilateral implantation, whether sequential or simultaneous, with a short interimplantation interval is that it ensures the matching of the devices and bilateral stimulation and development of the auditory system.[28] Research suggests that with unilateral cochlear implant use there may be a negative impact upon the bilateral auditory brainstem plasticity.[29] Moreover, if sequential implantation is pursued instead of simultaneous then consideration may need to be given to minimizing the time between implantation to decrease these negative effects. Mismatched timing of brainstem activity resolves within 9 months of bilateral cochlear implant use in children with 6 to 12 months of unilateral use, but persists with more prolonged unilateral use.

Some centers have been attempting to perform vestibular testing following cochlear implantation in an effort to delineate any potential impact upon balance. Vestibular testing can be challenging in the pediatric population and further studies are required to suggest the optimal technique for testing children and potential guidelines for or impact on bilateral cochlear implantation.

COCHLEAR IMPLANTATION OF MALFORMED COCHLEAE

GENERAL CONSIDERATIONS

Since the 1980s considerable experience has been amassed with pediatric cochlear implantation as this therapeutic intervention expands and is made available to increasing numbers of deaf children around the world. Children with cochleovestibular anomalies are not infrequently encountered in such cochlear implant programs considering that 20% of children with sensorineural hearing loss have associated radiologic anomalies of the temporal bone.[30] As radiologic imaging technology with CT and MRI continue to improve, more detailed information is garnered regarding cochleovestibular anatomy. Thus, cochleovestibular anomalies may be more frequently encountered than initial reports. In fact, there are reports that as many as 41% of children receiving cochlear implants at a major cochlear implant program have anomalous cochleovestibular anatomy in either the implanted or nonimplanted ear.[31] In ears with SNHL, the presence of a congenital syndrome significantly increased the risk of cochlear and vestibular abnormalities of the temporal bone (45% versus 14%; $p < 0.001$), including IAC abnormalities (30% versus 2%; $p < 0.001$), which overall were more commonly seen in children with (20%) versus without (3%) a congenital syndrome regardless of the presence of SNHL.[32] Previously, many of these children with anatomic anomalies may have been denied cochlear implants due to concerns regarding the probability of discrete current spread in an open, fluid-filled dysplastic cavity and the risk that facial nerve injury and meningitis might occur.[33] The first child with a cochleovestibular anomaly to receive a cochlear implant was in 1983.[34] Since that time there are reports from various cochlear implant programs describing successful cochlear implantation of these children discussing surgical techniques and audiologic outcomes. Familiarity with the unique anatomy and appropriately modifying surgical techniques are critical for performing safe implantation in children with cochleovestibular anomalies and producing audiologic gains.

COCHLEOVESTIBULAR ANOMALIES

It is believed that cochleovestibular anomalies result from an arrest of embryogenesis, abnormal development at some stage of fetal life, or genetic defects creating distinctive cochlear malformations. The thought that anomalies result from an arrest of development along a single developmental continuum is likely not entirely true; it is more likely that a number of distinct anomalous paths of development are possible arising in common from the otic placode.[31] CT imaging is helpful for detailing the bony structures of the inner ear and following the course of the facial nerve. MRI, specifically T2 fast-spin echo (FSE) and Fourier transformation constructive interference in the steady-state (FT-CISS) sequences, are commonly used to examine temporal bone anatomy and have become first-line imaging for cochlear implant candidates at some centers. MRI sequences can help delineate the IAC and the seventh-eighth nerve complexes, the membranous labyrinth, and intracavity soft tissue septations.[35] Jackler et al[30] described a classification scheme which included cochleovestibular aplasia (Michel's aplasia), common cavity (CC), hypoplastic cochlea (HC), and incomplete partition (IP). Several others have attempted to modify the classification scheme.[36–38] A useful classification scheme for clinical purposes describes cochleovestibular malformations (in descending order of severity) as follows: Michel deformity, cochlear aplasia, common cavity, IP-I (cystic cochleovestibular malformation), cochlear hypoplasia, and IP-II (Mondini deformity).[38] Table 8–1 outlines the various inner ear malformations that can be encountered.

Table 8–1. Inner Ear Malformations[38]

Cochlear Malformations
Michel Deformity
There is complete absence of all cochlear and vestibular structures. Not cochlear implant candidates.
Cochlear Aplasia
The cochlea is completely absent. Not cochlear implant candidates.
Common Cavity Deformity (CC)
There is a cystic cavity representing the cochlea and vestibule, but without showing any differentiation into cochlea and vestibule.
Incomplete Partition Type I (IP-I)
The cochlea is lacking the entire modiolus and cribriform area, resulting in a cystic appearance. This is accompanied by a large cystic vestibule.
Cochlear Hypoplasia (CH)
Malformation is further differentiated so that the cochlea and vestibule are separate from each other but their dimensions are smaller than normal. Hypoplastic cochlea resembles a small bud off the internal auditory canal (IAC).
Incomplete Partition Type II (IP-II) — Mondini Deformity
The cochlea consists of 1.5 turns, in which the middle and apical turns coalesce to form a cystic apex, accompanied by a dilated vestibule and enlarged VA.
Vestibular Malformations
Vestibular malformations include Michel deformity, common cavity, absent vestibule, hypoplastic vestibule, and dilated vestibule.
Semicircular Canal Malformations
Semicircular canal malformations are described as absent, hypoplastic, or enlarged.
Internal Auditory Canal Malformations
Internal auditory canal malformations are described as absent, narrow, or enlarged.
Vestibular and Cochlear Aqueduct Findings
Vestibular and cochlear aqueduct abnormalities are described as enlarged or normal.

A common cavity is present when the vestibule and cochlea are not separated and form a common cystic cavity (Fig 8–5A). A common cavity also results from the dilation of the ductus reunions, effectively making the cochlea and vestibule contiguous.[31] This is the second most common inner ear malformation reported by Jackler et al.[30] The IAC is frequently affected as well, with an enlarged IAC associated with a large CC and a narrow IAC with a small CC. Usually, the IAC enters the CC at its center and often the fundus of the IAC is thought to be defective.[38]

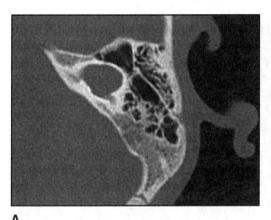
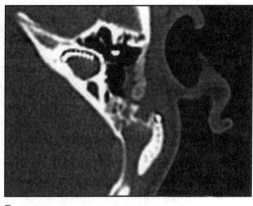

A   B

Figure 8–5. *Common cavity malformation.* **A.** *Patient with a common cavity malformation.* **B.** *Same patient after cochlear implantation. Note how the electrode array of the cochlear implant follows the contour of the outer wall of the common cavity where the neuroepithelium is located. Courtesy of Brian Dunham, MD.*

Incomplete partition deformities were collectively referred to previously as Mondini dysplasia; however, this was problematic due to a lack of specificity with which it was used in the literature. Sennaroglu et al have described two different types of incomplete partition: cystic cochleovestibular malformation (IP-I) and the classic Mondini deformity (IP-II). The type I malformation is less differentiated than the type II malformation. Classic Mondini deformity (IP-II) has three components (a cystic apex, dilated vestibule, and large vestibular aqueduct), whereas type I malformation has an empty, cystic cochlea and vestibule without an enlarged vestibular aqueduct.[38] IP-I is an empty cochlea due to the lack of a modiolus in its entire length from base to apex; IP-II has partial development of the modiolus near the base of the cochlea. Usually with IP-I, the cribriform area between the cochlea and IAC is defective and the IAC is enlarged. With IP-II the cochlea and vestibule are more normal in size, and the cochlea has 1.5 turns (Fig 8–6). As stated before, the

interscalar defect is at the apex with a normal basal modiolus. Furthermore, the IAC can be dilated in 60% of cases and an EVA is present.[38]

In cochlear hypoplasia, the cochlea and vestibule are differentiated, however the cochlea is smaller than normal in size. The cochlea may have a variety of abnormalities ranging from a rudimentary cochlear diverticulum to an incompletely formed cochlear bud measuring several millimeters.[39] The vestibule can be absent or hypoplastic and the IAC can be normal or narrower.

The vestibular aqueduct is considered enlarged when it measures >1.5 mm in diameter and has been found to account for 32% of the hearing loss in children who undergo CT of the temporal bone.[40] It is usually present bilaterally, although unilateral cases are less frequently seen. Progression of sensorineural hearing loss has been reported to occur in 11.8 to 60.9% of patients.[31] Although the exact mechanism of hearing loss is not known with enlarged vestibular aqueduct (EVA),

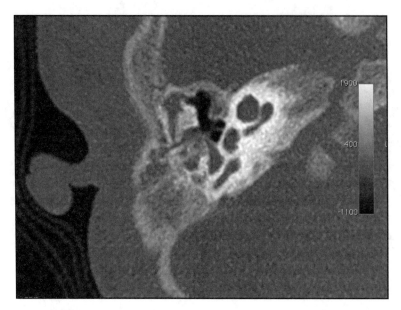

Figure 8–6. *Incomplete partition-II. Patient with 1.5 turns of the cochlea. Note basal turn of cochlea and a common cavity consisting of the middle and apical turns of the cochlea. A deficiency of the modiolus is present in the common cavity. Courtesy of John Germiller, MD.*

it is thought that EVA is an indicator of a congenital problem rather than the actual mechanism of hearing loss. The hearing loss associated with EVA may be a result of concomitant defects in the membranous labyrinth of the cochlea or defects on the cellular level. One study using CT imaging suggests that all cochlea associated with an EVA have an associated modiolar deficiency.[41] EVA is also known to be associated with Pendred syndrome and branchio-oto-renal syndrome. Patients with EVA can present a challenge during cochlear implantation, as many are associated with a CSF/perilymph "gusher."

The internal auditory canal can be malformed as well. The IAC can be abnormally narrow with an aplastic or hypoplastic cochlear nerve. Clearly, establishing the presence of a cochlear nerve is compulsory for successful cochlear implantation.

Moreover, the IAC can be "double," with a prominent crista falciformis; tapered towards the lamina cribrosa at its lateral end (associated with common cavity and spontaneous CSF fistula); and bulbous, as seen in X-linked deafness with a risk of surgically induced CSF gushers.[42] Papsin[31] reported on 11 children with narrowing of the IAC and all had other cochleovestibular anomalies (8 had HC, 1 child each had IP, CC, and EVA). Moreover, narrow IAC has been described with several syndromes such as Goldenhar, VATER-RAPADILLINO, Möbius, Okihiro, and, most notably, CHARGE.[31,43] Interestingly, a cochlear nerve can be absent even with a normal sized IAC and/or cochlea, and thus some believe that all pediatric cochlear implant candidates should undergo an MRI.[43,44] In patients for whom the cochlear nerve presence is questionable on MRI, promontory stimulation electrical auditory brainstem responses may be useful in determining cochlear nerve status and cochlear implant candidacy (Fig 8–7).[45]

SURGICAL IMPLICATIONS

The unique anatomy present in children with cochleovestibular anomalies requires the implant surgeon to make several special considerations in order to make cochlear implantation in this population safe and effective. Cochleovestibular anomalies previously precluded implantation due to surgical concerns about cochleostomy and electrode placement, electrode stability within the hypoplastic or dysplastic cochlea, risk of facial nerve injury from an aberrant course, the increased likelihood of perilymph/ CSF leak, potential for postimplantation bacterial meningitis, and potential misplacement of the electrode into the IAC.[31] Improvements in both radiologic imaging and surgical implantation techniques, and experience have helped to overcome many of these concerns.

The middle ear anatomy is often abnormal as well in children with cochleovestibular anomalies. Zheng et al[46] examined the histopathology of temporal bones with congenital cochlear malformations and found that 19% of ears had aplasia of the middle ear cavity; 67% had malformed ossicles, with the most common being stapes malformations; 57% had abnormal oval windows; and 29% had a closed or partially obstructed round window niche. These associated middle ear malformations can make recognition of traditional surgical landmarks and cochleostomy placement challenging.

An aberrant facial nerve course has been reported in 14 to 32% of patients with cochleovestibular anomalies at time of surgery; a temporal bone study reported a facial nerve anomaly in 43% of ears.[31,46–49] This range is much increased over the 0.3% prevalence rate of an aberrant facial nerve

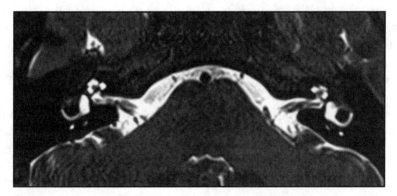

Figure 8–7. *Questionable cochlear nerve. This patient with profound sensorineural hearing loss was found on MR imaging to have normal-sized internal auditory canals; however, cochlear nerves could not be identified. Patient subsequently underwent promontory stimulation auditory brainstem response testing and was found to have robust cochlear nerve responses bilaterally without fatigue.*

in normal ears.[30] Facial nerve anomalies are more commonly encountered with semicircular canal aplasia, common cavity, hypoplastic cochlea, and coexistent craniofacial anomalies.[31,47] The aberrant nerve usually courses below the cochleariform process across the promontory and toward the round window and is thought to result from an anteromedial displacement of the second genu into the region of the oval or round window. Papsin reported that nearly all cases in which there was an anomalous facial nerve course, the stapes was absent or incomplete, suggesting that a normal stapes superstructure may be necessary for a normal facial nerve position.[31] Some children may have a facial nerve which splits, whereby a more anteriorly positioned nerve courses in conjunction with a normal facial nerve. This abnormal, anterior course of the facial nerve may obscure the round window and necessitate a more anteriorly placed cochleostomy on the promontory. In children with a common cavity, the facial nerve can be avoided entirely by performing a labyrinthotomy in the region of the horizontal semicircular canal or remnant, superior and posterior to the tympanic facial nerve.[47] Coelho et al[50] advocate for minimizing potential facial nerve problems when implanting common cavities by approaching through the mastoid antrum without performing a facial recess and making the cochleostomy laterally, at the inferior portion of the cavity. This part of the cavity bulges into the mastoid.[50] In some instances where the facial nerve and round window are not readily identified, a canal wall-down approach may be needed to facilitate better visualization and approach of middle and inner ear structures.[51] The canal can be reconstructed prior to closure. Facial nerve monitoring should be utilized in all cases. Facial nerve stimulation has been reported in 11 to 30% of implanted patients with cochleovestibular anomalies.[33,47] In general, it is believed to occur when current from the electrode stimulates nonauditory neural structures adjacent to the cochlea. Causes for this abnormal stimulation include an aberrant facial nerve course, location of the electrode in the deformed labyrinth, facial nerve dehiscence, or the proximity of the facial nerve to the electrode array.[33,52] In general, unwanted facial nerve stimulation is thought to occur more frequently in patients with cochleovestibular anomalies than normal patients. This problem may be remedied by selective deactivation of individual electrodes. However, intractable facial stimulation despite these efforts has been reported to result in revision surgery and nonuse of the implant.[47]

Intraoperative cerebrospinal fluid (CSF) or perilymph leaks can often be encountered in children with cochleovestibular anomalies. These CSF/perilymph gushers have been reported in as many as 50% of patients; however, there may be an overestimation in the reports as there is no standardization in what constitutes a gusher.[31,48] The likelihood of encountering a CSF/perilymph leak during surgery does not seem to correlate to the severity of cochleovestibular abnormality; CC is most commonly associated with a CSF/perilymph leak.[31] Intraoperative CSF/perilymph leakage after performing a cochleostomy is thought to occur as a result of a bony defect at the lateral end (fundus) of the IAC. Normally, the CSF in the subarachnoid space extends laterally into the IAC as far as the lateral fundus, where it is separated from the perilymph by the bony plate of the lamina cribrosa, by the nerves that pass through the lamina cribrosa, and by the spiral ganglion. Ears with cochleovestibular anomalies may have a deficiency in this barrier, allowing confluence between CSF and perilymph.[42] The presence of a cochleovestibular anomaly on radiologic imaging increases the likelihood of encountering an intraoperative CSF/perilymph leak.[42] Apart from this, a modiolar deficiency is not readily seen on CT or MR imaging sometimes. A modiolar defect is presumed to be present, even with normal appearing radiologic imaging, when a CSF/perilymph leak occurs intraoperatively in patients with cochleovestibular anomalies.[33] If a CSF/perilymph leak occurs after performing a cochleostomy, the head of the bed should be elevated and following electrode insertion, the cochleostomy should be plugged tightly with several pieces of temporalis fascia or muscle plugs, followed by a second layer with fibrin glue. Mannitol can be used intraoperatively as well. The patient is returned to a neutral position and observed for 10 to 15 minutes. Should a small CSF/perilymph leak continue, the cochleostomy should be bolstered with additional fascia and gelfoam and preparations should be made for placement of a lumbar drain for four days. Proper healing of the cochleostomy is critical because increased CSF pressure can dislodge the plug even after several years have elapsed, and children can present with late CSF/perilymph fistulas or recurrent meningitis.[31] Difficult to control leaks may require a subtotal petrosectomy, closing of the external auditory canal, blocking the eustachian tube, and obliteration of the middle ear and mastoid with soft tissue.[42,53] There is some debate whether it is better to drill a snug-fit or a bigger cochleostomy. Weber et al[49] believe that it is better to create a small cochleostomy that allows the electrode to partially block the CSF/perilymph flow

and reinforce with fascia or muscle.[49] Alternatively, Graham et al[42] advocate for creating a larger cochleostomy to facilitate packing of fascia or muscle inside the cochleostomy. When tightly packing the cochleostomy with fascia or muscle, one must always be aware of the course of the facial nerve. Facial nerve palsy has been described due to compression from a stack of soft tissue used to pack a cochleostomy tightly after a profuse CSF gusher was encountered intraoperatively.[38] Having fascia harvested and ready as well as noting the course of the facial nerve in relation to the cochleostomy prior to creating one can help the implant surgeon deal more efficiently and safely with CSF/perilymph leaks. Intraoperative imaging such as plain film x-ray, fluoroscopy, or intraoperative CT can be performed to evaluate that the electrode is not in the IAC.[54]

Electrode type and insertion technique may be influenced by the presence of cochleovestibular anomalies. Careful preoperative preparation can minimize the possibility of inserting the electrode into the IAC or carotid canal and maximize audiological outcomes. In CC deformity, it must be remembered that the modiolus and interscalar septum are absent and instead the neural tissue is located peripherally in the walls of the common cavity (Fig 8–5B). Therefore, the usual goal of a perimodiolar placement of the electrode does not apply and instead a straight electrode with circumferential electrodes (as opposed to modiolar oriented electrodes) is preferred.[50] McElveen et al[51] suggest using a precurved electrode to avoid insertion of the electrode into the IAC. Papsin[31] pushes a straight electrode gently against the promontory before inserting it into the cochlea to give a slight curve within the distal 3 to 5 electrodes. The curvature helps steer the electrode away from accidental insertion into the IAC. Alternatively, Coelho et al[50] use intraoperative fluoroscopic guidance to insert the electrode along the lateral wall, preventing kinking and bending, so that IAC placement is avoided. Others have described a double posterior labyrinthotomy or even a triple labyrinthotomy technique with custom electrodes and, in the latter technique, a third labyrinthotomy through which an endoscope could be used to position the electrode in close apposition to the neuroepithelium under direct visualization.[55,56] When implanting children with IP-I, the cochlea is empty and cystic and thus a circumferentially stimulating electrode is preferable.[38] Implanting children with IP-II is similar to normal cases employing a modiolar-hugging electrode.[38] In children with HC, there is danger of inserting the electrode array into the IAC due to the small space of the cochlea which prevents curling of the electrode array.[53] A shortened electrode array has the least likelihood of extending into the IAC and thus is a viable alternative employed by some. Full insertion is often possible in patients with cochleovestibular anomalies; however, caution should be observed as overly forceful attempts of electrode insertion can result in violation of a modiolar deficiency. In general, full insertion is more likely in patients with isolated EVA or IP-II and less possible in patients with CC, HC, or IP-I.

Recently, Chadha et al discussed their experience with bilateral cochlear implantation in children with cochleovestibular anomalies.[57] They report that all 10 children were detecting speech and most were developing good speech perception scores on closed-set and/or open-set tests. For bilateral simultaneous implantations, the second side was only pursued in the absence of an uncontrolled CSF/perilymph leak or concern about the facial nerve function after the first-side procedure. They also performed vestibular testing in between sequential implantation for some children. They found that none had any persistent imbalance after the second implant, although three patients had mild imbalance that resolved by 2 weeks postoperatively.

OUTCOMES IN CHILDREN WITH COCHLEOVESTIBULAR ANOMALIES

Several studies have shown that the audiologic benefits gained from cochlear implantation are similar between patients with cochleovestibular anomalies and normal cochleae.[31,33,52,53] These reports also highlight that open-set speech perception is possible in patients with cochleovestibular anomalies. Children with cochleovestibular anomalies may reach the same eventual audiologic outcomes with cochlear implants as children implanted with radiographically normal anatomy, but this may occur over a longer period of time.[58] This similar audiologic outcome between normal and anomalous anatomic patients may be a factor of electrical stimulation. Although the normal hearing patient has about 33,000 spiral ganglion cells and patients with Mondini dysplasia have been shown to have 7,600 to 16,000 ganglion cells, as few as 3,200 ganglion cells have been reported to be present in a cochlear implant user with average or above-average outcomes.[59,60] Patients with cochleovestibular anomalies may thus have enough spiral ganglion cells available for electrical stimulation. Regardless of the number of spiral ganglion cells, as the electrical stimulation provided by multichannel cochlear implants is relatively crude (compared to neural stimulation in a normal cochlea), it seems possible that the quality of the information presented to the auditory cortex by this simple system may be similar whether it is transmitted via a relatively intact spiral ganglion and afferent nerve population or by a depleted one.

Children with IP-II or isolated EVA tend to perform well on speech perception testing.[47,61] Children with CC and HC have been described as harder to program, which may be due to a poor or fluctuating contact between the electrode and the neuroepithelium in the walls of the cystic cavity. In general, patients with CC or HC tend to do poorer than other cochleovestibular anomalies.[31,47]

Children with narrow IAC deserve a special mention as they have been reported to perform at a significantly lower level as compared to patients with normal or other cochleovestibular anomalies.[31] Others have reported that children with narrow IAC have similar open-set sentence recognition as children with other cochleovestibular anomalies, but just with slower attainment.[45] MRI imaging and sometimes promontory stimulation testing may be necessary to confirm the presence of a cochlear nerve capable of transmitting an electrical stimulation. Further experience with this patient population will help elucidate outcomes.

REFERENCES

1. Bhatia K, Gibbin KP, Nikolopoulos TP, O'Donoghue GM. Surgical complications and their management in a series of 300 consecutive pediatric cochlear implantations. *Otol Neurotol.* 2004;25:730–739.

2. Cote M, Ferron P, Bergeron F, Bussieres R. Cochlear reimplantation: causes of failure, outcomes, and audiologic performance. *Laryngoscope.* 2007;117:1225–1235.

3. Cullen RD, Fayad JN, Luxford WM, Buchman CA. Revision cochlear implant surgery in children. *Otol Neurotol.* 2008;29: 214–220.

4. Hopfenspirger MT, Levine SC, Rimell FL. Infectious complications in pediatric cochlear implants. *Laryngoscope.* 2007; 117:1825–1829.

5. Davis BM, Labadie RF, McMenomey SO, Haynes DS. Cochlear implant fixation using polypropylene mesh and titanium screws. *Laryngoscope.* 2004;114:2116–2118.

6. Alexander NS, Caron E, Woolley AL. Fixation methods in pediatric cochlear implants: retrospective review of an evolution of 3 techniques. *Otolaryngol Head Neck Surg.* 2011;144:427–430.

7. Dodson KM, Maiberger PG, Sismanis A. Intracranial complications of cochlear implantation. *Otol Neurotol.* 2007;28:459–462.

8. Adunka OF, Buchman CA. Cochlear implant fixation in children using periosteal sutures. *Otol Neurotol.* 2007;28:768–770.

9. Balkany TJ, Whitley M, Shapira, et al. The temporalis pocket technique for cochlear implantation: an anatomic and clinical study. *Otol Neurotol.* 2009;30:903–907.

10. Davids T, Ramsden JD, Gordon KA, James AL, Papsin BC. Soft tissue complications after small incision pediatric cochlear implantation. *Laryngoscope.* 2009;119:980–983.

11. O'Donoghue GM, Nikolopoulos TP. Minimal access surgery for pediatric cochlear implantation. *Otol Neurotol.* 2002;23: 891–894.

12. James AL, Papsin BC. Device fixation and small incision access for pediatric cochlear implants. *Int J Pediatr Otorhinolaryngol.* 2004;68:1017–1022.

13. Campisi P, James A, Hayward L, Blaser S, Papsin B. Cochlear implant positioning in children: a survey of patient satisfaction.

Int J Pediatr Otorhinolaryngol. 2004;68: 1289–1293.

14. Kronenberg J, Migirov L, Dagan T. Suprameatal approach: new surgical approach for cochlear implantation. *J Laryngol Otol.* 2001;115:283–285.

15. Migirov L, Carmel E, Kronenberg J. Cochlear implantation in infants: special surgical and medical aspects. *Laryngoscope.* 2008; 118:2024–2027.

16. Postelmans JT, Grolman W, Tange RA, Stokroos RJ. Comparison of two approaches to the surgical management of cochlear implantation. *Laryngoscope.* 2009;119: 1571–1578.

17. Postelmans JT, Tange RA, Stokroos RJ, Grolman W. The suprameatal approach: a safe alternative surgical technique for cochlear implantation. *Otol Neurotol.* 2010; 31:196–203.

18. Johr M, Ho A, Wagner CS, Linder T. Ear surgery in infants under one year of age: its risks and implications for cochlear implant surgery. *Otol Neurotol.* 2008;29:310–313.

19. Colletti L. Long-term follow-up of infants (4–11 months) fitted with cochlear implants. *Acta Otolaryngol.* 2009;129:361–366.

20. James AL, Papsin BC. Cochlear implant surgery at 12 months of age or younger. *Laryngoscope.* 2004;114:2191–2195.

21. Roland JT, Jr., Cosetti M, Wang KH, Immerman S, Waltzman SB. Cochlear implantation in the very young child: long-term safety and efficacy. *Laryngoscope.* 2009; 119:2205–2210.

22. Colletti V, Carner M, Miorelli V, Guida M, Colletti L, Fiorino FG. Cochlear implantation at under 12 months: report on 10 patients. *Laryngoscope.* 2005;115:445–449.

23. Brown RF, Hullar TE, Cadieux JH, Chole RA. Residual hearing preservation after pediatric cochlear implantation. *Otol Neurotol.* 2010;31:1221–1226.

24. Friedland DR, Runge-Samuelson C. Soft cochlear implantation: rationale for the surgical approach. *Trends Amplif.* 2009;13:124–138.

25. Skarzynski H, Lorens A, Piotrowska A, Anderson I. Partial deafness cochlear implantation in children. *Int J Pediatr Otorhinolaryngol.* 2007;71:1407–1413.

26. Gantz BJ, Dunn CC, Walker EA, et al. Bilateral cochlear implants in infants: a new approach—Nucleus Hybrid S12 project. *Otol Neurotol.* 2010;31:1300–1309.

27. Ramsden JD, Papsin BC, Leung R, James A, Gordon KA. Bilateral simultaneous cochlear implantation in children: our first 50 cases. *Laryngoscope.* 2009;119:2444–2448.

28. Basura GJ, Eapen R, Buchman CA. Bilateral cochlear implantation: current concepts, indications, and results. *Laryngoscope.* 2009;119:2395–2401.

29. Gordon KA, Valero J, Papsin BC. Auditory brainstem activity in children with 9–30 months of bilateral cochlear implant use. *Hear Res.* 2007;233:97–107.

30. Jackler RK, Luxford WM, House WF. Congenital malformations of the inner ear: a classification based on embryogenesis. *Laryngoscope.* 1987;97:2–14.

31. Papsin BC. Cochlear implantation in children with anomalous cochleovestibular anatomy. *Laryngoscope.* 2005;115:1–26.

32. McClay JE, Tandy R, Grundfast K, et al. Major and minor temporal bone abnormalities in children with and without congenital sensorineural hearing loss. *Arch Otolaryngol Head Neck Surg.* 2002;128:664–671.

33. Luntz M, Balkany T, Hodges AV, Telischi FF. Cochlear implants in children with congenital inner ear malformations. *Arch Otolaryngol Head Neck Surg.* 1997;123:974–977.

34. Mangabeira-Albernaz PL. The Mondini dysplasia—from early diagnosis to cochlear implant. *Acta Otolaryngol.* 1983; 95:627–631.

35. Parry DA, Booth T, Roland PS. Advantages of magnetic resonance imaging over computed tomography in preoperative evaluation of pediatric cochlear implant candidates. *Otol Neurotol.* 2005;26:976–982.

36. Phelps PD. The basal turn of the cochlea. *Br J Radiol.* 1992;65:370–374.

37. Zheng Y, Schachern PA, Cureoglu S, Mutlu C, Dijalilian H, Paparella MM. The shortened cochlea: its classification and histo-

pathologic features. *Int J Pediatr Otorhinolaryngol.* 2002;63:29–39.

38. Sennaroglu L, Saatci I. A new classification for cochleovestibular malformations. *Laryngoscope.* 2002;112:2230–2241.

39. Incesulu A, Vural M, Erkam U, Kocaturk S. Cochlear implantation in children with inner ear malformations: report of two cases. *Int J Pediatr Otorhinolaryngol.* 2002;65:171–179.

40. Lee KH, Lee J, Isaacson B, Kutz JW, Roland PS. Cochlear implantation in children with enlarged vestibular aqueduct. *Laryngoscope.* 2010;120:1675–1681.

41. Lemmerling MM, Mancuso AA, Antonelli PJ, Kubilis PS. Normal modiolus: CT appearance in patients with a large vestibular aqueduct. *Radiology.* 1997;204:213–219.

42. Graham JM, Phelps PD, Michaels L. Congenital malformations of the ear and cochlear implantation in children: review and temporal bone report of common cavity. *J Laryngol Otol* (suppl). 2000;25:1–14.

43. Bamiou DE, Worth S, Phelps P, Sirimanna T, Rajput K. Eighth nerve aplasia and hypoplasia in cochlear implant candidates: the clinical perspective. *Otol Neurotol.* 2001; 22:492–496.

44. Casselman JW, Offeciers FE, Govaerts PJ, et al. Aplasia and hypoplasia of the vestibulocochlear nerve: diagnosis with MR imaging. *Radiology.* 1997;202:773–781.

45. Kim AH, Kileny PR, Arts HA, El-Kashlan HK, Telian SA, Zwolan TA. Role of electrically evoked auditory brainstem response in cochlear implantation of children with inner ear malformations. *Otol Neurotol.* 2008;29:626–634.

46. Zheng Y, Schachern PA, Djalilian HR, Paparella MM. Temporal bone histopathology related to cochlear implantation in congenital malformation of the bony cochlea. *Otol Neurotol.* 2002;23:181–186.

47. Buchman CA, Copeland BJ, Yu KK, Brown CJ, Carrasco VN, Pillsbury HC 3rd. Cochlear implantation in children with congenital inner ear malformations. *Laryngoscope.* 2004;114:309–316.

48. Loundon N, Rouillon I, Munier N, Marlin S, Roger G, Garabedian EN. Cochlear implantation in children with internal ear malformations. *Otol Neurotol.* 2005;26: 668–673.

49. Weber BP, Dillo W, Dietrich B, Maneke I, Bertram B, Lenarz T. Pediatric cochlear implantation in cochlear malformations. *Am J Otol.* 1998;19:747–753.

50. Coelho DH, Waltzman SB, Roland JT Jr. Implanting common cavity malformations using intraoperative fluoroscopy. *Otol Neurotol.* 2008;29:914–919.

51. McElveen JT Jr., Carrasco VN, Miyamoto RT, Linthicum FH Jr. Cochlear implantation in common cavity malformations using a transmastoid labyrinthotomy approach. *Laryngoscope.* 1997;107:1032–1036.

52. Arnoldner C, Baumgartner WD, Gstoettner W, et al. Audiological performance after cochlear implantation in children with inner ear malformations. *Int J Pediatr Otorhinolaryngol.* 2004;68:457–467.

53. Tucci DL, Telian SA, Zimmerman-Phillips S, Zwolan TA, Kileny PR. Cochlear implantation in patients with cochlear malformations. *Arch Otolaryngol Head Neck Surg.* 1995;121:833–838.

54. Bloom JD, Rizzi MD, Germiller JA. Real-time intraoperative computed tomography to assist cochlear implant placement in the malformed inner ear. *Otol Neurotol.* 2009;30:23–26.

55. Beltrame MA, Bonfioli F, Frau GN. Cochlear implant in inner ear malformation: double posterior labyrinthotomy approach to common cavity. *Adv Otorhinolaryngol.* 2000; 57:113–119.

56. Manolidis S, Tonini R, Spitzer J. Endoscopically guided placement of prefabricated cochlear implant electrodes in a common cavity malformation. *Int J Pediatr Otorhinolaryngol.* 2006;70:591–596.

57. Chadha NK, James AL, Gordon KA, Blaser S, Papsin BC. Bilateral cochlear implantation in children with anomalous cochleovestibular anatomy. *Arch Otolaryngol Head Neck Surg.* 2009;135:903–909.

58. Eisenman DJ, Ashbaugh C, Zwolan TA, Arts HA, Telian SA. Implantation of the malformed cochlea. *Otol Neurotol.* 2001; 22:834–841.

59. Linthicum FH Jr., Fayad J, Otto S, Galey FR, House WF. Inner ear morphologic changes resulting from cochlear implantation. *Am J Otol.* 1991;12 (suppl):8–10; discussion 18–21.

60. Schmidt JM. Cochlear neuronal populations in developmental defects of the inner ear. Implications for cochlear implantation. *Acta Otolaryngol.* 1985;99:14–20.

61. Bent JP 3rd, Chute P, Parisier SC. Cochlear implantation in children with enlarged vestibular aqueducts. *Laryngoscope.* 1999; 109:1019–1022.

Chapter 9

The Suprameatal Approach: An Alternative Surgical Technique for Cochlear Implantation

LELA MIGIROV AND JONA KRONENBERG

INTRODUCTION

The mastoidectomy with posterior tympanotomy approach (MPTA) was proposed initially for cholesteatoma surgery and was adopted for cochlear implantation (CI) thereafter.[1] The early attempts to introduce the electrode into the cochlea transmeatally resulted in infection and electrode extrusion due to the placement of the electroe directly underneath the skin of the external auditory canal.[2-4] During the last decade the MPTA was less utilized for cholesteatoma surgery due to the use of endoscopes and mastoid obliteration techniques as well as for CI due to the development of various alternative approaches.[5-15] CI is a safe surgical procedure that, however, bears the risks of complications associated with performing of posterior tympanotomy approach. The MPTA provides access to the middle ear through the facial recess that matures fully to a mean width of 4.11 mm at the age of 2 years.[16] It may occasionally be a narrow "keyhole," especially when the facial nerve is anteriorly located or when the recess is not yet developed, as in young children under two years of age. Working through a narrow "keyhole" may lead to difficulties in identifying the landmarks used for cochleostomy drilling. Thus, the facial recess approach can result in such surgical complications as damage to the facial nerve and chorda tympani, and electrode misplacement.[17-32] Anteriorly based sigmoid sinus can limit an adequate surgical access.[35-37] Mastoidectomy changes the mastoid physiology and can lead to mastoiditis and subperiosteal abscess in the implanted children.[21-22,33,34]

The suprameatal approach (SMA) was developed as an alternative to the traditional MPTA with the intent to simplify the surgical procedure and to avoid damage to the facial nerve and chorda tympani.[7,8]

SURGICAL TECHNIQUE

The patient is placed in a supine position as for mastoid surgery. Any skin incision used for cochlear implantation can be used for this approach. The skin incision is performed in the hair line between the area over the temporal line and the area over the mastoid tip. The anterior skin cut should be high enough and anterior over the root of the zigoma alowing exposition of the suprameatal area and preventing bulky flaps.

A skin flap and a large periosteal flap are elevated (Fig 9–1). A bony well is drilled in the parietal bone for implant fixation. A superior and posterior subperiosteal pouch are prepared to accommodate the body of the implant and the ground electrode (when relevant). Fixation of the implant is important to prevent migration and two tie-down holes should be drilled for implant fixation. The posterior pouch should be deep enough to accommodate the implant body (see Fig 9–1). The skin of the posterior wall of the

external auditory canal is incised horizontally, 4 to 5 mm lateral to the annulus and is retracted anteriorly with a one-quarter inch Penrose drain. A 6 o'clock vertical incision is made in the meatal skin and a tympanomeatal flap is elevated to expose the middle ear cavity. The 6 o'clock vertical incision should be done close to the anulus and start at about 5 o'clock in order to prevent tension on the tympanic membrane during elevation (Fig 9–2).

A wide exposure of the middle ear is achieved. The chorda tympani is exposed and a 1-mm long groove is drilled in the wall of the middle ear cavity posterosuperior to the chorda tympani, lateral to the body of the incus untill the long process of the incus is well seen. The visualization of the incus serves as a target for drilling and prevents injury to the facial nerve located medially to the incus. In certain cases there is no need in groove drilling since it is already exist (Fig 9–3). The suprameatal tunnel is drilled posterosuperiorly to the external auditory meatus at 1 o'clock position in relation to the external auditory canal. This closed tunnel

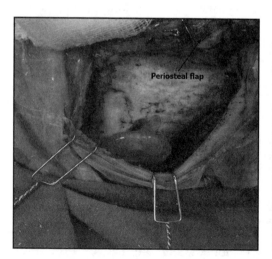

Figure 9–1. *Elevated periosteal flap and a demo placed in the posterior pouch.*

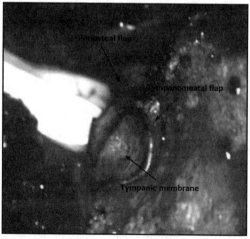

Figure 9–2. *Anterior displacement of the tympanomeatal flap.*

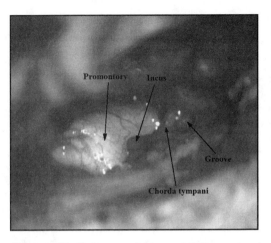

Figure 9–3. *View of the middle ear and promontory.*

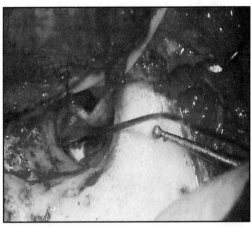

Figure 9–4. *Location of tunnel opening in the suprameatal area and direction of the drilling.*

supposed to prevent contact of the electrode with the skin of the external auditory canal or with the tympanic membrane. Suction tip can be used for localization of the tunnel opening. An immaginary line should connect the cochleostomy site, groove, and the suprameatal area (Fig 9–4). The end of the tunnel and entrance to the middle ear should be medial to the chorda tympani and lateral to the incus body. Preoperative coronal CT scan of the temporal bones can predict the position of the middle fossa dura. Very low-set dura is a contraindication for this approach. Once the dura has been visualized, a 1.5-mm cutting bur followed by a 2-mm diamond bur are used to create the tunnel. The tunnel is drilled inferior to the dura, with a mean length of 13 mm in adults and 7 mm in children. Care should be taken to maintain a safe distance between the tunnel and the bony external auditory canal wall which may vary between 3 and 7 mm. Drilling is performed in an oblique line from posterosuperior to anteroinferior ending in the groove, lateral to the incus. The direction of drilling is adjusted by aiming to the groove, untill bone dust is appearing

(see Fig 9–4). The bone dust should be washed out the tunnel by water irrigation. The width of the tunnel is a matter of personal preferance, some surgeon like it wide and some narrow. In a wide tunnel the incus and chorda tympani may be seen.

The cochleostomy is drilled in the promontory using a 0.8-mm diamond bur, close to the round window niche, and in case of nicely seen round window membrane a small incision of the membrane can be sufficient for the electrode insertion into the scala tympani. The implant is placed into the posterior pouch, the ball electrode (when relevant) is positioned underneath the temporalis muscle and the electrodes are passed through the suprameatal tunnel and groove into the cochleostomy (Fig 9–5). Small pieces of temporalis fascia are used for meticulous sealing of the cochleostomy. The tympanomeatal flap is placed back and fixed by small pieces of Gelfoam. The subperiosteal flap is used to cover the electrode.

In the SMA technique, cochleostomy and electrode insertion are performed through the external auditory canal following elevation of a tympanomeatal flap,

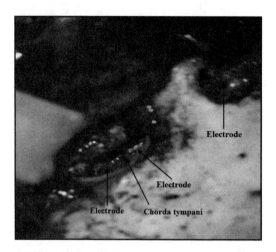

Figure 9–5. *The electrodes are inserted into the lateral opening of the suprameatal tunnel and through the groove medial to the chorda tympani into the cochleostomy.*

which provides a wide exposure of the middle ear and promontory. In the SMA, the facial nerve is not in the path of drilling and the tunnel which is created for electrode insertion is in a safe distance from the course of the facial nerve both in its tympanic and mastoidal segments. In addition, the facial nerve is protected by the body of the incus. The chorda tympani nerve is exposed and preserved, and there is no need in sacrificing the nerve in order to obtain adequate access to the middle ear and cochlea.[25] Damage to chorda timpani had become very important issue since the number of bilaterally implanted patients increased. The benefits of avoiding the risk of damage to the facial nerve and chorda tympani as well as minimizing the risk of electrode misplacement have made the non-mastoidectomy techniques routine approaches for cochlear implantation in more than 20 centers worldwide.

The exclusion of mastoidectomy in the SMA implies less drill work. Therefore, the duration of surgery is shortened

and, thus, the SMA is a preferable technique for bilateral simultaneous CI.[38] The added benefit of decreased bony drilling may be the future application of this surgical technique in local anesthesia and the immediate intraoperative hearing testing.

The SMA is a safe technique for cochlear implantations, especially bilateral simultaneous procedures in young children with undeveloped mastoid and narrow facial recess, in patients with malformed inner ears or ossified cochlea, and in CI candidates with food, smell or taste-related occupations or in people for whom the taste of food contributes appreciably to their quality of life. In addition the SMA can be recommended in cases of protruding sigmoid sinus and narrow antrum. The suprameatal approach is a very precise technique for carrying out a safe cochleostomy and gentle electrode insertion into the scala tympani.

REFERENCES

1. House WF. Cochlear implant. *Ann Otol Rhinol Laryngol.* 1976;85(suppl) 27:2–6.
2. Banfai P, Kubik G, Hortmann G. Our extra-scala operating method of cochlear implantation. Experience with 46 cases. *Acta Otolaryngol.* (suppl) 1983;411:9–12.
3. Schindler RA. Surgical consideration for multichannel cochlear implants. In: Schindler RA, Merzinich MM, eds. *Cochlear Implants.* New York, NY: Raven Press; 1985: 417–420.
4. Chouard CH, MacLeod P. Implantation of multiple intracochlear electrodes for rehabilitation of total deafness: preliminary report. *Laryngoscope.* 1976;86:1743–1751.
5. Gantz BJ, Wilkinson EP, Hansen MR. Canal wall reconstruction tympanomastoidectomy with mastoid obliteration. *Laryngoscope.* 2005;115:1734–1740.

6. Tarabichi M. Endoscopic management of cholesteatoma: long-term results. *Otolaryngol Head Neck Surg*. 2000;122:874–881.

7. Kronenberg J, Migirov L. How we do it? The suprameatal approach—an alternative surgical technique for cochlear implantation. *Cochlear Implants Int*. 2006; 7:142–147.

8. Kronenberg J, Migirov L, Dagan T. Suprameatal approach: new surgical approach for cochlear implantation. *J Laryngol Otol*. 2001;115:283–285.

9. Kiratzidis T, Iliades T, Arnold W. Veria operation. II. Surgical results from 101 cases. *ORL J Otorhinolaryngol Relat Spec*. 2002;64:413–416.

10. Häusler R. Cochlear implantation without mastoidectomy: the pericanal electrode insertion technique. *Acta Otolaryngol*. 2002;122:715–719.

11. Arnoldner C, Baumgartner WD, Gctoettner W, Hamzavi J. Surgical considerations in cochlear implantation in children and adults: a review of 342 cases in Vienna. *Acta Otolaryngol*. 2005;125:228–234.

12. Yin S, Chen Z, Wu Y, et al. Suprameatal approach for cochlear implantation in 45 Chinese children. *Int J Pediatr Otorhinolaryngol*. 2008;72:397–403.

13. Taibah K. The transmeatal approach: a new technique in cochlear and middle ear implants. *Cochlear Implants Int*. 2009;10: 218–228.

14. Postelmans JT, Grolman W, Tange RA, Stokroos RJ. Comparison of two approaches to the surgical management of cochlear implantation. *Laryngoscope*. 2009; 119:1571–1578.

15. Guevara N, Bailleux S, Santini J, Castillo L, Gahide I. Cochlear implantation surgery without posterior tympanotomy: can we still improve it? *Acta Otolaryngol*. 2010; 130:37–41.

16. Su WY, Marion MS, Hinolosa P, Matz GJ. Anatomical measurements of the cochlear aqueduct, round window membrane, round window niche, and facial recess. *Laryngoscope*. 1982;92:483–486.

17. Hou JH, Zhao SP, Ning F, Rao SQ, Han DY. Postoperative complications in patients with cochlear implants and impacts of nursing intervention. *Acta Otolaryngol*. 2010;130:687–695.

18. Joseph ST, Vishwakarma R, Ramani MK, Aurora R. Cochlear implant and delayed facial palsy. *Cochlear Implants Int*. 2009; 10:229–236.

19. Kandogan T, Levent O, Gurol G. Complications of paediatric cochlear implantation: experience in Izmir. *J Laryngol Otol*. 2005;119:606–610.

20. Li Y, Zhang D. Perioperative complications of 1396 patients with cochlear implantation [in Chinese]. *Lin Chung Er Bi Yan Hou Tou Jing Wai Ke Za Zhi*. 2010;24:433–435.

21. Ramos A, Charlone R, de Miguel I, Valdivielso A, Cuyas JM, Pérez D, Vasallo JR. Complications in cochlear implantation [in Spanish]. *Acta Otorrinolaringol Esp*. 2006;57:122–125.

22. Stratigoueleas ED, Perry BP, King SM, Syms CA III. Complication rate of minimally invasive cochlear implantation. *Otolaryngol Head Neck Surg*. 2006;135:383–386.

23. Lin YS, Lee FP, Peng SC. Complications in children with long-term cochlear implants. *ORL J Otorhinolaryngol Relat Spec*. 2006;68:237–242.

24. Hansen S, Anthonsen K, Stangerup SE, Jensen JH, Thomsen J, Cayé-Thomasen P. Unexpected findings and surgical complications in 505 consecutive cochlear implantations: a proposal for reporting consensus. *Acta Otolaryngol*. 2010;130: 540–549.

25. Migirov L, Drendel M, Kronenberg J. Taste changes in patients who underwent cochlear implantation by the nonmastoidectomy approach. *ORL J Otorhinolaryngol Relat Spec*. 2009;71:66–69.

26. Orús Dotú C, Venegas Pizarro Mdel P, De Juan Beltrán J, De Juan Delago M. Cochlear reimplantation in the same ear: Findings, peculiarities of the surgical technique and complications [in Spanish]. *Acta Otorrinolaringol Esp*. 2010;61:106–117.

27. Kim CS, Oh SH, Chang SO, Kim HM, Hur DG. Management of complications in cochlear implantation. *Acta Otolaryngol.* 2008;128:408–414.

28. Loundon N, Blanchard M, Roger G, Denoyelle F, Garabedian EN. Medical and surgical complications in pediatric cochlear implantation. *Arch Otolaryngol Head Neck Surg.* 2010;136:12–15.

29. Sorrentino T, Coté M, Eter E, et al. Cochlear reimplantations: technical and surgical failures. *Acta Otolaryngol.* 2009;129:380–384.

30. Migirov L, Yakirevitch A, Kronenberg J. Surgical and medical complications following cochlear implantation: comparison of two surgical approaches. *ORL J Otorhinolaryngol Relat Spec.* 2006;68:213–219.

31. Mueller CA, Khatib S, Temmel AFP, Baumgartner WD, Hummel T. Effects of cochlear implantation on gustatory function. *Ann Otol Rhinol Laryngol.* 2007;116:498–501.

32. Lloyd S, Meerton L, Di Cuffa R, Lavy J, Graham J. Taste change following cochlear implantation. *Cochlear Implants Int.* 2007; 8:203–210.

33. Rodríguez V, Cavallé L, De Paula C, Morera C. Treatment of acute mastoiditis in children with cochlear implants [in Spanish]. *Acta Otorrinolaringol Esp.* 2010;61:180–183.

34. Migirov L, Yakirevitch A, Henkin Y, Kaplan-Neeman R, Kronenberg J. Acute otitis media and mastoiditis following cochlear implantation. *Int J Pediatr Otorhinolaryngol.* 2006;70:899–903.

35. Leung R, Briggs RJ. Indications for and outcomes of mastoid obliteration in cochlear implantation. *Otol Neurotol.* 2007; 28:330–334.

36. Ma X, Zhang D, Zhang Y. Cochlear implant approach in children patients with sigmoid sinus antedisplacement [in Chinese]. *Lin Chung Er Bi Yan Hou Tou Jing Wai Ke Za Zhi.* 2008;22:885–887.

37. Carfrae MJ, Foyt D. Intact meatal skin, canal wall down approach for difficult cochlear implantation. *J Laryngol Otol.* 2009;123:903–906.

38. Migirov L, Kronenberg J. Bilateral, simultaneous cochlear implantation in children: surgical considerations. *J Laryngol Otol.* 2009;123:837–839.

Chapter 10

Hearing Preservation: Cochlear Implantation and Electroacoustic Stimulation

SANDRA PRENTISS AND HINRICH STAECKER

INTRODUCTION

It is estimated that more than 31 million Americans are hearing impaired, most of whom do not have profound sensorineural hearing loss (SNHL) (MarkeTrak Survey, 2004). The most common form of hearing loss in adults is high frequency SNHL, which makes it difficult to distinguish speech sounds, particularly consonants in background noise. These patients are often frustrated with hearing aids or do not benefit from them due to poor word understanding abilities. Cochlear implants are a useful tool for the treatment and rehabilitation of severe to profound hearing losses. Those with good low-frequency hearing and poor high-frequency hearing and marginal discrimination were initially not considered cochlear implant candidates. This was due to the idea that preservation of residual hearing was not thought to be possible as well the possibility that the brain could not reconcile acoustic and electric input.

Improvements in electrode design and adjustment of surgical technique have now made preservation of residual hearing possible. This allows the expansion of cochlear implantation to those who have essentially good, or aid-able, low-frequency hearing and severe high-frequency loss above 1000 Hz with poor speech discrimination (Fig 10–1). With a less traumatic surgical approach, low frequency hearing can be preserved resulting in combined low frequency auditory perception and mid- to high-frequency electric perception (Fig 10–2).[1–10]

In this patient group, it has been observed that patients who hear via a combination of low frequency acoustic hearing and mid to high frequency stimulation with a cochlear implant perform better in background noise than patients using a hearing aid alone or a cochlear implant alone. This effect can be achieved both with ipsilateral acoustic and electric stimulation (EAS) or electrical stimulation with contralateral acoustic stimulation (bimodal).[11–15] This represents a

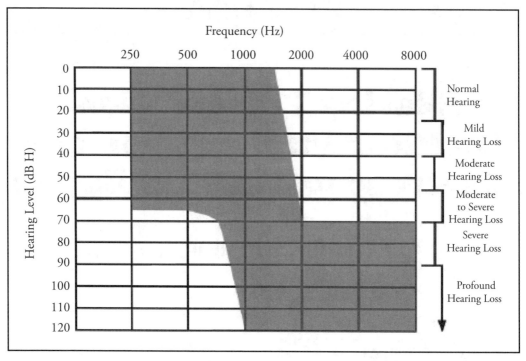

Figure 10–1. *The shaded region of this audiogram represents the thresholds of the ideal candidate for hearing preservation cochlear implantation. If thresholds in the low frequencies are decreased, amplification is provided in this frequency region. Some patients will present with normal hearing at 250 to1000 Hz and these patients can be treated with electrical stimulation of the basal half of the cochlea. Current studies are evaluating patients with SD scores as high as 70% in the nonimplanted ear. (Image courtesy of MED-EL, Gmbh. Innsbruck, Austria. FlexEAS implant and DUET sound processor are investigational and limited by US law to investigational use.)*

significant change in our understanding of cochlear implantation. We now know that it is possible to reliably access the inner ear and preserve residual hearing and have come to appreciate the ability of the brain to integrate acoustic and electrical percepts. This combination of acoustic hearing allows patients to function better in background noise and potentially also aids with sound localization and music understanding. Additional theoretical benefits include preservation of spiral ganglion cells and prevention of vestibular damage.

RATIONALE OF HEARING PRESERVATION SURGERY

Histopathologic evaluations of temporal bones from implant patients have shown damage to cochlear structures following insertion of an electrode.[16,17] Structures affected have included the basilar membrane, osseous spiral lamina, spiral ligament, Reissner's membrane, and loss of spiral ganglion cells.[18–21] Hearing preservation cochlear implantation originated from a desire to avoid these side effects of

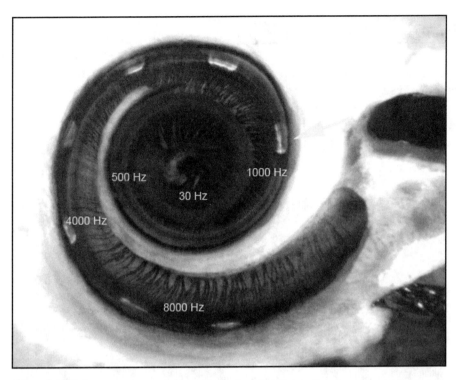

Figure 10–2. *Electroacoustic stimulation (EAS) implies insertion of an electrode into the basal, damaged portion of the cochlea, with electrical stimulation of the mid- to high-frequency spiral ganglion cells. Surviving hair cells in the apical region of the cochlea the patient with acoustic hearing in the low frequency domain. As seen in this temporal bone specimen, an implant electrode has been inserted approximately 20 mm to the 1000-Hz region. Hearing is intact apically from this point.*

implantation. The idea of a less traumatic "soft" surgical approach originated with Lehnhardt who modified the standard cochleostomy by placing it anteriorly to the round window region thereby, reducing trauma to the cochlea and surrounding structures.[22] The ability to manipulate and instrument the inner ear was then confirmed in animal models. Additional theoretical benefits of soft surgical approaches are the potential for preservation of structures apical to the implant. Temporal bone histopathology studies have demonstrated degeneration of both supporting cells and spiral ganglion neu-

rons apical to the tip of an implant when compared to the contralateral unimplanted side.[23] If an implant electrode migrates through the scala media to the scala vestibule as suggested by Finley et al,[24] the resulting damage may result in degeneration of residual functioning portions of the cochlea and poorer outcomes. Some animal studies also suggested that traumatic insertions affected spiral ganglion survival.[25] Atraumatic insertion of the implant should therefore lead to long term better outcomes and the ability to replace the implant several times during the life span of the patient.

SURGICAL TECHNIQUE

Hearing preservation implantation can be carried out via several approaches. When looking at the human temporal bones, the round window membrane is much easier to view when the overhang of the round window niche is drilled away, allowing for easier insertion of the implant into the scala tympani.[26] This approach allows for certain access to the scala tympani without violating the basilar membrane, which is a key feature of consistently preserving hearing. As can be seen in Figure 10–3, a standard cochleostomy has

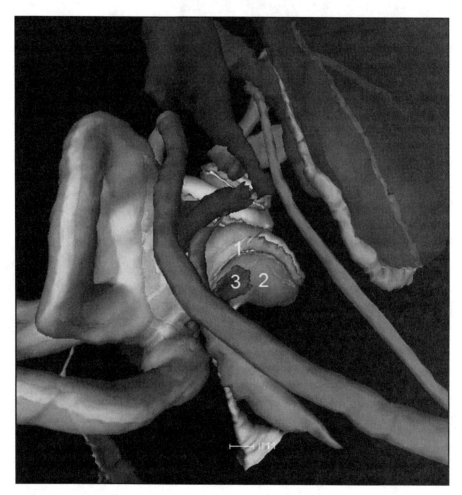

Figure 10–3. *Reconstruction of a human temporal bone demonstrates differences in cochleostomy design. Traditional cochleostomies anterior to the round window (1) have the potential of violating the scala media resulting in hearing loss. Alternative approaches include placing the cochleostomy inferior to the round window (2) or using a direct round window insertion (3). Adapted from https://research.meei.harvard.edu/otopathology/3dmodels.*

the potential of violating the scala media, resulting in loss of residual hearing. This has led many surgeons to adopt a cochleostomy that is located anterior inferior to the round window. This requires careful drilling and exposure of the scala tympani endosteum. The endosteum is then punctured and the electrode carefully inserted. A potential alternative approach is to insert the electrode through the round window. Round window insertions were used early in the history of cochlear implantation but then abandoned due to the difficulty of passing the older large electrodes through the hook region. The extended round window approach overcomes many of these problems. After performance of a mastoidectomy and facial recess (posterior tympanotomy) approach to the middle ear, all bone dust is irrigated out of the wound. Hemostasis is obtained and all excess blood is removed from the area.

Animal studies have demonstrated that intrascalar blood results in sensorineural hearing loss.[27,28] Many studies advocate application of steroids to the round window prior to implantation based on animal studies that demonstrate protection of hearing in a variety of implant models.[28–31] Human study have demonstrated improvement of impedances with preimplant treatment with steroids.[32–35] We currently apply 0.5 cc of decadron 10 mg/mL to the round window niche as soon as the facial recess is opened. The implant bed is then drilled to give the steroids some time to diffuse through the round window. To expose the round window the bony overhang of the round window niche is removed with a 1-mm diamond bur and the round window clearly visualized by testing the round window reflex. If a round window reflex cannot be estab-

lished it is due to the presence of a pseudomembrane which needs to be removed with a fine pick. For the extended round window approach the bone anterior inferior to the round window is removed, keeping the scala tympani endosteum intact. The wound is once again irrigated and Healon™ is used to cover the round window and endosteum. The endosteum is then opened with a small pick and the implant electrode is carefully inserted. With the newer more flexible electrodes, atraumatically advancing the electrode via this approach is easy. Some surgeons additionally advocate coating the electrode in healon or steroids although there is no current evidence to support either method. This approach has the advantage of clearly defining the scala tympani and removing the crista fenestra, a small ridge of bone at the anterior end of the round window, that can interfere with implant insertion. In some cases the position of the round window is favorable allowing direct insertion of the implant through an incision in the anterior mid portion of the round window (Fig 10–4). In some cases the positioning of the round window is unfavorable and exposure via a facial recess cannot be obtained.[36] Some studies have attempted direct comparisons of different surgical approaches.

Berrettini et al (2008)[19] conducted a retrospective study on implant recipients undergoing different surgical techniques. Thirty recipients, all of whom had residual hearing prior to surgery, were selected and divided into three groups. The first group was implanted via standard cochleostomy. Group two underwent surgery with the soft-surgical approach with a standard cochleostomy, and the third group's technique involved a cochleostomy drilled anteroinferior to the round

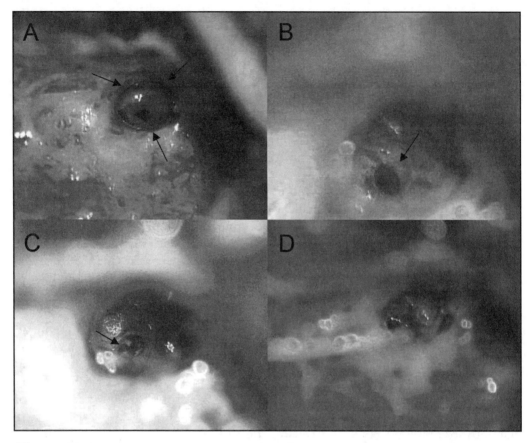

Figure 10–4. *Insertion through the round window. Effective round window insertion requires a wide facial recess (**A**). The bone of the round window niche is then carefully removed with a small diamond burr (**B**). After identifying the round window through confirmation of the round window reflex, the round window is covered in Healon ® and carefully incised (**C**). The electrode is then carefully inserted (**D**).*

window niche. The surgical technique used for group three was found to preserve the most hearing in the low-mid frequencies.[19] Studies using vestibular measures as an outcome suggest that the round window approach is less traumic to the inner ear than a standard cochleostomy.[37] Even with these modifications to surgical technique careful psychophysical testing does suggest that there are subtle changes in auditory function associated with hearing preservation surgery.[38]

OUTCOMES OF HEARING PRESERVATION AND EAS

Beyond altering the surgical approach, the design and length of the implant electrode influence outcomes. Initially, shorter electrode arrays or partial insertions were used to prevent cochlear damage. Gantz et al, used a 10-mm electrode to demonstrate the feasibility of hearing preservation in cochlear implantation. In this initial study 13 volunteers were implanted to a depth of 6 to 10 mm from the cochleostomy. [5,39] Following implantation, their ability to recognize familiar melodies was significantly more accurate than the standard cochlear implant users (who did not have or lost residual low-frequency hearing. Furthermore, they performed better in speech in noise than the standard implant users. Skarzynski[40–44] implanted 10 subjects, all of which had significant residual low frequency hearing. Partial insertion using the of the MED-EL Combi 40+ was completed using the soft surgical technique allowing up to 8 electrodes to be inserted depending on the amount of residual hearing. All but one had preserved hearing following surgery and 12 months post surgery. Several studies have shown that patients listening in the electroacoustic condition (EAS) perform better in background noise and have improved music appreciation as compared to those in the implant only condition.[5,40–44] Another study done by James et al showed improved speech recognition in noise with the EAS approach. The Nucleus® Contour Advance™ was implanted in 12 patients with insertion depths ranging between 17 to 19 mm. An in-the-ear hearing aid (ITE) was fit in the ipsilateral ear to amplify the preserved low frequencies. They measured a 20% improvement with speech in quiet along with a 3 dB improvement in signal to noise ratio. Subjectively, patients were very satisfied with the bimodal hearing.[45] Garcia-Ibanez et al[46] implanted the Nucleus® Contour Advance™ up to 17 mm for the purpose of preserving residual hearing. They found that hearing thresholds were measurable postoperatively in 71 to 86% of their subjects. Thirty-six percent of these patients had preservation of thresholds within 10 dB of their preoperative thresholds and

approximately 67% within 20 dB HL of the preoperative thresholds.[46] Hearing preservation was thus attainable with a variety of different electrode designs with insertion depths to approximately the 1000 Hz region of the cochlea. An example of hearing preservation and speech outcomes is seen in Figure 10–5.

One of the major concerns with hearing preservation cochlear implantation is that residual hearing is lost over time, resulting in a partially implanted and stimulated cochlea. Deeper implantation with sequential activation of apical electrodes presents a potential solution to this dilemma. Although short electrodes have been shown to be beneficial for speech understanding, deep insertions also have advantages, even for hearing preservation candidates. With limited access to the apical regions, the implant may be less effective in the event that the residual hearing is lost as the apical region activates more spiral ganglia, which can provide a broader spectrum of hearing, and in turn, result in more speech and pitch information.[47] Most electrodes arrays are approximately inserted 18 to 24 mm when inserted and cover about 1.5 turns of the cochlea. MED-EL electrodes are designed for insertions of up to 31 mm; however, when fully inserted, reaches approximately a 630-degree turn, which is still significantly shorter than the length of the cochlea as spiral ganglion neurons extend to 720 degrees with an approximate frequency of 58 Hz.[48] Frequency allocations may be reassigned to the apical end; however, Reiss et al suggests that it may require a significant amount of time for the users to adjust to the frequency shift.[49,50] Furthermore, temporal bone studies have shown that insertions extending beyond 360 degrees (about 20 mm) showed increased cochlear trauma.[6]

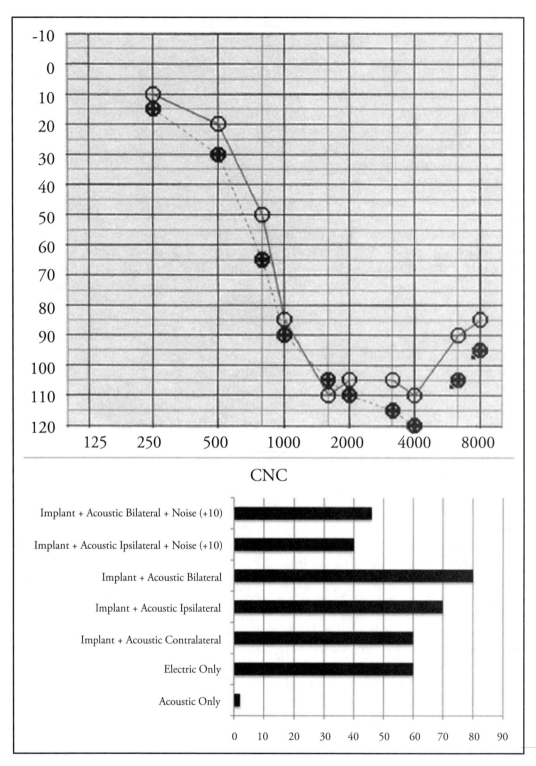

Figure 10–5. Pre- and postoperative audio from a patient with a right 20-mm insertion of a MED-EL "M" electrode, demonstrating preservation of hearing. Testing of the patient in multiple listening conditions demonstrates superior hearing in background noise when low-frequency acoustic information is used to supplement electrical stimulation.

Preservation of hearing with deeper insertions implies that it is possible to maintain the integrity of the apical structures of the cochlea while being able to electrically stimulate the basal region of the cochlea. From a hearing outcomes perspective, low pitch acoustic hearing is important to preserve as it gives the listener cues for localization and pitch.[51–53] Sound localization is governed by interaural time differences between when the sound reaches the ears. Those changes are detectable when they are about 10 microseconds apart and this processing begins to "break down" with sinusoids above 1500 Hz. Additionally, the acoustic hearing entails fine spectral resolution, which is not entirely replicated in the current processing strategies. This results in poor abilities to detect pitch frequency changes and pitch patterns for standard implants. Preserving low-frequency hearing helps patients maintain better localization and hearing in background, especially when aids are worn binaurally. Currently, both MED-EL and Cochlear Corp produce speech processors that combine a hearing aid with the implant processor.

Newer electrode designs aim to allow atraumatic insertion with implantation to at least 20 mm. Potentially, even deeper insertion into the cochlea with limited damage is possible. Baumgartner et al[54] implanted 23 adults with a specialized flexible 31 mm electrode manufactured by MED-EL. The electrode features five single contacts in the apical end and seven pairs across the rest of the array. With this design, the apical end is much thinner. Hearing preservation was achieved in four cases up to 12 months. Improvements were seen with monosyllabic words, as well as hearing in noise (+10 db signal to noise ratio) with mean scores of 54 and 57%, respectively. Gstoettner et al[8] also

found that deeper insertions could indeed be achieved with the MED-EL electrode arrays. This is significant as implantation to 20 mm is predicted to give patients electrical hearing through the 1000-Hz range, leaving the apical, hearing portion of the cochlea intact. Twenty-one patients were implanted with insertions depths ranging from 18 to 24 mm. Hearing was successfully preserved in 85.7% of the patients. When compared to the electric-only condition, all patients performed better in the EAS condition. A key component to preserving hearing in these cases was found to be an atraumatic ("soft") surgical approach.[8] Prentiss et al[55] further supported this with the ability to achieve insertions of up to 28 mm with preservation of hearing using the MED-EL Pulsar ti100 and Sonata ti100 implants. Evaluation of 25 cases that have been implanted with soft surgical techniques via a round window or extended round window approach show no correlation between insertion depth and change in hearing, suggesting that electrode choice and atraumatic technique can allow extensive frequency range coverage (Fig 10–6). In this patient population there was significant improvement of hearing both for electric only and EAS hearing.[55]

Recent publications of multicenter studies from centers implanting the MED-EL device suggest that hearing preservation can be stable and achieved independent of site. As in previous studies, this trial demonstrated an improvement of hearing in background noise for the EAS condition versus the electric only listening condition. Review of the results from the U.S. Hybrid trial, carried out with the Nucleus device similarly report stable hearing outcomes for a large patient population. Additionally besides demonstrating augmented hearing in background

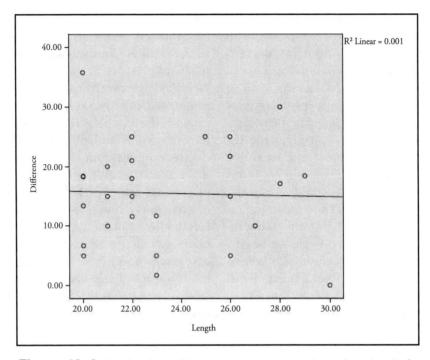

Figure 10–6. *Evaluation of hearing loss versus insertion depth for a population of patients implanted with MED-EL electrodes. Hearing change is listed as change in pure-tone average (PTA) as patients in this group had only low frequency hearing. There was no correlation between insertion depth and change in hearing with insertions up to 30 mm.*

noise, this study also demonstrated the potential for patients to centrally alter pitch perception over time. This opens the possibility of improving hearing through implant as well as rehabilitative strategies. Current research is focusing on optimizing the depth of implantation, developing customized processing strategies for this group of patients, and enhancing our ability to ensure acute and chronic stability of acoustic hearing after implantation.

PROGRAMMING PATIENTS WITH RESIDUAL ACOUSTIC HEARING

Programming these patients can often be complicated due to the overlap between

acoustic and electric stimulation. Finding the low frequency cutoff is often very difficult as the pitch perception of these patients does not always correlate with the center frequency of the electrodes, especially in the apical end of the cochlea. Programming patients follows standard implant programming. Most comfortable loudness (MCL) levels are measured for each electrode. Often times, patients will tend to undershoot these levels, meaning that when the implant is initially activated, the volume is subdued. The levels are then increased until the patient hears sounds at an adequate volume. This process is repeated at every programming session. Although the same methods are used to program every electrode, EAS patients are often more complicated due to the overlap between acoustic and electric stimulation. One of the most important parameters to consider is the frequency range assigned over the implanted electrodes. This controls which frequencies of a signal are allowed to pass through the device effectively. The boundaries are set at 70 to 8500 Hz; however, they can be manipulated to decrease low frequency input by changing the range to 350 to 8500 Hz. Finding where to program the boundaries can be very difficult as we are not always certain where the overlap between the acoustic and electric signals occur. Furthermore, pitch perception of these patients is often mismatched, meaning the frequency presented may not be the frequency the listener perceives. This mismatch is more apparent in the apical end of the cochlea. It is important to note that the audiogram cannot be used to identify frequency boundaries.

Finding the low frequency cutoff is often very difficult as the pitch perception of these patients does not always correlate with the center frequency of the electrodes, especially in the apical end of the cochlea. Interestingly, the full frequency range is preferred for music appreciation.

Outcomes are measured by calculating word discrimination scores with CNC word lists and HINT sentences at 70 dB SPL. Measures are recorded at 3, 6, and 12 month postinitial activation. Hearing preservation patients are tested in a variety of conditions: (1) electric only, (2) EAS, and, if possible, (3) EAS in the ipsilateral ear + acoustic contralateral ear. Patients tend to show rapid improvement after activation; however, subjectively, these patients will often report disappointment in the sound quality. In our experience, patients are much more pleased with the sound quality right around the 12-month mark, although their word understanding scores have not changed much as compared to the 6-month mark. With two different

modes of stimulation, it may require the brain more time to learn how to integrate the two different signals. In addition, the more shallow insertions may give way to the unnatural sound or distortion of higher frequencies that seem to resolve over time as the brain compensates.[56] This memory of "normal" hearing can lead to unrealistic expectations of the implants capabilities. Counseling these patients is time consuming and crucial to their success and satisfaction of their performance.

CAN WE PREDICT VARIABILITY IN OUTCOMES?

Several variables can play a role in patient performance. Gifford et al studied the effects of the electrode insertion on cochlear function and the nonlinearity of the cochlea. Nonlinear function of the cochlea are responsible for hearing sensitivity, acuity, and enhanced spectral purity. This study included nine subjects with insertions ranging from 10 to 20 mm. To assess the nonlinearity, the Shroeder phase effects were measured at 250 and 500 Hz. All subjects but one demonstrated abnormal nonlinear cochlear function suggesting that the electrode disturbs the natural nonlinearity of the cochlea and cochlear mechanics.[38] Adunka et al[47] also studied the comparison of EAS versus electric stimulation alone in the ipsilateral ear to determine if the acoustic residual hearing is truly more beneficial than conventional implants. Using a within subjects design, the addition of acoustic hearing provided significantly better speech understanding than with electric hearing alone at both 3- and 6-month postoperative measurements; however, when compared to conventional CI users, the electric only scores were very comparable. As mentioned above, this continues to suggest that the apical region of the cochlea provides important spectral cues to discriminate speech.[47]

As seen with several studies, the addition of low frequency acoustic input to electric stimulation has shown significant improvements in speech understanding; however, there are still those patients who are not performing as well. To truly predict the performance of a candidate, more physiologic aspects of the auditory nerve and neural pathways should be considered. Electrically evoked potentials may give way to understanding the underlying pathways of sound and perhaps even how plasticity takes effect after extended use of the cochlear implant.

CONCLUSIONS

Treatment for severe high-frequency hearing loss has expanded beyond hearing aids. The instigation of less invasive electrodes and advances in surgical technique have allowed us to preserve useable, residual hearing. The addition of acoustic hearing to electric hearing has shown and continues to show enhanced benefits over electric stimulation alone in terms of speech discrimination. Interestingly, the length of insertion has no correlation to amount of hearing preservation. Hearing preservation has also extended to the pediatric population and similar results have been noted.[57] Preservation of cochlear structures may result not only in hearing, but also in balance. Further research will determine optimal candidacy criteria and define the depth of insertion needed for optimal outcomes.

REFERENCES

1. Gantz BJ, Hansen MR, Turner CW, Oleson JJ, Reiss LA, Parkinson AJ. Hybrid 10 clinical trial: preliminary results. *Audiol Neurootol.* 2009;14(suppl 1):32–38.
2. Gantz BJ, Turner C, Gfeller K. Expanding cochlear implant technology: combined electrical and acoustical speech processing. *Cochlear Implants Int.* 2004;(5 suppl) 1:8–14.
3. Gantz BJ, Turner C, Gfeller KE. Acoustic plus electric speech processing: preliminary results of a multicenter clinical trial of the Iowa/Nucleus Hybrid implant. *Audiol Neurootol.* 2006;11(suppl 1):63–68.
4. Turner CW, Reiss LA, Gantz BJ. Combined acoustic and electric hearing: preserving residual acoustic hearing. *Hear Res.* 2008; 242:164–171.
5. Turner CW, Gantz BJ, Vidal C, Behrens A, Henry BA. Speech recognition in noise for cochlear implant listeners: benefits of residual acoustic hearing. *J Acoust Soc Am.* 2004;115:1729–1735.
6. Adunka O, Kiefer J. Impact of electrode insertion depth on intracochlear trauma. *Otolaryngol Head Neck Surg.* 2006;135: 374–382.
7. Adunka O, Gstoettner W, Hambek M, Unkelbach MH, Radeloff A, Kiefer J. Preservation of basal inner ear structures in cochlear implantation. *ORL J Otorhinolaryngol Relat Spec.* 2004;66:306–312.
8. Gstoettner W, Kiefer J, Baumgartner WD, Pok S, Peters S, Adunka O. Hearing preservation in cochlear implantation for electric acoustic stimulation. *Acta Otolaryngol.* 2004;124:348–352.
9. Gstoettner WK, van de Heyning P, O'Connor AF, et al. Electric acoustic stimulation of the auditory system: results of a multi-centre investigation. *Acta Otolaryngol.* 2008;128: 968–975.
10. Kiefer J, Gstoettner W, Baumgartner W, et al. Conservation of low-frequency hearing in cochlear implantation. *Acta Otolaryngol.* 2004;124:272–280.

11. Dorman MF, Gifford RH. Combining acoustic and electric stimulation in the service of speech recognition. *Int J Audiol.* 2010; 49:912–919.

12. Dorman MF, Gifford R, Lewis K, et al. Word recognition following implantation of conventional and 10-mm hybrid electrodes. *Audiol Neurootol.* 2009;14:181–189.

13. Dorman MF, Gifford RH, Spahr AJ, McKarns SA. The benefits of combining acoustic and electric stimulation for the recognition of speech, voice and melodies. *Audiol Neurootol.* 2008;13:105–112.

14. Gifford RH, Dorman MF, Brown CA. Psychophysical properties of low-frequency hearing: implications for perceiving speech and music via electric and acoustic stimulation. *Adv Otorhinolaryngol.* 2010;67:51–60.

15. Gifford RH, Dorman MF, McKarns SA, Spahr AJ. Combined electric and contralateral acoustic hearing: word and sentence recognition with bimodal hearing. *J Speech Lang Hear Res.* 2007;50:835–843.

16. Handzel O, Burgess BJ, Nadol JB Jr. Histopathology of the peripheral vestibular system after cochlear implantation in the human. *Otol Neurotol.* 2006;27:57–64.

17. Khan AM, Handzel O, Damian D, Eddington DK, Nadol JB Jr. Effect of cochlear implantation on residual spiral ganglion cell count as determined by comparison with the contralateral nonimplanted inner ear in humans. *Ann Otol Rhinol Laryngol.* 2005;114:381–385.

18. Rossi G, Bisetti MS. Cochlear implant and traumatic lesions secondary to electrode insertion. *Rev Laryngol Otol Rhinol (Bord).* 1998;119:317–322.

19. Berrettini S, Forli F, Passetti S. Preservation of residual hearing following cochlear implantation: comparison between three surgical techniques. *J Laryngol Otol.* 2008; 122:246–252.

20. Chao TK, Burgess BJ, Eddington DK, Nadol JB Jr. Morphometric changes in the cochlear nucleus in patients who had undergone cochlear implantation for bilateral profound deafness. *Hear Res.* 2002; 174:196–205.

21. Nadol JB, Jr., Ketten DR, Burgess BJ. Otopathology in a case of multichannel cochlear implantation. *Laryngoscope.* 1994; 104:299–303.

22. Cohen NL. Cochlear implant soft surgery: fact or fantasy? *Otolaryngol Head Neck Surg.* 1997;117:214–216.

23. Khan AM, Handzel O, Damian D, Eddington DK, Nadol JB Jr. Effect of cochlear implantation on residual spiral ganglion cell count as determined by comparison with the contralateral nonimplanted inner ear in humans. *Ann Otol Rhinol Laryngol.* 2005;114:381–385.

24. Finley CC, Holden TA, Holden LK, et al. Role of electrode placement as a contributor to variability in cochlear implant outcomes. *Otol Neurotol.* 2008;29:920–928.

25. Leake PA, Stakhovskaya O, Hradek GT, Hetherington AM. Factors influencing neurotrophic effects of electrical stimulation in the deafened developing auditory system. *Hear Res.* 2008;242:86–99.

26. Roland PS, Wright CG, Isaacson B. Cochlear implant electrode insertion: the round window revisited. *Laryngoscope.* 2007;117:1397–1402.

27. Radeloff A, Unkelbach MH, Tillein J, et al. Impact of intrascalar blood on hearing. *Laryngoscope.* 2007;117:58–62.

28. Maini S, Lisnichuk H, Eastwood H, et al. Targeted therapy of the inner ear. *Audiol Neurootol.* 2009;14:402–410.

29. Connolly TM, Eastwood H, Kel G, Lisnichuk H, Richardson R, O'Leary S. Pre-operative intravenous dexamethasone prevents auditory threshold shift in a guinea pig model of cochlear implantation. *Audiol Neurootol.* 2011;16:137–144.

30. Eastwood H, Chang A, Kel G, Sly D, Richardson R, O'Leary SJ. Round window delivery of dexamethasone ameliorates local and remote hearing loss produced by cochlear implantation into the second turn of the guinea pig cochlea. *Hear Res.* 2010;265:25–29.

31. James DP, Eastwood H, Richardson RT, O'Leary SJ. Effects of round window dexamethasone on residual hearing in a

Guinea pig model of cochlear implantation. *Audiol Neurootol.* 2008;13:86–96.

32. Paasche G, Tasche C, Stover T, Lesinski-Schiedat A, Lenarz T. The long-term effects of modified electrode surfaces and intracochlear corticosteroids on postoperative impedances in cochlear implant patients. *Otol Neurotol.* 2009;30:592–598.

33. Huang CQ, Tykocinski M, Stathopoulos D, Cowan R. Effects of steroids and lubricants on electrical impedance and tissue response following cochlear implantation. *Cochlear Implants Int.* 2007;8:123–147.

34. Paasche G, Bockel F, Tasche C, Lesinski-Schiedat A, Lenarz T. Changes of postoperative impedances in cochlear implant patients: the short-term effects of modified electrode surfaces and intracochlear corticosteroids. *Otol Neurotol.* 2006;27:639–647.

35. De CG, Johnson S, Yperman M, et al. Long-term evaluation of the effect of intracochlear steroid deposition on electrode impedance in cochlear implant patients. *Otol Neurotol.* 2003;24:769–774.

36. Roland PS, Wright CG, Isaacson B. Cochlear implant electrode insertion: the round window revisited. *Laryngoscope.* 2007;117:1397–1402.

37. Basta D, Todt I, Goepel F, Ernst A. Loss of saccular function after cochlear implantation: the diagnostic impact of intracochlear electrically elicited vestibular evoked myogenic potentials. *Audiol Neurootol.* 2008;13:187–192.

38. Gifford RH, Dorman MF, Spahr AJ, Bacon SP, Skarzynski H, Lorens A. Hearing preservation surgery: psychophysical estimates of cochlear damage in recipients of a short electrode array. *J Acoust Soc Am.* 2008;124:2164–2173.

39. Gantz BJ, Turner CW. Combining acoustic and electrical hearing. *Laryngoscope.* 2003;113:1726–1730.

40. Skarzynski H, Lorens A, Piotrowska A, Skarzynski PH. Hearing preservation in partial deafness treatment. *Med Sci Monit.* 2010;16:CR555–CR562.

41. Skarzynski H, Lorens A, Piotrowska A, Podskarbi-Fayette R. Results of partial deafness cochlear implantation using various electrode designs. *Audiol Neurootol.* 2009;14 (suppl) 1:39–45.

42. Skarzynski H, Lorens A, Piotrowska A, Anderson I. Preservation of low frequency hearing in partial deafness cochlear implantation (PDCI) using the round window surgical approach. *Acta Otolaryngol.* 2007;127:41–48.

43. Skarzynski H, Lorens A, Piotrowska A, Anderson I. Partial deafness cochlear implantation provides benefit to a new population of individuals with hearing loss. *Acta Otolaryngol.* 2006;126:934–940.

44. Skarzynski H, Lorens A, D'Haese P, et al. Preservation of residual hearing in children and post-lingually deafened adults after cochlear implantation: an initial study. *ORL J Otorhinolaryngol Relat Spec.* 2002;64:247–253.

45. James C, Albegger K, Battmer R, et al. Preservation of residual hearing with cochlear implantation: how and why. *Acta Otolaryngol.* 2005;125:481–491.

46. Garcia-Ibanez L, Macias AR, Morera C, et al. An evaluation of the preservation of residual hearing with the Nucleus Contour Advance electrode. *Acta Otolaryngol.* 2009;129:651–664.

47. Adunka OF, Pillsbury HC, Adunka MC, Buchman CA. Is electric acoustic stimulation better than conventional cochlear implantation for speech perception in quiet? *Otol Neurotol.* 2010;31:1049–1054.

48. Boyd PJ. Potential benefits from deeply inserted cochlear implant electrodes. *Ear Hear.* 2011;32(4):411–427

49. Reiss LA, Lowder MW, Karsten SA, Turner CW, Gantz BJ. Effects of extreme tonotopic mismatches between bilateral cochlear implants on electric pitch perception: a case study. *Ear Hear.* 2011;32(4):536–540

50. Reiss LA, Gantz BJ, Turner CW. Cochlear implant speech processor frequency allocations may influence pitch perception. *Otol Neurotol.* 2008;29:160–167.

51. Gantz BJ, Turner C, Gfeller KE, Lowder MW. Preservation of hearing in cochlear implant surgery: advantages of combined electrical and acoustical speech processing. *Laryngoscope.* 2005;115:796–802.

52. Francart T, Brokx J, Wouters J. Sensitivity to interaural time differences with combined cochlear implant and acoustic stimulation. *J Assoc Res Otolaryngol.* 2009; 10:131–141.

53. Francart T, Brokx J, Wouters J. Sensitivity to interaural level difference and loudness growth with bilateral bimodal stimulation. *Audiol Neurootol.* 2008;13:309–319.

54. Baumgartner WD, Jappel A, Morera C, et al. Outcomes in adults implanted with the FLEXsoft electrode. *Acta Otolaryngol.* 2007;127:579–586.

55. Prentiss S, Sykes K, Staecker H. Partial deafness cochlear implantation at the University of Kansas: techniques and outcomes. *J Am Acad Audiol.* 2010;21:197–203.

56. Dorman MF, Loizou PC, Rainey D. Simulating the effect of cochlear-implant electrode insertion depth on speech understanding. *J Acoust Soc Am.* 1997;102:2993–2996.

57. Skarzynski H, Lorens A, Piotrowska A, Anderson I. Partial deafness cochlear implantation in children. *Int J Pediatr Otorhinolaryngol.* 2007;71:1407–1413.

Chapter 11

Bilateral Cochlear Implantation

ROBERT R. PETERS

INTRODUCTION

The fact that serious discussion is warranted concerning the bilateral application of cochlear implants (CI) is testimony to this technology's revolutionary success. Although there is little remaining debate concerning the benefits of unilateral CI for the treatment of appropriate patients with severe to profound sensorineural hearing loss, bilateral application has been far from intuitive and has been approached with caution. In fact, the 15 to 20 years it has taken from the time unilateral cochlear implantation was introduced until broad acceptance of its bilateral application is a significantly longer time period than that of other major hearing interventions in the past (such as the stapedectomy procedure that was applied bilaterally only 2 to 3 years after its introduction—personal communication with Dr. John Shea). As touched on in this chapter, bilateral cochlear implantation (BCI) has added another layer of complexity to the CI decision process, requiring judgments to be made about two ears with varying amounts of residual hearing and possibly quite different hearing histories in the same patient. Such decisions must be made with a critical mind toward what technologic options the future may bring.

HISTORY

In 1972 the House 3M single-channel CI became the first commercially available device in the United States. Although over 1,000 of these devices were implanted between 1972 and the early 1980s, the auditory benefits realized by recipients (albeit revolutionary in their time) were relatively modest. The development of multichannel cochlear implants and more robust processing strategies were anticipated to be major advances with regard to auditory performance, but this remained to be clarified. The first published report of a patient undergoing BCI was in 1988 by Balkany et al.[1] The focus of the report was the performance comparison of these 2 different CI technologies in each ear, that is, single channel versus the newer multichannel devices. Such comparison of older and newer CI technologies in the opposite ears of the same patient continued to be the main point of interest for many years and for which BCI provided the most useful opportunity for study.[2]

Once multichannel CIs established themselves as the superior technology, interest in answering the question of which ear of a patient would perform best with a CI was studied with BCI.[3] It became evident that existing predictive patient criteria were not always accurate in choosing the better ear for unilateral CI. BCI ensured "capture" of the better performing ear. In this light the main goal was to ensure that each patient had at least one CI with good auditory performance.

It is only since the late 1990s that research has focused on the development and/or restoration of binaural auditory mechanisms through BCI: the benefits of two ears working together over just one alone.[4,5] Even though earlier published reports alluded to anecdotal binaural benefits in some of their BCI subjects, there was no concerted effort to analyze these quantitatively. The prospect of broad application of BCI to the general CI candidate population raised several concerns among surgeons and researchers, such as the safety of BCI surgery in children, the potential negative vestibular effects, the need to preserve one ear for future technology, and the cost effectiveness of the second CI. Interestingly, the earliest large series of BCI patients appears to be in children coming out of Europe. By the year 2000 Dr. J. Mueller at the University of Wurzburg began reporting his experience with close to 200 BCI children.[6] Although no safety concerns were reported from his series, a quantitative analysis evaluating the efficacy of BCI was not quickly forthcoming.

In the United States, the safety concerns mentioned above led to initial BCI research being focused on adults. The inaugural multicenter US BCI study was the "Nucleus Simultaneous Bilateral Cochlear Implantation in Adults" project sponsored by Cochlear Americas.[7] This was followed soon after by multicenter adult studies sponsored by the other 2 major CI manufactures (MED-EL Corp and Advanced Bionics Corporation).[8,9] The positive results of these studies eased some of the safety concerns and raised interest in evaluating BCI in children in greater detail. The Nucleus Sequential BCI study in children provided the earliest prospective multicenter US analysis of auditory BCI performance in a larger group of children ($n = 30$).[10] In this study, early unilaterally implanted children (<3 years of age at first CI) who were various ages at the time of their second CI, showed significant binaural benefits for speech perception tasks. In addition, this study was the first to demonstrate an "age affect" for the second CI in these congenitally deafened children; the younger the child at the time of their second CI the better the speech discrimination ability of that ear. What has followed is not only the expansion of BCI to younger and younger children, and that increasingly in simultaneous surgery, but also a great expansion in knowledge on the practical implications of critical periods and age-related neural plasticity in the central auditory system (CAS) serving both ears.[11]

Worldwide experience with BCI is now quite extensive. As can be seen from Table 11–1 there are nearly 22,000 BCI patients worldwide as of the end of 2010, representing 11% of the CI population, up from only 5% just 3 years ago.[11] Although there has been a 29% increase in CI recip-

Table 11–1. CI and BCI Population Statistics As of Year-End 2010 From the Databases of Advanced Bionics Corp., Cochlear Corp., and MED-EL Corp. Percentages are for proportion of adults versus children for each region.

December 31, 2010 3 Manufacturers	Total Worldwide	US	Non-US
Total CI	153,000	59,670	93,330
Adults	81,090 (54%)	36,398 (61%)	48,516 (52%)
Children	71,910 (46%)	23,272 (39%)	44,814 (48%)
Total BCI	8042	4182	3860
Adults	3056 (38%)	1882 (45%)	1174 (30%)
Children	2686 (62%)	2300(55%)	2686 (70%)

ients in the last 3 years, there has been a 173% increase in BCI recipients.[11] The differences in how both CI and BCI are applied to adults and children in the US versus all other non-US countries is noteworthy. The United States has a greater percentage of adults than children in its general CI population and a higher percentage of adults receive BCIs in the US than in other non-US countries. However the majority of BCIs are being done in children worldwide.

RATIONALE

Cochlear implant recipients are unable to hear "normally" in all of the listening environments found in typical day to day living. This fact has spurred the impressive improvements of increasing sophistication of implant devices and processing strategies seen over the past 20 years. However, extrapolation from what is known about single-sided deafness (normal hearing in one ear and profound hearing loss in the other) indicates that even if a CI was able to provide "normal" hearing, deficits in day to day listening would persist in unilaterally implanted subjects. Psychoacoustical research has shown that this fact is due to the inability of monaural listeners to benefit from certain binaural auditory mechanisms, those designed to greatly assist listening in more adverse environments.[12] These mechanisms are the head shadow effect, binaural redundancy, binaural squelch, and sound localization.[13]

The "head shadow effect" is a physical phenomenon that is the result of the head acting as an acoustic barrier to sounds coming from different locations in space. In Figure 11–1, head shadow effect is measured with a speech signal originating either from right or left speaker with noise interferer originating from opposite speaker. In a patient with normal hearing in both ears who is in a noisy environment, the ear farthest from the noise source will have a more advantageous signal-to-noise ratio (SNR) to listen to the sound of interest than the ear closest

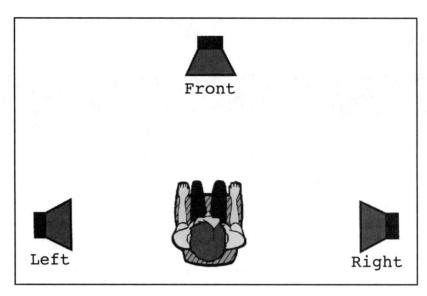

Figure 11–1. *Speaker test arrangement. Speech signal and noise interferer can be varied between front, left, and right speaker for measuring head shadow, redundancy, and squelch effects. (Image by permission of Cochlear Ltd.)*

to the noise source. This effect results in an average of 6.4 dB of noise attenuation but can be as high as 20 dB for high frequency speech sounds.[14,15] This may not seem significant but increasing the SNR by that amount can result in substantial improvements in speech intelligibility, in some listening environments by as much as 50%.[12,14] Interestingly, in patients with unilateral hearing loss, an aspect of the head shadow effect still occurs but in their case can be a detriment if speech originates on the opposite side of the head from their only hearing ear.[12]

Binaural redundancy and squelch are true central nervous system (CNS) auditory processes. Redundancy improves on the distinct acoustic signals arriving at each ear even when the signals are the same. In Figure 11–1, redundancy is measured with the speech signal originating from the front speaker, with or without noise originating from the same speaker.

A summation effect results from enhanced brainstem and midbrain response in the binaural condition, resulting in a perceived 10 dB increase or a near doubling of sound intensity. Binaural redundancy can be thought of as the advantage to be derived from listening in noise with two ears over one alone when the signal is in front of the listener.[17] In such a case, binaural hearing affords a 1 to 2 dB advantage in terms of SNR, compared with the monaural condition.

If, however, the speech and noise signals are from spatially separated sources, the binaural squelch effect comes into play (Fig 11–2). When speech and noise are spatially separated, each ear receives the signal at a different SNR. Binaural squelch allows the listener to attend to the ear with the better SNR, in essence suppressing the ear with the poorer SNR. An improvement of 3dB on average is possible when compared to just listening

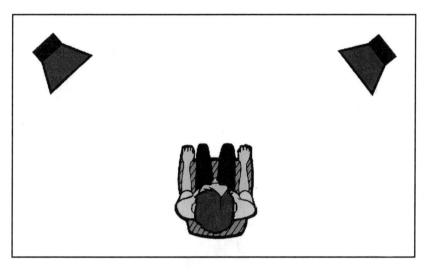

Figure 11–2. *Alternative speaker arrangement for measuring binaural squelch. Speech signal and noise interferer can be alternated between speakers. (Image by permission of Cochlear Ltd.)*

to the ear receiving the better SNR.[17] In effect, the SNR can be about 3dB worse for a binaural listener and still achieve the same speech understanding as a monaural listener via the squelch effect. Through these binaural mechanisms (head shadow, redundancy, and squelch) the binaural listener is able to understand speech in the presence of a more adverse SNR than a monaural listener.[13,18]

Sound localization ability is made possible by the central auditory system's amazing ability to calculate minute differences in the characteristics of sound arriving at each ear (Fig 11–3). Differences in sound intensity, phase, frequency spectrum, and arrival time are calculated for each ear to determine the origin of sound.[12,18,19] The normal human auditory system can distinguish as little as a 1-dB difference in sound intensity between each ear and 0.1-msec difference in arrival time.[18,19] Frequency spectrum differences are created by the variable effect of attenuation from head shadowing and the

shape of the pinna on different frequencies. The central auditory system, "knowing" these spectral effects, can calculate the origin of sound in both the horizontal and vertical planes. These mechanisms are so accurate that the normal-hearing binaural listener can have accuracy down to 1 degree for identifying a sound source.

These binaural mechanisms enhance an individual's ability to understand speech in quiet, but are particularly beneficial in the presence of background noise, in some instances improving speech understanding by as much as 60% when compared to the monaural condition.[12] It is through these mechanisms that the mature auditory system is able to process the time and intensity cues of the auditory percept arriving at each ear for optimal hearing in adverse listening environments such as noisy restaurants, classrooms, and group meetings. Individuals with monaural hearing are, for the most part, unable to utilize these binaural mechanisms that are important for effective hearing in typical

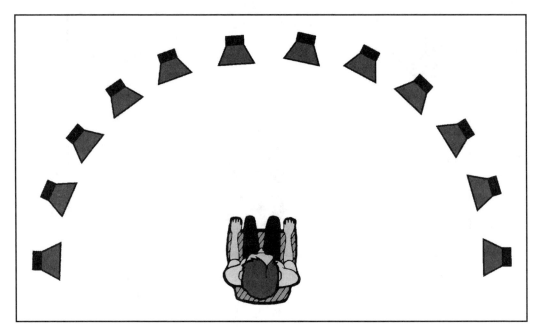

Figure 11–3. *Twelve speaker arrangement for sound localization testing. (Image by permission of Cochlear Ltd.)*

everyday life.[12,21] Even with many years of experience with unilateral hearing loss, central auditory mechanisms are unable to fully compensate for one-sided auditory deprivation.[22] The question of interest to this discussion is to what degree does BCI enable recipients to benefit from these mechanisms, a question that has been the topic of extensive research over the past 10 years.

RESEARCH FINDINGS

ADULTS

In patients who first acquire hearing loss in adult life, BCI has been shown capable of providing some degree of all of the binaural hearing mechanisms described above, despite the psychoacoustic limi-tations of current CI processor arrange-ments and strategies.[5,7,8,20,23–27] Some ben-efits also have been shown in prelingually deafened adults. These adult BCI studies have looked at various aspects of BCI per-formance which will only be summarized here. The current understandings about adult BCI characteristics are:

1. The binaural mechanism providing the greatest measurable binaural gain is the head shadow effect.
2. Binaural squelch and redundancy also provide statistically significant binaural gains in some subjects but to a smaller degree and with less consistency among BCI users than the head shadow effect.
3. Sound localization ability is signifi-cantly enhanced with 2 implants over one CI alone but does not achieve the accuracy of normal hearing listeners.

4. BCI users benefit primarily from inter-aural level (or amplitude) differences (ILD) with the clinical processors currently available. BCI users are not able to benefit significantly from interaural timing differences (ITD) with these processor arrangements (which cannot reproduce the time-dependent synchronization seen in normal-hearing listeners). This explains why BCI users perform better in situations where they can make use of the head shadow effect (which is more dependent on ILD) rather than from the squelch effect (which is more dependent on ITD). Postlingually deafened adults have been shown capable of benefiting from ITDs with synchronized research processors.[28]

5. Prelingually deafened adults demonstrate ability to benefit from BCI. Speech perception performance typically plateaus well below that of postlingually deafened adults.[28,30] The age at which an adult becomes deaf appears to be a predictor of how well they are able to utilize binaural cues, particularly ITDs provided by research processors.[28]

6. Improved health related quality of life and favorable cost utility has been demonstrated for the second CI in adult BCI patients.[31]

In summary, pre- and postlingually deafened adults as a group demonstrate significant benefit from BCI.

CHILDREN

There are several studies that have shown a significant binaural advantage for speech perception in quiet and in noise for BCI children.[10,32–36] These studies have usually been a comparison of the bilateral and unilateral conditions within the same subject. What has been most desired is longitudinal comparison of speech and language acquisition between cohorts of age-matched early unilateral CI and BCI children. Some studies did set out to compare early simultaneous BCI children to early unilateral CI peers longitudinally so that the BCI children were not serving as their own controls. A major obstacle encountered in such studies has been that when parents of children in the unilateral CI control group heard and read about emerging BCI benefits they tended to select out of the study in order to have their child implanted in the other ear.[37] As more evidence has emerged showing the importance of early second ear implantation on optimal second ear auditory capabilities, such controlled, longitudinal studies seem more difficult to sustain. Although it is not a study of early simultaneous BCI, Sparreboom et al (2010)[38] recently compared sequentially implanted BCI children of various ages at the time of their second CI with unilateral CI peers, showing significant advantages for speech in noise and sound localization ability in the BCI children.

From the studies published to date the following characteristics of BCI in children can be enumerated:

1. The younger a child receives both cochlear implants the better the outcome is likely to be with regard to speech perception ability in each ear and benefit from binaural cues.[10,39–42]

2. BCI surgery in children under 12 months of age in experienced hands is safe and well tolerated.[40,41]

3. There appear to be neurodevelopmental advantages to simultaneous

BCI (or at least short sequential with <3 months interimplant interval) in young children with regard to brainstem binaural integration when compared to more delayed sequential surgery.[42]

4. Children who have their first CI at a young age (<3 years of age) but do not receive their second CI until a few years later are likely to have permanent first ear objective and subjective dominance with regard to auditory abilities and preference.[43]

5. Older sequentially implanted children who have lengthy interimplant intervals can still benefit from a second CI but a successful outcome requires strong motivation on the part of the child and parents as well as focused second CI therapy.[10,43]

6. Sound localization and spatial hearing ability in profoundly deaf children is very dependent upon them receiving BCI. Spatial hearing abilities appear to be related to the age at which BCI is provided and number of years of BCI experience.[44,45]

7. Benefits from a second CI emerge over time and may continue to improve for several years with consistent BCI experience.[10,45]

8. Cost-effectiveness data for BCI in children are still emerging, as are the improved benefits seen with earlier unilateral implantation, but to date is positive.[46] It is expected that the noted trend toward simultaneous BCI will show cost savings with regard to a single operation and reduced programming and therapy costs when compared to long-interval sequential BCI. This combined with the number of benefit years characteristic of children is likely to produce a large

Quality Adjusted Life Years (QALYs) rating.

An extensive body of research continues to accrue with regard to the neurodevelopmental aspects of BCI.[47-50] Certain measures of central auditory development have been shown to be good correlates of binaural hearing abilities in children.[49,50] Almost invariably they indicate that the earlier each ear receives a CI the more likely that these central auditory measures are to normalize. Many of these studies appear to be a major impetus behind the worldwide trend toward early simultaneous BCI in children.[11]

CANDIDACY

Based on professional society position statements and worldwide trends of BCI application, the provision of binaural hearing as a standard of care can now be argued to include cochlear implant treatment, just as it exists for hearing aids and other ear and hearing-related interventions.[11,51-54] However, as is true for all medical interventions, the most conservative treatment that can provide binaural benefit is preferable, which in some cases may be partially provided with bimodal hearing (CI + contralateral HA). Therefore, it should not be assumed that just because a patient is a candidate for unilateral implantation, bilateral implantation should automatically follow. At a minimum this stated philosophy encourages planning for the most effective use of both ears instead of limiting the focus to one cochlear implant.

An evidenced-based medicine approach to BCI now permits for some defining of candidate groups based on several patient specific characteristics including:*

➤ Age at presentation for each CI (in children the younger the better for both ears)

➤ Duration of profound hearing loss for each ear (the shorter duration the better)

➤ Residual hearing in the better ear and anticipated benefit of bimodal hearing (CI+ contralateral hearing aid).[55] If significant bimodal benefit is expected or demonstrated after the first CI, a decision may be made to delay a second CI.

➤ Patient/parent's perception of residual hearing in each ear (ie, does the patient or parent perceive that useful residual hearing still exists in one ear)

➤ Progressive and/or fluctuating hearing loss (a decision must be made as to when is the proper time in the progression of hearing loss to proceed with CI and BCI)

➤ Central auditory development measures in children (ie, cortical auditory evoked potentials). These are currently not widely available but in the future may be found useful in determining timing of CI and BCI in children.[56]

➤ Vestibular history (should give careful consideration when there is a history of conditions such as Ménière's disease, prior vestibular neurectomy, etc).

➤ Anatomic abnormalities (ie, cochlear malformations, open mastoid cavities, congenital aural atresia—these con-ditions make a sequential approach preferred)

➤ Comorbid or complicating conditions (ie, auditory neuropathy, other neurologic disorders, chronic otitis media-make a sequential approach preferred)

➤ History of meningitis (implant both ears as soon as possible when indicated)

➤ Degree of success with the first CI (capture of a better performing ear with BCI can be carefully considered even if first CI performance is below expectations)

➤ Patient/parent treatment philosophy/motivation (BCI is a more comprehensive CI approach with which patients/parents must be in agreement).

Each of these factors may affect the decision as to whether BCI is appropriate, and if so whether a sequential or simultaneous approach is best.

SURGICAL ISSUES

Cochlear implant surgery in experienced hands has been refined to involve smaller incisions, shorter operating time, and a low complication rate. Device manufacturers have responded to the need for lower profile implants that minimize tissue disruption and simplify surgical steps, particularly for surgery in children. Nonetheless, a highly experienced surgical team remains an important determinant of outcomes. The addition of second ear surgery with BCI involves a few additional caveats.

---

*For a more detailed analysis of BCI candidacy criteria in children and adults see "Worldwide Trends in Bilateral Cochlear Implantation, Appendix II," *Laryngoscope Suppl.* 120, May 2010, pp. 38–41.

SIMULTANEOUS SURGERY IN THE VERY YOUNG CHILD

It can be argued that the current evidenced based standard of care is to provide binaural hearing at as early an age as possible, even if it requires BCI. Children under 3 years of age represent the fastest growing BCI demographic among experienced clinics worldwide.[11] They are also the only age group to date in which simultaneous surgeries outnumber sequentials. With early hearing loss diagnosis made possible by universal newborn screening, the opportunity for BCI under 12 months of age more commonly presents itself. This raises the question as to how much surgery is a reasonable risk in a child of this age. Studies in unilateral CI suggest that in experienced hands CI surgery is well tolerated at least down to 6 months of age. Adding a second-ear CI surgery at the same sitting increases anesthetic time and blood loss. Issues therefore that may affect the decision to perform simultaneous BCI in children under 12 months of age include the surgeon's proficiency (surgical times for one CI can vary dramatically between surgeons, from 1 hour up to 4 hours), the child's weight (which is a better determinant of a child's tolerance of blood loss than age), and any other comorbid medical conditions that may affect the child. If any of these variables raise additional concerns, a short sequential approach (6 to 12 weeks between operations) may be preferred.

SINGLE OR DOUBLE PREP IN SIMULTANEOUS SURGERY

There are two options with differing pros and cons in regard to sterile prep and drape in simultaneous BCI surgery. Approaching an ear with a separate prep and drape is the standard approach to almost all other otologic surgery and is most familiar to the surgical team. With this approach planning is needed to maintain sterility of the instrument table and surgical components that connect off the sterile field (such as power drills, camera cables, etc) when removing the drapes after completion of the first side and for preparation of the second side. This approach requires additional time for the transition process and uses 2 sets of drapes but has the advantage of allowing for utilization of one set of facial monitoring electrodes for both sides and a simpler draping layout around the ear. A second option is to prepare both ears into a single sterile field. This requires placing a set of facial monitoring sensors on both sides of the face at the beginning of the procedure and a more complex draping process that allows access to both ears while maintaining sterility. The advantage is some time savings and the use of only one set of drapes. This setup is less familiar to an otologic surgical team but is used frequently by our plastic surgical colleagues in operations such as microtia reconstruction and otoplasty.

SYMMETRY OF PLACEMENT

Of primarily aesthetic interest is the surgical placement of each CI device so that the locations of the antenna coils during later CI use are not strikingly dissimilar. Such asymmetry would be more apparent in short haired individuals, particularly when viewed from behind. The best option is for the surgeon to use his/her own consistent method for judging the location of the receiver when operating on each ear. One method of small incision surgery is to elevate periosteum to form a tight pocket without bone fixation of the device. The subperiosteal pocket is raised between the periosteal attachments to the temperoparietal and lamdoid sutures that serve as anchors of the periosteum. This or another method to place the devices at a consistent angle relative to pinna landmarks should provide reasonable symmetry.

HEMOSTASIS DURING SECOND EAR SURGERY

Whether BCI is being done sequentially or simultaneously, once the first CI is in place, monopolar cautery can no longer be used in the head and neck region so as to avoid electrical trauma to the device or cochlea. This fact requires the most significant modification of surgical technique related to BCI surgery. One option is to use bipolar cautery to control bleeding in conjunction with traditional sharp instrumentation when doing the second ear surgery. Another method is to use thermal cutting instruments that do not produce electrical current, such as the Shaw Scalpel©. Once familiarized with their most efficient use, these do an excellent job of speeding the dissection process while controlling bleeding.

UNUSUAL CASES

At times, unexpected findings during surgery may prompt altering the original plan for simultaneous BCI. Encountering unexpected alterations of anatomy, middle ear effusion/ infection, or a significant cerebrospinal fluid leak during first ear surgery may make a sequential approach advisable in order to assess the outcome before proceeding with second ear surgery.

PROGRAMMING ISSUES

Programming cochlear implant processors has become an audiologic specialty in and of itself that is both art and science. The addition of a second implant introduces considerations that vary depending on whether the addition is simultaneous or sequential. Only a few general principles can be mentioned in this discussion with regard to issues unique to programming a patient with BCI.

As a rule, patients with BCI should initially have each implant programmed separately from one another. It is more important that each processor be optimized for individual ear implant performance than it is to have the same pulse width, pulse rate, or stimulation mode on each side. When programmed separately it is unlikely that the programs will be identical for each ear. We are thankful that manufacturers have responded to the increasing application of BCI by developing electronic implant identification technology that prevents a processor from being used on the wrong ear. Once programmed individually, both implants are subsequently turned on together. There will likely be the need to decrease loudness growth on each side by approximately 10% due to the summation effect.

Bilateral balancing is then achieved by adjusting the processors so that each ear sounds equally loud to the patient. Balancing is important with regard to optimization of sound localization ability. Such balancing is easier in patients who have undergone simultaneous BCI, both ears having equal implant experience. Sequentially implanted patients have varying degrees of difficulty achieving this goal. In particular, sequentially implanted children, depending on their length of interimplant interval, may have permanent first ear dominance that forever prevents effective balancing. In adults, immediate subjective feedback clarifies this process greatly. Young children however require an ongoing multivisit proccss that must involve the feedback of parents, therapists, and the behavioral response of the child. Regardless of whether it is an adult or child, programming for optimal performance with BCIs is an incremental process best served by patience, experience, and close observation.

REHABILITATION IN BCI

Aural rehabilitation therapy is an essential part of cochlear implant treatment for patients of all ages. In prelingually deafened children it serves a crucial role in helping the auditorially immature brain acclimate to and make use of the new cochlear implant signal, ultimately leading to language acquisition. Even in postlingually deafened adults it hastens the transition from acoustic to electrical hearing, supporting the patient through an often difficult period that could be the difference between success and failure. BCI adds a few unique considerations.

In simultaneously implanted subjects the therapist should attend to the progress of each ear individually in addition to the patient as a whole. This is particularly true in children where the therapist provides important input with regard to auditory-verbal progress for the programming audiologist. It cannot be assumed

that each ear in a simultaneous BCI child is making equal progress, is optimally programmed, or even that the equipment is working correctly. Therefore, the therapist should at times assess the auditory performance of each ear individually and solicit the feedback of parents with regard to the child's preference or avoidance of one implant over the other. Postlingually deafened adults with simultaneous BCI are able to provide more useful subjective feedback in this regard, but at times the auditory progress may vary between ears, requiring more focused attention on rehabilitation of a particular side.

Sequentially implanted subjects can present a more challenging situation for the auditory-verbal therapist. The candidate for sequential BCI is likely doing very well with their first implant and often has "graduated" from AV therapy for that ear. The patient or parent must be convinced preoperatively that the second CI necessitates reentering therapy for optimal progress with the newly implanted ear, even though they are an experienced CI user. Such counsel is often met with skepticism and resistance. However, it is exactly because the patient now has a higher performing ear with which to compare the new CI (a situation quite dissimilar from the circumstances at the time of first CI surgery) that they may be disappointed and frustrated with the second side, often forgetting the adjustment process they went through after the first implant. The experienced therapist plays an important role in mitigating these difficulties with therapy techniques, home program suggestions, and patient/parent education.

Prelingually deafened, sequentially implanted BCI children present the most unique rehabilitative challenge of all candidate groups. There are age-dependant neurodevelopmental processes at work in these children that play a major role in the variable outcome between ears implanted at different ages.[10] In this regard the auditory-verbal therapist is presented with the sometimes arduous task of encouraging use and optimizing performance of the second CI in the face of a highly dominant first CI. If the child had early first ear implantation (prior to 3 years of age) the difficulty of adjusting to the second CI will be related to the interimplant interval and age at the time of second CI.[10,43] When such a child has an interimplant interval of even just a few years, first ear dominance appears to be permanent in the majority of cases.[43] However, the second ear can still achieve significant gains and develop open-set speech discrimination abilities of its own with persistence. The best therapy techniques for achieving optimal performance of the second ear in these older sequentially implanted children are still being clarified. Experience on the part of the author as well as data published in the ophthalmologic literature with regard to the correlative childhood problem of amblyopia suggest that sensory deprivation of the dominant side while selectively stimulating the new side achieves the greatest gains in second side performance.[43,57] However, asking an older child to do without their first implant for extended periods of time is usually met with stiff resistance from the patient, as they are very dependent on the hearing from their first ear for day to day functioning. There are exceptions to this of course, and some preschoolers and school-aged children have integrated the signal from the second implant without the use of special strategies. The therapist must reach a compromise of what is necessary and logistically feasible for each patient and monitor the progress of each ear.

THE FUTURE

A prominent concern which has been raised from the beginning of any discussion related to BCI is the likely exclusion from use of future technologic advancements of BCI recipients. In particular, the main concern relates primarily to inner ear hair cell research. CI recipients will likely always be candidates for future advances in CI devices, as surgical replacement of an implant is currently done with some frequency and can be done without loss of performance. However, the intracochlear changes caused by a cochlear implant are likely to make therapies such as hair cell regeneration ineffective or at least less effective in CI recipients. Thus, the question is raised as to whether we should "save" at least one ear of CI recipients so they may benefit from such future treatments. Although research developments in hair cell regeneration are exciting and hopeful, the verdict is still out as to whether or not such a therapy will ever find useful application in humans, if so whether the auditory benefits will exceed that of the CI technology that exists at that time, and what time frame we are likely to encounter before its introduction. In light of what we know about the age-dependent critical period limitations on auditory performance in children, saving one ear of a child for future, uncertain technology seems ill advised. Even in adults it is a question of whether to proceed with current proven benefit or to wait for future uncertain technology. At a minimum, there should be open discussion about this dilemma with parents and/or patients.

There remains potential for improving the binaural benefit of BCI users with advances in processor technology and programming strategies. Current processor arrangements lack the time-dependent synchronization between ears needed to allow recipients to fully benefit from ITDs. In addition processing strategies need to more effectively retain fine structure, low frequency information that contains important cues for full functioning of central binaural mechanisms.[58] There needs to be greater understanding of how to make the most use of programming parameters (such as pulse rate, pulse width, and stimulation mode) between ears. Research processors have already shown the ability to more precisely synchronize pairs of electrodes in each ear as well as reproduce fine structure cues, allowing more effective use of ITDs and spectral information.[29] Further research will help clarify ways to maximize the real-world, everyday auditory abilities of BCI users.

REFERENCES

1. Balkany T, Boggess W, Dinner B. Binaural cochlear implantation: comparison of 3M/House and Nucleus 22 devices with evidence of sensory integration. *Laryngoscope.* 1988;98(10):1040–1043.

2. Green Jr JD, Mills DM, Bell BA, Luxford WM, Tonokawa LL. Binaural cochlear implants. *Amer J Otol.* Nov 1992;13(6):502–506.

3. Ramsden, R, Greenhan, P, O'Driscoll M, et al. Evaluation of bilaterally implanted adult subjects with the Nucleus 24 cochlear implant system. *Otol Neurotol.* 2005; 26:988–998.

4. Mawman DJ, Ramsden RT, O'Driscoll M, et al. Bilateral cochlear implants controlled by a single speech processor. *Amer J Otol.* 2000;19(6):758–761.

5. Muller, J, Schoen, F, Helms, J. Speech understanding in quiet and noise in bilateral users of the Med-El COMBI 40/40+

6. Muller J, Schoen F, Helms J. *Bilateral cochlear implantation in children—simultaneous or non-simultaneous implantation. Some conclusions after five years experience with bilateral cochlear implantation in children.* 9th Symposium on Cochlear Implants In Children, Washington, DC, 2003.

7. Litovsky R, Parkinson A, Acaroli J, Sammeth C. Simultaneous bilateral cochlear implantation in adults: a multicentre study. *Ear Hear.* 2006 Dec;27(6):714–731.

8. Buss E, Pillsbury H, Buchman C, et al. Multicenter U.S. bilateral MED-EL cochlear implantation study: speech perception over the first year of use. *Ear Hear.* 2008; 29:20–32.

9. Peters BR, Lake J. HiRes Benefit in a bilaterally implanted adult. *Auditory Research Bulletin, Biennial Edition.* Advanced Bionics Corporation;2005:150–151.

10. Peters BR, Litovsky R, Parkinson A, Lake, J. Importance of age and postimplantation experience on speech perception measures in children with sequential bilateral cochlear implants. *Otol Neurotol.* 2007;28(649):657.

11. Peters B, Wyss J, Manrique M. Worldwide trends in bilateral cochlear implantation. *Laryngoscope Suppl.* May 2010;120(5).

12. Welsh L, Rosen L, Welsh J, Dragonette J. Functional impairments due to unilateral deafness. *Ann Otol Rhinol Laryngol.* 2004;113:987–993.

13. Moore DR. Anatomy and physiology of binaural hearing. *Audiology.* 1991;30: 125–134.

14. Tillman TW, Kasten RN, Horner IS. Effect of head shadow on reception of speech. *ASHA.* 1963;5:778–779.

15. Markides A. Advantages of binaural hearing over monaural hearing. In: Markides A, ed. *Binaural Hearing Aids.* London, UK: Academic Press; 1977.

16. Dillon H. *Hearing Aids.* Turramurra, NSW: Boomerang Press; 2001.

cochlear implant system. *Ear Hear.* 2002; 23:198–206.

17. Marks L. Binaural summation of the loudness of pure tones. *J Acoust Soc Am.* 1978; 64:107–113.

18. Palmer C. Fitting strategies for patients with symmetrical hearing loss. In: *Strategies for Selecting and Verifying Hearing Aid Fittings*, 2nd ed. 2002:202–220.

19. Moore DR. Anatomy and physiology of binaural hearing. *Audiology.* 1991;30: 125–134.

20. Senn P, Kompis M, Vischer M, Haeusler R. Minimum audible angle, Just noticeable interaural differences and speech intelligibility with bilateral cochlear implants using clinical speech processors. *Audiol Neurotol.* 2005;10:342–352.

21. Cox R, Bisset J. Relationship between two measures of aided binaural advantage. *J Speech Hear Res.* 1984;49:399–408.

22. Colletti V, Fiorino F, Carner M, Rizzi R. Investigation of the long-term effects of unilateral hearing loss in adults. *Br J Audiol.* 1988;22:113–118.

23. Murphy J, O'Donoghue G. Bilateral cochlear implantation: an evidence-based medicine evaluation. *Laryngoscope.* 2007; 117(8):1412–1418.

24. Tyler RS, Dunn CC, Witt SA, Noble WG. Speech perception and localization with adults with bilateral sequential cochlear implants. *Ear Hear.* 2007;28(2 suppl): 86S–90S.

25. Neuman AC, Haravon A, Sislian N, Waltzman, SB. Sound-direction identification with bilateral cochlear implants. *Ear Hear.* 2007;28(1), 73–82.

26. Schleich P, Nopp P, D'Haese P. Head shadow, squelch, and summation effects in bilateral users of the Med-El COMBI 40/40+ cochlear implant. *Ear Hear.* Jun 2007;25(3):197–204.

27. Nopp, P, Schleich, P, D'Haese, P. Sound localization in bilateral users of Med-El COMBI 40/40+ cochlear implants. *Ear Hear.* Jun 2007;25(3):205–214.

28. Litovsky RY, Jones GL, Agrawal S, van Hoesel R. Effect of age at onset of deafness on binaural sensitivity in electric hearing in humans. *J Acoust Soc Am.* Jan 2010;127(1):400–414.

29. Litovsky R, Bilateral cochlear implants: are two ears better than one? http://www.asha. org/Publications/leader/2010/100216/ BilateralCochlearImplants.htm

30. Bassim MK, Buss E, Clark MS, et al. MED-EL Combi40+ cochlear implantation in adults. *Laryngoscope.* Sep 2005;115(9):1568–1573.

31. Bichey BG, Miyamto RT. Outcomes in bilateral cochlear implantation. *Otolaryngol Head Neck Surg.* 2008;138:655–661.

32. Papsin BC, Gordon KA. Bilateral cochlear implants should be the standard for children with bilateral sensorineural deafness. *Curr Opin Otolaryngol Head Neck Surg.* 2008;16:69–74.

33. Steffens T, Lesinski-Schiedat A, Strutz J, et al. The benefits of sequential bilateral cochlear implantation for hearing-impaired children. *Acta Otolaryngol.* 2008;128:164–176.

34. Manrique M, Huarte A, Valdivieso A, Perez B. Bilateral sequential implantation in children. *Audiol Med.* 2007;5:224–231.

35. Beijen J, Snik AM, Mylanus EM. Sound localization ability of young children with bilateral cochlear implants. *Otol Neurotol.* 2007;28:479–485.

36. Galvin KL, Mok M, Dowell RC. Perceptual benefit and functional outcomes for children using sequential bilateral cochlear implants. *Ear Hear.* 2007;28:470–482.

37. Peters B. *Prospective evaluation of bilateral cochlear implant performance in young deaf children: study design considerations.* CI 2007, Charlotte, North Carolina, April 13, 2007.

38. Sparreboom M, Snik AF, Mylanus EA. Sequential bilateral cochlear implantation in BPchildren: development of the primary auditory abilities of bilateral stimulation. *Audiol Neurotol.* 2010 October 27;16(4):203–213.

39. Wolfe J, Baker S, Caraway T, et al. 1-year postactivation results for sequentially implanted bilateral cochlear implant users. *Otol Neurotol.* 2007;28(5), 589–596.

40. Dettman SJ, Pinder D, Briggs RJ, Dowell RC, Leigh JR. Communication development in children who receive the cochlear implant younger than 12 months: risks versus benefits. *Ear Hear.* 2007 Apr;28(2 suppl):11S–18S.

41. Waltzman SB, Roland JT Jr. Cochlear implantation in children younger than 12 months. *Pediatrics.* 2005 Oct;116(4): e487–e493.

42. Gordon KA, Valero J, Papsin BC. Auditory brainstem activity in children with 9–30 months of bilateral cochlear implant use. *Hear Res.* 2007;233(1–2):97–107.

43. Peters B, Parkinson A, Lianos L. Long-term wearing patterns and speech perception performance in bilateral sequentially implanted older children. San Diego, CA, April 11, 2008.

44. Grieco-Calub TM, Litovsky RY. Sound localization skills in children who use bilateral cochlear implants and in children with normal acoustic hearing. *Ear Hear.* 2010 Oct;31(5):645–656.

45. Godar SP, Litovsky RY. Experience with bilateral cochlear implants improves sound localization acuity in children. *Otol Neurotol.* 2010 Oct;31(8):1287–292.

46. Summerfield AQ, Lovett RE, Bellenger H, et al. Estimates of the cost-effectiveness of pediatric bilateral cochlear implantation. *Ear Hear.* 2010 Oct;31(5):611–624.

47. Sharma A, Dorman MF, Kral A. The influence of a sensitive period on central auditory development in children with unilateral and bilateral cochlear implants. *Hear Res.* 2005;203(1–2):134–143.

48. Sharma A, Gilley PM, Martin K, Roland P, Bauer P, Dorman M. Simultaneous versus sequential bilateral implantation in young children: effects on central auditory system development and plasticity. *Audiol Med.* 2007;5(4):218–223.

49. Nash A, Sharma A, Martin K, Biever A. (2008). Clinical applications of the P1 cortical auditory evoked potential (CAEP) biomarker. *A Sound Foundation Through Early Amplification: Proceedings of a Fourth International Conference.* Chicago, IL, 2007.

50. Sharma A, Gilley PM, Dorman MF, Baldwin R. Deprivation-induced cortical reorganization in children with cochlear implants. *Int J Audiol.* 2007;46(9), 494–499.

51. Balkany T, Hodges A, Telischi F, et al. William House Cochlear Implant Study Group position statement on bilateral cochlear implants. *Otol Neurotol.* 2008 Feb;29:107–108.

52. American Academy of Otolaryngology-Head and Neck Surgery Cochlear Implant Policy Statement, Revised 12/27/2007. http://www.entnet.org/Practice/policy CochlearImplants.cfm

53. BCIG position paper on bilateral cochlear implants. Revised May 2008. http://www .bcig.org.uk/downloads/pdfs/BCIG%20 position%20statement%20-%20Bilateral %20Cochlear%20Implantation%20May% 2007.pdf

54. Offeciers E, Morera C, Muller J, et al. International consensus on bilateral cochlear implants and bimodal stimulation. *Acta Otolaryngol.* 2005 Sep;125(9):918–919.

55. Potts LG, Skinner MW, Litovsky RA, Strube MJ, Kuk F. Recognition and localization of speech by adult cochlear implant recipients wearing a digital hearing aid in the nonimplanted ear (bimodal hearing). *J Am Acad Audiol.* 2009 Jun;20(6):353–373.

56. Sharma A, Nash A. Brain maturation in children with cochlear implants. Retrieved 1/16/2010 from http://www.asha.org/Pub lications/leader/2009/090414/f090414b. htm .

57. Holmes J, Repka M, Kraker R, Clarke M. The treatment of amblyopia. *Strabismus.* 2006;15(1):37–42.

58. van Hoesel RJ, Jones GL, Litovsky RY. Interaural time-delay sensitivity in bilateral cochlear implant users: effects of pulse rate, modulation rate, and place of stimulation. *J Assoc Res Otolaryngol.* 2009 Dec; 10(4):557–567. Epub 2009 Jun 10.

Chapter 12

Adult Cochlear Implant Programming: A Basic Introduction

MICHELLE L. MONTES AND JENNIFER ROTZ

INTRODUCTION

The goal of cochlear implant programming is to code or transform an acoustic signal of varying intensities from 0 to 120 dB into an electrical signal of 20 dB. Characteristics of the acoustic signal that are coded into a recipient's program or "map" are intensity (ie, loudness), frequency (ie, pitch), and timing (ie, duration). This chapter provides the reader with an overview of programming in the adult cochlear implant recipient.

PROGRAMMING APPROACHES

Programming can involve obtaining some type of behavioral response from the patient or employing objective measures utilizing no or limited response from the patient initially. Philosophies vary as to whether behavioral, objective, or combined behavioral and objective approaches yield better patient outcomes. Our clinical experience has led us to use a combination of behavioral and objective measures when programming our adult implant patients. However, this topic remains subject to debate.

BEHAVIORAL MEASURES

Psychophysical measures can be used to obtain a patient's electrical dynamic range for an individual or group of electrodes. Measurement stimuli for psychophysical testing can include live voice, tonal, or "noise" stimuli. These measures may include obtaining "threshold" as well as maximum or most comfortable listening level for the stimulus. The lower and upper limits of the electrical dynamic range are defined differently across implant manufacturers.

True threshold is accepted to mean the level at which the stimulus is identified fifty per cent of the time. Practically defined, it is the level at which the individual can just begin to hear the stimulus. For example, Cochlear Corporation utilizes *true* threshold in their programming. Advanced Bionics and MED-EL Corporations recommend setting the lower limits of the patient's programming to default at 10% of the electrical dynamic range.

The patient's listening program must also specify an upper limit of stimulation. Again, this level is defined within the context of the manufacturers' software. Cochlear Corporation and MED-EL both utilize *maximum* comfortable listening level as the upper limit of stimulation. Advanced Bionics defines the upper limits of stimulation as the *most* comfortable listening level. That being said, all manufacturer software allows for manipulation of dynamic range parameters at the clinician's discretion.

OBJECTIVE PHYSIOLOGIC MEASURES

Objective measures allow for programming in the absence of a patient response. The programming audiologist may use this approach based on their own clinical preference. Alternatively, objective measures may be employed when a patient is unable to provide reliable behavioral information. Current implant technologies allows for delivery of a stimulus as well as a telemetry mechanism to allow for objective feedback of electrical activity in the form of impedances and auditory neural responses. Common objective measures used in programming are the electrically evoked compound action potential (ECAP) thresholds, the electri-

cal evoked stapedial reflex thresholds (ESRT), and the electrically evoked auditory brainstem response (EABR).

Electrically Evoked Compound Action Potential-ECAP

The electrically evoked compound action potential recording demonstrates the synchronous firing of auditory nerve fibers. This measure is comparable to electrocochleography (ECoG) which is recorded with an acoustic stimulus. ECAP threshold testing involves delivering an electrical stimulus to the patient and looking for the lowest stimulation level at which the auditory nerve is observed to fire. As indicated previously, the implant itself can both deliver the stimulus as well as measure the neural response. Intraoperatively, the observation of the ECAP may suggest that stimulation through the implant is effectively eliciting a physiologic response. This response, however, does not serve as a predictor of patient performance. Postoperatively, the ECAP response may be used for programming. Measures are easily obtained, even in the nonquiescent individual. Although it is accepted that the patient's ECAP threshold will occur within the individual's electrical dynamic range, the use of the ECAP alone for programming is discouraged in recent literature.[1,2] Instead, behavioral measures or a combination of behavioral and ECAP measures may produce a more optimal program or map. Once the ECAP threshold is obtained, there are a variety of methods that can be applied to set the upper and lower limits of the patient's electrical range of hearing.

The nomenclature referencing the ECAP varies across implant manufacturers. Advanced Bionics refers to their ECAP measurements as Neural Response

Imaging (NRI). Neural Response Telemetry (NRT) is the term used to define the measure by Cochlear Corporation. MED-EL refers to their measures as Auditory Nerve Response Testing (ART). Regardless of the acronym these tests all reflect the electrically evoked compound action potential.

Electrical Stapedial Reflex Threshold-ESRT

ESRT represents the lowest level at which the stapedial reflex is elicited to electrical stimulation. While introducing an electrical stimulus through the implant, the middle ear stapedial reflex is measured using a conventional acoustic immittance meter. A strong relationship has been demonstrated between ESRT and maximum comfort levels,[3,4] potentially making it more useful in programming than ECAP alone. Potential limiting factors in ESRT acquisition are the level of patient myogenic activity or history of middle ear dysfunction which may confound reliable measurement.

Electrical Auditory Brainstem Response-EABR

The electrically evoked auditory brainstem response, while not identical is much like its acoustic counterpart, the auditory brainstem response. It represents the function of the auditory brainstem pathway. The measure offers information related to the peripheral auditory neural pathways and may be conducted intraoperatively or during programming. This measure tends to be used less often clinically than either ECAP or the ESRT largely because of the time involved in test setup and administration. Also, as we saw with the ESRT recording the EABR may be confounded by patient variables such as the level of myogenic activity.

PROGRAMMING PARAMETERS

As previously noted, the goal of cochlear implant programming is to transform the important intensity, frequency, and timing information of the acoustic signal into a meaningful electrical signal. The clinician must make some preliminary decisions about fundamental map parameters at the time of initial implant activation.

SPEECH CODING STRATEGIES

The first decision the clinician must make when creating a listening program is how timing, pitch, and intensity will be manipulated by the speech processor to provide the most meaningful signal to the patient. This is accomplished by way of applying a mathematical formula or algorithm known as the *coding strategy*. Speech coding strategies have evolved as technology has advanced. Table 12–1 provides a list of the speech coding strategies that are currently offered in the programming software. Each manufacturer offers a limited selection of speech coding strategies based on their philosophy of sound coding and how their device is designed to function. Clinicians may opt for specific speech coding strategies based on factors including: patient performance, available number of electrodes, and listening preferences.

Once a speech-coding strategy has been selected, there are other general parameters that may be manipulated during programming. The challenge in providing programming overviews across manufacturers is that certain parameters are clinician manipulated whereas others are automatically manipulated within the

Table 12–1. Current Speech-Coding Strategies Available

Manufacturer	Advanced Bionics	Cochlear Corporation	MED-EL Corporation
Default Coding Strategy	HiRes S	ACE	FSP
Alternate Coding Strategies Available	HiRes P	CIS	HCCIS
	HiRes S with Fidelity 120	Speak	CIS+
	HiRes P with Fidelity 120		
	CIS		
	MPS		

software based on patient responses. The specific programming parameters available for clinical manipulation are documented in the reference manuals provided by each of the manufacturers. The basic parameters to consider include: stimulus duration (sometimes referred to as pulse width), stimulus rate, and the frequency range to be delivered to the implant.

STIMULUS DURATION-PULSE WIDTH

The loudness of the stimulus is determined by a combination of stimulus duration and stimulus rate. Stimulus duration or "pulse width" may be a fixed number or may vary depending on the patient's electrical dynamic range on any given electrode. A narrower pulse width may be more desirable to provide increased stimulation rates. Narrower pulse widths also offer the advantage of more efficient power consumption. That said, wider pulse widths are sometimes necessary to effectively stimulate at the upper limits of the patient's electrical dynamic range. Manufacturers provide default pulse width starting

points. Cochlear Corporation allows the clinician to select from a variety of pulse widths. Alternatively, Advanced Bionics and MED-EL pulse widths are varied automatically by the software as a function of the patient's most comfortable or maximum comfort levels, respectively.

STIMULUS RATE

Stimulus or channel rate refers to the number of electrical pulses per second that are delivered to the electrode array. The stimulation rate may be reported on a per channel basis or as an overall stimulation rate which includes all the electrodes collectively. Stimulation rate can impact a patient's perception of both pitch and loudness. Additionally, the stimulation rate contributes to the implant user's perception of temporal information in the speech signal. Again, the availability of different stimulation rates will vary with the speech coding philosophy embraced by the implant manufacturer. Theoretical arguments can be made that faster stimulation rates provide the listener with the speech signal that is most like the acoustic speech signal. The neural firing of the human auditory system in response to a speech signal is stochastic or random in nature. A high stimulation rate (above 2500 Hz) is needed to achieve stochastic neural firing. Increased stimulation rates may also result in perceptions of increased loudness or increased higher frequency sound quality. However, in reality not all patients perform optimally at high stimulation rates.[5] Lower stimulation rates result in synchronous neural activity. A number of factors specific to the individual (etiology of deafness, duration of deafness, neural survival) may explain why a faster stimulation rate isn't necessarily better. Some clinicians will provide new users with programs of differing stimulation rates, programming patients according to subjective preferences for sound quality and loudness.

FREQUENCY ALLOCATION

The frequency range or frequency allocation of stimuli delivered to the implant is typically set at the outset of programming with modifications commonly applied based on the patient's subjective reaction to sound quality. Default frequency ranges are provided by the manufacturers based on their sound coding philosophies. Across companies, frequency limits may range from 63 Hz to 8700 Hz. Frequency assignment across individual electrodes or channels is typically assigned by the software based on the number of available electrodes.

FINE TUNING

The goal of fine tuning is to optimize the patient's sound quality and clarity. Suc-cessful fine tuning is dependant upon the patient's ability to discriminate small change in sound. Fine-tuning approaches will vary across clinics, clinicians, and patient population.

Once the fundamental map parameters (strategy, rate, pulse duration, frequency boundaries) have been established and the electrical dynamic range has been established, a personal listening program can be created.

BALANCING AND SWEEPING

Balancing loudness percepts across the electrode array when possible is an important tool to avoid loudness spikes which can be uncomfortable to the listener. The objective of balancing is to provide the listener with an equal sense of loudness across the array. Differences in relative loudness across electrodes can result in discomfort in some cases and negative sound quality in others. Balancing electrodes for loudness can be accomplished using as few as two electrodes at a time or multiple electrodes in a sweep. Sweeping refers to stimulating several successive electrodes. When stimulated at the maximum electrical dynamic range, the listener is instructed to report the "offending" electrode so that its stimulation level may be increased or decreased to be more comparable with adjacent electrodes. The clinician may also sweep and balance at an intermediate level (eg, 50%) within the dynamic range. This facilitates fine tuning of thresholds levels resulting in improved sound quality and loudness growth within the dynamic range. Successful balancing and sweeping is dependent on the patient's ability to provide reliable subjective comparisons between electrodes.

FREQUENCY CONSIDERATIONS

Intuitively, providing the patient with the broadest frequency range gives them access to the greatest amount of available auditory information. As most clinician's recognize, subjective responses to the broadest range may be negative. The following is a brief discussion of techniques available to optimize the frequency parameters for an individual.

Modification of the Frequency Boundaries

An individual's subjective response to the sound quality of the program may direct the clinician to make modifications to the frequency response parameters. Although high frequency information is critical to the recognition of speech, not all implant recipients can utilize the broadest available frequency range. This may result from a distorted percept from having been deprived of this frequency of stimulation for a prolonged period or poor neural survival at the location of the electrode contact. In these cases, it may be necessary to lower the high frequency boundary of the most basal electrode(s).

Low-frequency information provides the listener with fine structure information that contributes to the quality of individual pitches. This information is thought to be especially important for appreciation of music and for localizing sound.[6] It follows then that providing the greatest amount of low frequency information should provide the greatest benefit to the implant user. Most hearing loss occurs in the high frequencies initially. Consequently, lower frequency sounds are the most familiar and are often better

tolerated by new implant users. However, just as some patients are unable to appreciate very high frequency information others report deleterious effects from too much low frequency information. Patients commonly complain of their voice sounding "boomy" or ambient noise being too pervasive. This may direct the clinician to reduce lower frequency stimulation by increasing the low frequency limit of the most apical electrode. The programming audiologist must walk a fine line when adjusting the frequency range provided to the patient. Ideally, small changes to the frequency response will correct for the negative patient percept without taking away from speech discrimination and overall sound appreciation.

Frequency Shaping

Frequency shaping can be accomplished by gain modifications or by adjusting the upper limits of the dynamic range. The programming software of Cochlear Corporation and Advanced Bionics allow for modification of the gain parameter on a group of successive or individual electrodes, respectively. When modifying gains, the clinician is adjusting the amplitude of the signal prior to the output stage.

Both Cochlear and MED-EL software allows the clinician to shape the frequency response by applying global modifications to the electrical dynamic ranges (ie, "tilting") or individual electrode modifications, respectively. For example, in the Cochlear software, the clinician may elect to provide the patient with an upward tilting electrical dynamic range generally meaning that progressively increased stimulation will be delivered to the basal electrodes. Concomitantly, progressively lower electrical stimulation will be delivered the apical electrodes. This may be done when the patient has difficulty tolerating their own voice or requires enhancement to effectively discriminate higher frequency consonants. Conversely, an individual with longer term deafness who is most accustomed to traditional amplification of lower frequencies may have difficulty adapting to the higher frequency sounds provided by a cochlear implant. In this case, it may be beneficial to provide a tilt with increased low and reduced high frequency stimulation. Gradual flattening of this tilt may be introduced as the individual becomes more accepting of higher frequency stimuli. Separate from gain changes to the entire electrode array, Advanced Bionics software provides for more discreet frequency shaping by allowing gain modifications to individual electrodes at the clinician's discretion. Cochlear software, on the other hand, allows for modification of basal, mid, or apical electrodes as a group.

INPUT DYNAMIC RANGE

Input dynamic range (IDR) defines the electrical dynamic range or "window of sound" provided to the user. Philosophies vary as to the appropriate input dynamic range across manufacturers. Advanced Bionics favors use of a broad IDR (up to 80 dB) to preserve the relative relationship between soft, medium, and loud sounds. That said, a 60 dB range is the recommended setting for general use. Cochlear Corporation offers an IDR range of 20 to 75 dB, most commonly spanning 25 to 65 dB. By use of Auto Sensitivity and Instantaneous Input Dynamic Range settings, the incoming signal selected for

delivery represents the dynamic range of soft to loud speech rather than background noise. MED-EL offers a 75 dB IDR using a 55 dB sound window that "roves" between 25 to 100 dB. This allows for mapping of the broader incoming signal into the recipient's narrow electrical dynamic range.

Clinicians have the latitude to set the IDR relative to user needs. A broader IDR may be more desirable for a dynamic acoustic signal such as music where there is interest in preserving the relationship between particularly diverse intensity signals. Narrowing the IDR may be useful when the recipient complains that lower intensity background sounds or environmental noise are intrusive. This would result in the mapping these sounds lower in the recipient's electrical dynamic range softening these sounds from the user's perspective.

ASSESSING INTERNAL HARDWARE FUNCTION

Proper internal device function is integral to a patient's success with their cochlear implant system. Monitoring internal device function is an ongoing process. Tools available include implant telemetry testing by the clinician and integrity testing with manufacturer support when indicated.

IMPEDANCE TELEMETRY TESTING

Current implant technologies allows for delivery of a stimulus as well as a *telemetry* mechanism to allow for feedback of electrical activity information in the form of impedances and/or auditory neural responses. Implant telemetry testing or impedance testing should always be conducted at the outset of patient programming. Impedance refers to resistance to the flow of current through the electrode/internal hardware and through the patient's tissue. Particularly at the time of initial activation, impedance telemetry testing can provide information as to the viability of individual electrodes. For example, the internal array can demonstrate open electrodes which may require deactivation prior to stimulation. Shorted electrodes will be identified as well and deactivated or maintained based on patient percept. High impedances may result in decreased compliance levels. Compliance is the inverse measure of impedance, reflecting the ease of current flow and the ability of the electrode to deliver the desired stimulation level. Compliance values are electrode specific. If compliance levels are exceeded, the clinician cannot be assured that the system is providing the desired levels of stimulation given the predefined mapping parameters.

IMPEDANCE TELEMETRY MEASURES

Impedance generally refers to the opposition or resistance to the flow of energy. Information regarding the electrical impedance of the electrode is desirable as it can provide feedback regarding the function of the electrodes and their ability to deliver the stimulation sufficiently to the surviving neural elements. High impedance measures may result from open circuits (eg, a break in the electrode wiring), air bubbles, extracochlear placement, or excessive intracochlear tissue growth.

High impedances can sometimes necessitate deactivation of electrodes in question or a change in the stimulation mode (ie, the relationship between the active and indifferent electrode). Unusually low impedance measures may indicate a short circuit (ie, direct physical contact) between two electrodes or their wiring. Deactivation of shorted electrodes is often based on patient sound quality percepts with and without inclusion of the offenders in a patient's program or map.

INTEGRITY TESTING

Integrity testing is a specialized test battery completed by a clinical specialist representing the implant manufacturer. This testing is indicated when a patient's performance is poorer than expected, declines unexplainably, or when the patient experiences atypical percepts. Integrity testing allows for a more thorough investigation of implant function than is available clinically. Device function is assessed via far-field scalp recordings. Measurements look at a variety of implant characteristics including: electrode current flow, amplitude growth functions, pulse duration growth functions, intermittencies, device power-up, and function of the receiver/stimulator. The results of the integrity test provide information about whether the device is functioning according to the manufacturer's specifications.

SPECIAL PROGRAMMING NEEDS

Occasionally, the function of the implant will result in programming needs that go beyond the routine fine-tuning that most implant patients receive. The clinician may be called upon to manipulate the electrical signal in a more detailed manner than is typically required. Implant programming can be especially challenging in these cases.

IMPEDANCE/COMPLIANCE ISSUES

As previously discussed, telemetry measures provide information regarding the electrical impedance of the electrode. High electrode impedances and consequent low electrode compliance values may confound programming efforts. The challenge that arises when compliance levels are exceeded is that the maximum implant voltage cannot generate the desired current level. The patient experience is inadequate or no loudness growth. To achieve maximum /most comfortable listening, the electrodes may be managed by modifying map parameters such as the rate of stimulation and pulse duration. A necessary alternative may be deactivation of the offending electrode entirely.

FACIAL STIMULATION

Occasionally stimulation of the cochlear implant will result in the patient reporting a sensation other than hearing. These sensations are referred to as "nonauditory percepts." Facial stimulation is one of if not the most common form of nonauditory percept. The proximity of the facial nerve to the auditory nerve leaves it vulnerable to unwanted spread of electrical stimulation from the cochlear implant. The degree of stimulation varies in its presentation. Facial stimulation can range from a light twitch that is felt but not visible to

severe facial grimacing. Regardless of its presentation, facial nerve stimulation is bothersome to the patient and should be managed through programming.

Nonauditory percept of this form can result from a single electrode, a group of adjacent electrodes, or from cumulative stimulation of the entire array. Psychophysical measurements may be used to identify the offending electrode(s). The clinician may stimulate discreet electrodes at the patient's maximum levels and monitor for any aversive nonauditory percepts. It may not be possible to identify a single or group of electrodes causing the problem. A number of management options are available when nonauditory percepts are present. These include: reduction of the maximum stimulation level, peak-clipping, increasing the pulse duration, and, if necessary, deactivation of one or several electrodes. The effect of increasing the pulse duration or widening the pulse width is to allow for comparable loudness percept at a reduced current level, thus lessening the likelihood of unwanted current spread.

LIMITED ELECTRODE AVAILABILITY

Electrode availability may be limited by factors such as partial insertion of the array or internal device anomalies (eg, shorts or open circuits). The anatomical condition of the cochlea (dysmorphology or ossification) may preclude complete insertion of the electrode array. The risk of partial insertion may be known prior to surgery via imaging studies. It should be evident in all cases at the time of surgery. It is helpful for the programming audiologist to be aware of a partial insertion prior to activation of the implant. This will allow the clinician to avoid stimulating extracochlear electrodes which can elicit uncomfortable, nonauditory percepts. The topic of shorted electrodes or open circuits were addressed previously (see Impedance Telemetry Testing). When the number of viable electrodes is severely limited, the patient's speech recognition can be compromised. There are programming techniques which maximize patient benefit in these situations.

As discussed earlier, there are a number of speech coding strategies available to the programming audiologist. When faced with the dilemma of a limited number of electrodes the audiologist may opt to use a strategy that better utilizes a lesser number of electrodes. This option will be limited by the number of speech coding strategies which are made available in the individual manufacturer's software.

Historically, a second programming option was employed in cases of limited electrode availability. This method, known as double channel mapping, involved the assigning of multiple frequency bands to a single electrode, thus creating a double channel of stimulation. This allowed for a wider frequency allocation then was delivered by single channel mapping with a reduced number of electrodes. Currently, the programming software from the three manufacturers automatically reassigns frequency allocation based on the number of available electrodes, making double channel mapping unnecessary.

ness, age of onset of deafness, duration of deafness, experience with or benefit from amplification, tinnitus) collectively can contribute to their success and satisfaction with a cochlear implant. At the time of activation, it is not only essential to provide the patient with an appropriate program but to counsel them also about realistic expectations. The auditory signal through the implant can be very disparate from what they remember. Consequently, their initial listening experience can be challenging. Patients must understand the importance of daily use and practice. Programming the adult patient is most successful when done collaboratively. They should be encouraged to actively participate in the process by providing both positive and negative feedback on what they are hearing.

The frequency with which patients return for programming varies from clinic to clinic. Our approach is to see patients for a series of 3 to 4 appointments, spread over a 4- to 6-week period either weekly or biweekly. Because the patient may experience significant changes in hearing during the initial weeks of use, more frequent appointments may be necessary to maintain appropriate programming. As hearing stabilizes, the need for reprogramming lessens. Return appointments are spaced over several month intervals. After one year, patients are followed for annual evaluation. Interim programming is managed on an as needed basis.

FREQUENCY OF PROGRAMMING/PATIENT VARIABLES

Perhaps the greatest variables in programming are the patient themselves. Their hearing history (eg, etiology of deaf-

CONCLUSION

Cochlear implant programming has become increasingly streamlined providing the clinician with numerous tools to effectively transform an acoustic signal into something electrically functional for the patient. A good understanding of the parameters available, their functions, and their interactions is integral in providing the patient with an optimal outcome. There are a number of excellent texts available that explore the different aspects of cochlear implantation on a much more detailed level than is presented here.[7–9] The reader is referred to the Web sites of the implant manufacturers for additional information about their individual philosophies of cochlear implant programming.[10–12]

REFERENCES

1. Holstad BA, Sonneveldt VG, Fears BT, et al. Relation of electrically evoked compound action potential thresholds to behvioral T- and C-levels in children with cochlear implants. *Ear Hear.* 2009;30:115–127.
2. Potts LG, Skinner MW, Gotter BD, Strube MJ, Brenner CA. Relation between neural response telemetry thresholds, T- and C-levels, and loudness judgments in 12 adult nucleus 24 cochlear implant recipients. *Ear Hear.* 2007;28:495–511.
3. Hodges AV, Balkany TJ, Ruth RA, Lambert PR, Dolan-Ash S, Schloffman JJ. Electrical middle ear muscle reflex: use in cochlear implant programming. *Otolaryngol Head Neck Surg.* 1997;117:255–261.
4. Bresnihan M, Norman G, Scott F, Viani L. Measurement of comfort levels by means of electrical stapedial reflex in children. *Arch Otolaryngol Head Neck Surg.* 2001; 127:963–966.
5. Shannon RV, Cruz RJ, Galvin JJ. Effect of stimulation rate on cochlear implant users' phoneme, word and sentence recognition in quiet and in noise. *Audiol Neurotol.* 2011;16:113–123.
6. Smith ZM, Delbutte B, Oxenham AJ. Chimaeric sounds reveal dichotomies in auditory perception. *Nature.* 2002;416:87.
7. Cullington H, ed. *Cochlear Implants Objective Measures.* London and Philadelphia: Whurr Publishers; 2003.
8. Niparko JK. *Cochlear Implants Principles and Practices.* 2nd ed. Philadelphia, PA: Wolters Kluwer/Lippincott Williams & Wilkins; 2009.
9. Wolfe J, Schafer EC. *Programming Cochlear Implants.* San Diego, CA: Plural Publishing; 2010.
10. Advanced Bionics. Retrieved March 24, 2011 from http://www.advancedbionics.com/For_Professionals/?langid=1
11. Cochlear Corporation. Retrieved March 13, 2011 from http://professionals.cochlear.com/
12. MED-EL Corporation. Retrieved March 13, 2011 from http://www.medel.com/us/index/indes/id/1/title/home

Chapter 13

Pediatric Cochlear Implant Programming: A Basic Introduction

MICHAEL F. JACKSON

INTRODUCTION

To make appropriate adjustments to a cochlear implantation the pediatric population, it is critical to understand auditory skill development as well as the technology. Extrapolating the combination of behavioral responses, clinical observations, parent observation, and school reports shape a child's cochlear implant program. A program, or "map," is a set of clinician-determined parameters that control how sound is manipulated into an electrical signal presented through a finite number of electrodes. Observing how a child's behaviors direct further adjustments are equally as important as understanding how elements of timing, intensity and pitch construct a cochlear implant program. A young child may not be able to give direct feedback in the form of a hand raise or a yes-no response to a question. Moreover, although a cochlear implant can provide near immediate access to sound (ie, the sense of hearing), success with an implant is gauged in how a child is able to use that sound meaningfully (ie, the skill of listening and understanding).

THE PREOPERATIVE EVALUATION

A child's ability to utilize electrical stimulation for understanding speech is dependent on many factors. Some include: age of onset of hearing loss, previous experience with hearing aids, present auditory skills, language and/or intellectual abilities, cochlear anatomy, family structure and support, and educational program. With appropriate medical and clinical evaluations, many of these factors may be evident during determination of cochlear implant candidacy. Programming considerations are dependent on the best possible understanding of a child's abilities and challenges. A comprehensive preoperative evaluation is critical to determine understanding and predicting a child's postoperative needs. The Children's Implant Profile (ChIP) is an effective tool in understanding a child's specific strengths and areas of concern preoperatively. [1-4] Many centers use their own modified version of the ChIP (mChIP) specific for their population. The profile lists criteria from different disciplines (ie, audiology, speech language pathology, social work, and education). Concerns raised in any of these areas may impact cochlear implant outcomes. For example, audiologic factors that influence outcome with a cochlear implant may include: preoperative test reliability, attention/behavior, hearing aid use, parental compliance with previous recommendations, hearing aid benefit (amount of residual hearing), auditory skills given chronologic age, duration of deafness, as well as other disabilities. Although one purpose of the ChIP or mChIP is to determine if a child will obtain enough benefit with a cochlear implant to justify surgery, the other purpose is to proactively identify concerns that may arise during postoperative programming. Counseling about these issues is critical for parents, patient, family, and educators in order to proactively address areas of concern and appropriate expectations.

EQUIPMENT ORIENTATION

The introduction of a cochlear implant is the start of many expectations, both for the child and their parents. First, the child must acclimate to wearing the speech processor on the ear. For those with limited hearing aid experience, this can be a difficult transition. For children under the age of six, some centers provide families the cochlear implant equipment prior to ini-

tial activation. The equipment orientation allows parents to familiarize themselves with the speech processor and additional equipment. Parents can review the manufacturer materials to better prepare themselves to support, as well as advocate for their child once they use the device daily. The child can practice wearing the speech processor and parents can trial different speech processor retention tools, either from the manufacturer or purchased by the parents. (eg, cotton "pilot" cap or bonnet). Men's toupee tape can be effective for processor retention. Toupee tape should be restricted in the weeks following surgery as its application could irritate the healing surgical site. For children over the age of 6, the equipment orientation and initial activation can be performed on the same day at the discretion of the clinician.

SETTING UP THE ROOM FOR PROGRAMMING

For children, especially younger children, the setup of the room is a critical component of effective cochlear implant programming. As the child will be returning for many programming visits over the years, the room should be inviting, comfortable, but structured for the purpose of listening. Toys should be kept out of sight, but easily available as needed. Children will more likely respond to sound when comfortable; so having a variety of seating arrangements is preferable. Although the parent's lap is sometimes the best choice for the child to sit based on their comfort and age, the child should also be provided other options to promote independent listening during the programming session. A high chair, a small table and chair, and larger chairs for older children and adults, should all be available. The back of a high chair has a tendency to brush off a child's coil during programming. A small, firm pillow to bolster the child's back is helpful in positioning the child for proper coil retention.

Some clinics have the availability of two clinicians, or an audiologist and trained support staff, to serve as programmer and assistant. While the audiologist works behind the computer screen, the assistant can keep the child occupied and on task. Two audiologists or an audiologist and a trained assistant are ideal, but sometimes are not available in a busy clinic setting. If support staff is not available, a "one clinician" setup can be utilized. With some practice, the clinician can have access to the keyboard and mouse while still being within arm's reach of the child. The parent, at the clinician's discretion, can also be used as an assistant. With instruction and continued clinician observation, many parents can provide useful support in redirecting a child to the programming tasks.

INITIAL ACTIVATION

The initial activation process is typically performed over one or two consecutive days, followed by anappointment after-one or two weeks. The most fluctuation in program levels occurs in the first three months of continued implant use, but especially in the first week. Allowing a child to return a week or two following the initial activation, allows for electrode conditioning, as well as increased experience with sound, increasing the likelihood of meaningful behavioral feedback.

The child may not have seen the implanting surgeon since implantation. At the initial activation, the implant site should be inspected for any atypical appearance. This inspection should in no way replace the necessary post operative medical examination, but an experienced clinician should be aware of red flags such as redness, swelling, continued complaints of pain, or dizziness. Even minor concerns should be immediately relayed to the child's surgeon as to prevent further escalation. Moving forward, this inspection should be a part of each subsequent programming visit.

The clinician should offer the weakest magnet necessary to consistently affix the headpiece to the site. Excessive magnet strength may lead to skin problems requiring the child to discontinue use of processor while the magnet site heals. It is helpful to have a variety of magnets in stock to choose the most appropriate fit for a child.

MEASURING IMPEDANCES

The following is a summary of programming protocols at initial activation as well as any subsequent programming appointment. After connecting the speech processor to the programming computer and placing the processor over the implant, the clinician first measures the impedance levels of each channel. The impedance levels measure a channel's resistance to electrical flow. If any electrodes are not functioning properly, such as with open (very high impedance) or shorted circuits (very low impedance), those channels or stimulation modes should be deactivated from future programs. Use of shorted or open circuits may present a distorted, unpredictable signal to the child. Given the implant has not been stimulated in 3 to 4 weeks following surgery, impedance levels will be higher than at later programming sessions. Conversely, compliance levels for each channel will be lower than for long-term users. Compliance is the estimation of how much current a channel is capable to provide. This fluctuation is due to several factors, including the need for the electrodes to stimulate and condition to electric stimulation. With continued implant use, impedance levels will decrease. Therefore, children may experience fluctuations in volume with initial programs, without changes to the mapping parameters. Over time, loudness and mapping parameters should stabilize.

SPEECH-CODING STRATEGIES

Choosing the speech-coding strategy, or how the processor uses the elements of pitch, timing, and intensity to create an electrical signal, is an important consideration. Children, unlike adults, do not have the ability to trial various strategies to determine the optimal choice. Variability across clinics exists in which coding strategy, rate, or manufacturer proprietary parameters to use at initial activation. This choice will depend on current clinical practice, available electrodes, anatomic considerations as well as the speech-coding strategy used in the opposite ear if the patient receives a sequential bilateral cochlear implant. Clinicians should consult with the cochlear implant manufacturers for the current recommendations for initial speech-coding strategies.

If a child is appearing to meet appropriate speech and language goals, little change may required to the program parameters beyond continued psychophysical measurements. Until the child can provide feedback regarding sound quality, the clinician should minimize arbitrary changes to programming parameters without confidence that the sound quality will be improved. If through audiologic and speech-language assessment, poor progress is noted, a change to signal coding strategy may be considered. Although the speech-coding strategy is important, a more critical factor is appropriate psychophysical measurements within the chosen processing strategy. The first goal in programming is to provide comfortable audibility. This is done through measurement of individual channel threshold levels (as with Cochlear Corporation software), or by globally increasing stimulation with the microphone active (as with Advanced Bionics and MED-EL software) The need to measure threshold levels, or the level at which a child begins to consistently perceive a sound, is dependent on which speech-coding strategy is utilized. If other changes are made to the program (eg gain or maxima adjustments), the changes should be small, deliberate, and monitored at subsequent programming visits to ascertain effect on performance.

PSYCHOPHYSICAL AND OBJECTIVE MEASUREMENTS

Children arrive to the initial activation appointment with a great variability in previous auditory experience. This variability may present with additional challenges to the clinician in determining how the child will give feedback allowing for optimal cochlear implant programming. Some have used hearing aids with success, others have used hearing aids but given severity of hearing loss, have only attained the ability to detect, rather than discriminate speech. Others may have had little to no auditory experience due to severity of hearing loss or lack of consistent hearing aid use. The greater exposure to meaningful sound predisposes a child for improved speech perception outcomes with a cochlear implant.[5] The primary objective in cochlear implant programming is determining how much electrical current provides the most appropriate, comfortable access to sound. An adult, as described in Chapter 12, can provide direct, verbal feedback. However, for young children other ways to determine programming parameters are required.

VISUAL REINFORCEMENT AUDIOMETRY

Visual reinforcement audiometry (VRA) is an effective method in measuring hearing sensitivity for children between 6 months and 2 and a half years of age. Visual reinforcement uses operant conditioning techniques to teach a child to look to an object (eg, a lighted, animated, mechanical toy) whenever they hear a sound. When the audiologist provides the stimulus, either a specific electrode, group of electrodes, or live voice such as with the Ling sounds, the child's eye shift or head turn response is rewarded by activation of the toy. The child's attention is then distracted back to midline. Once the child can respond to stimuli at suprathreshold levels, a clinician can reduce the level of the stimulus to effectively measure threshold levels using traditional audiometric bracketing technique.

CONDITIONED PLAY AUDIOMETRY

Once the child nears 30 months of age, he or she may begin to tire of the reinforcing toy and need more engaging games. Although VRA is a more passive activity, conditioned play audiometry is a tool to allow a child a more active role in their programming by making a game out of listening. A variety of toys can be used wherein a child is conditioned to respond to an auditory stimulus. Examples of effective conditioned play games for programming are throwing blocks in a bucket, placing large beads on a string, putting stickers on a piece of paper, or inserting coins in a piggy bank. Once the child is conditioned, the audiologist can use traditional audiometric bracketing technique to obtain threshold measurements. These games should be engaging, but not too exciting, as the child may not be inclined to listen, but rather just play with the toy. Several games may be required to complete one programming session. Children with cochlear implants will be performing these tasks often, so it is important to keep a good supply of varied toys for rotation.

Responses obtained solely through VRA or CPA methods are a critical component of programming children, but often are not enough to create the most appropriate map for a child. A child in the beginning stages of learning to listen may provide very limited feedback with VRA or CPA tools. A child with profound hearing loss may have difficulty understanding expectations of the task. The ability of a child to adopt the "listening posture" necessary to respond to sound may be unrefined. Sitting quietly, following an adult led game, and just the act of listening, may be developing skills for a young child. A child may respond to a novel sound once, but not again. A child may quickly grow tired of a game and not want to participate. Unsuccessful attempts at obtaining these conditioned responses are however not without purpose. In these cases, visual reinforcement and conditioned play are important routines for the child to learn for future programming sessions. Practicing these psychophysical measurement techniques can also be addressed in the child's regular sessions with their early interventionist, speech-language pathologist, itinerant hearing support teacher, or teacher of the deaf.

BEHAVIORAL OBSERVATION

For children not yet able to master VRA or CPA, observation of nonconditioned behavioral responses may indicate a sound is audible, or possibly uncomfortable: a cocked eyebrow, stilling, changes in sucking pattern of a pacifier, eye shift, crying, or looking to a parent for reassurance. In the first few months with a cochlear implant however, a young child may be unable to show a consistent behavioral response to sound at threshold or suprathreshold levels. Behavioral observation is an informal, but useful method when used in conjunction with other objective and behavioral programming methods. Use of BO requires other crosscheck procedures. Elements of behavioral observation, although not a formal technique, help guide the clinician along with other methods in determination of appropriate parameters. A clinician should note these responses during programming and evaluation, but clearly document that these are observations of behavior and not necessarily indicative of threshold measurement.

ESTIMATING LOUDNESS LEVELS

Although establishing threshold is a more concrete concept, determination of "How loud is loud enough?" can be more abstract. Controlling loudness, or the maximal stimulation of each channel can be a challenging part of programming children. Balancing audibility and comfort is a difficult concept for anyone with a cochlear implant, but especially a young child. With continued implant use, current needs will change, but in the beginning tolerance for electricity will likely be low. Although adults can provide direct feedback to determine what is too soft or too loud, children cannot provide such feedback. Behavioral observation can be used to ascertain comfort with stimulation of both individual channels or in live voice. Other, more objective, methods are also available.

The Electrically Evoked Middle Ear Reflex

The electrically evoked middle ear muscle reflex, or EMEMR, is a commonly used tool in setting upper comfort levels.[6,7] To measure EMEMR, the clinician places an immittance probe in the ear opposite the cochlear implant. The probe is placed in the contralateral ear because, although the middle ear muscle reflex is bilateral, it is more likely to be observed in the nonsurgical ear. While the acoustic admittance is being recorded, the clinician chooses a channel and presents the electrical stimulus in an ascending manner. The middle ear muscle reflex will be observed when the stimulus reaches the EMEMR level, and the response will be absent at presentation levels below EMEMR. EMEMR can be measured on multiple channels and comfort levels for unmeasured channels can be interpolated. As with any objective measurement, comfort levels should be decreased from EMEMR determined levels, prior to activation of the microphone.

Once the live program is determined to be comfortable, the comfort levels can be globally increased with the clinician observing the child's behavior for signs of discomfort.

The Electrically Evoked Compound Action Potential

Another objective, but less effective method to measure loudness is the ECAP, or electrically evoked compound action potential. Depending on the manufacturer used, this neural response measurement goes by different terminology (NRI, NRT, ART). Although useful in the operating room to determine appropriate device function, or postoperatively to confirm audibility on tested channels, there can be considerable patient variability in threshold and comfort levels as compared to ECAP thresholds. ECAP thresholds should not be used as a primary measurement to estimate loudness. Along with threshold measurement, behavioral observation, EMEMR, and loudness scaling, it should serve as a cross-check component to establish a contour of how much current may be required across the array.[8]

Behavioral Measurements of Loudness

Before a child leaves the programming session, the audiologist should verify that the newly created program presents all sounds at a comfortable level. This can be performed by "sweeping" the electrodes. Sweeping electrodes presents each channel at a percentage up to its maximal level of the dynamic range. Although a young child will not be able to make loudness judgments, the clinician should observe any apparent discomfort or facial stimulation related to individual channel stimu-

lation. Older children, typically around 8 years of age, may be able to discriminate loudness between channels. This method is called "balancing" and addresses the establishment of equal loudness across the array.

Following electrode sweeping and balancing, the program should be activated to live voice. The clinician should quickly spot check Ling sound detection[9] ("ah," "ee," "oo," "sh," "ss," "mm"), watching for discomfort as well as to confirm detection. If the child is older, the clinician can ask the child to informally repeat words to see if performance meets previously established levels. The purpose of this quick listening check is to look for sound confusions or sound omissions prior to disconnecting the processor from the computer. Some phoneme confusions can be addressed with mapping changes. For example, if a child demonstrates high frequency phoneme confusion, they may benefit from a high-frequency emphasis program. Information from parents regarding speech errors or discomfort with certain sounds may mandate changes in the program.

Around the age of 5 or 6, children can transition from conditioned play games to more traditional hand raising testing techniques. Still, they are by no means small adults. A 5-year-old, although often more compliant than a younger toddler, still may have difficulty providing feedback for the purposes of making programming changes. It is not until children are approximately 8 years of age wherein they can reliably provide consistent loudness discrimination. Judging loudness can be a difficult concept for a child with the cochlear implant because if comfort levels have been programmed appropriately, no sound they have experienced should be "too loud." Some children with limited language may also have difficulty making qualitative distinctions. Pointing to picture cards showing animated concepts of "too soft," "good," and "too loud" can be used. These cards may use graphic representations of loudness such as happy and sad faces familiar to children.

SOUND QUALITY AT INITIAL ACTIVATION

Performance at initial activation is highly variable and not necessarily indicative of long-term outcomes. Sound quality at initial activation can be quite poor, but will improve with continued wear and regular programming. A child's ability to tolerate electrical current is much lower in the initial weeks and months following initial activation. With limited feedback from the child, it is important to program conservatively in the initial programming sessions. The activation of the speech processor may be the first significant exposure a child has to sound. Reactions of fear, crying, or laughter are typical and should be expected. Given the lack of meaningful exposure to sound, the child may have no reaction at all. Parents should be counseled as to the range of possible reactions. The goal of the initial activation is to provide a comfortable program for the child to go home and wear the speech processor with consistency. Once an initial program is created, the clinician should provide the parents with a range of volume control so that, when they place the processor on their child's head, it will be not be too loud. Parents are instructed that after the child is wearing the device and appears to be acclimated to the loudness, to increase the volume of the program. Current speech

processors can hold either three or four programs. The clinician should provide multiple programs of slightly increased loudness (ie, higher current). Once at home, parents can access these programs by adjusting controls on the processor as their child's tolerance allows.

Following activation of the processor microphone, the clinician can perform a listening check, either in a sound booth or informally in the programming room. Many clinicians use the "Ling" sounds to provide an estimate of detection across the speech frequency spectrum. Often, children are not able to show consistent awareness given their previous limited exposure to meaningful sound. Older children with greater auditory abilities may be able to begin to discriminate closed set words, or even open set words or sentences.

Even with a successful equipment orientation, families may not be fully transitioned in adopting this new technology into their lives. Parents are told the child should wear the processor during all waking hours, which can be a struggle. Conservatively programming the device in the initial program visits allows for the child to more easily bond with the device without risk of sound being uncomfortably loud. Parents should be counseled that "louder is not necessarily better" and arbitrarily raising stimulation levels might not expedite habilitation.

THE FIRST THREE MONTHS AND BEYOND

Following the initial appointment and 1-week follow-up, the child should return for continued programming approximately one month following initial activation. Postoperative appointment schedules vary by clinic. Families generally should return every month for the first 3 months postactivation. Following the 3-month appointment, the child should return every 3 months until the one-year anniversary of the device activation. Following this time, children may return on an as needed basis, but no longer than every 6 months until the clinician, parent, and educators are comfortable that the child's program progress is stable. Typically, this can take several years. Following that point, the child should return annually for reprogramming, evaluation, and equipment status check.

Every postactivation appointment should begin with a brief history from the parent followed by an audiometric evaluation. The components of the audiogram will vary based on the age and auditory skill level of the child but could be composed of a combination of the following:

1. A speech awareness threshold to Ling sounds.
2. A speech reception threshold to familiarized spondee words, either closed set or open set based on child's auditory skill level.
3. A measurement of frequency specific thresholds to FM stimuli in the sound field, 0.25 to 4 kHz. Elevated thresholds measured in the sound field may be due to a variety of factors: a need to increase current levels in the program, an impaired microphone, or a child's inattentiveness to sound.
4. Discrimination testing to the child's abilities. This may include closed or open set discrimination, in quiet or noise. If a child has two cochlear implants, or a cochlear implant and a hearing aid, unilateral and bilateral testing should be attempted. A full battery of testing may not be possible given time constraints, the child's age, mood, or auditory abilities.

Initial audiograms following cochlear implant activation are unlikely to be optimal. Behavioral responses are likely elevated as compared to long-term implant users. As children acclimate to the electric signal, they will be able to respond to softer sounds. Within the first 2 to 3 months, a child's audiogram should approach optimal sound field responses to speech and FM tones between 20 to 25 dB HL or even lower. These levels are measurements of hearing sensitivity and not indicative of speech reception or understanding.

Following audiologic booth testing, the psychophysical programming measurements made at the previous session should be reassessed. This procedure is similar to the procedure described at the initial activation. However, the child presents with the auditory skills gained in the previous weeks or months. Testing methods will change as the child matures, moving from visual reinforcement tasks, to conditioned play tasks to more traditional adult (hand-raising) techniques. The objective is however the same: optimize psychophysical parameters (ie, threshold and comfort levels). The audiologist should confer with the other professionals working with the child to confirm appropriate auditory, speech, or language milestones are being reached. If not, further changes to programming parameters may be necessary.

Equipment status is an important factor in how a child is hearing especially if the child has shown a recent regression in performance. An impaired microphone, intermittent cable coil, faulty processor can have significant impact on a child's performance. A well-stocked troubleshooting kit is a critical tool during programming sessions. The kit should contain a spare processor, monitor earphones, and accessories for each of the speech processors the clinician may encounter.

THE AUDITORY HIERARCHY

Parents and professionals working with this population should have an understanding of auditory skill development. It is effective for development of listening and spoken language or auditory function .It encourages exposure to meaningful communication accessible at the child's skill level. Children's discrimination abilities move from closed set to open set; children understand shorter, then longer utterances. Many models have been offered on auditory skill development, usually comprised of at least four main stages[10,11]:

1. Detection: Showing awareness to voice, environmental sounds, or Ling sounds. Children at initial activation and the weeks following generally demonstrate this response to sound with behaviors such as stilling, eye widening, or crying. Later, detection can be observed with visual reinforcement, conditioned play, or traditional hand-raising techniques.

2. Discrimination: Perceiving similarities or differences between two or more speech stimuli or sounds. The child is able to attend to differences among sounds and respond differently (eg, "mmmm" versus "no no no," or "ball" and "shoe").

3. Identification: Using awareness to associate the stimulus with previous experiences, world knowledge. (eg, hearing a word and pointing to a picture, imitating a word presented).

4. Comprehension: Demonstrating understanding of a language concept and relating it to other concepts (eg, answering a question through auditory input only).

Depending on their auditory skill and their language base, children with cochlear implants could present at any of these stages. For those with prior auditory skill development, progression through the beginning stages may be faster than for those with no prior auditory experience. Understanding these stages gives parents the structure to work on developmentally appropriate skills and see goals achieved as they happen. A child's current auditory skill will affect their ability to participate in programming as well as performance evaluation tasks. For more information on development of auditory skills, please refer to the works cited at the end of the chapter.[9]

PROGRAMMING CHILDREN WITH MALFORMED ANATOMY

Review of the operative report as well as continued collaboration with the cochlear implant surgeon is critical, especially when working with a child with abnormal anatomy or incomplete electrode insertion. The electrode placement, verified by postoperative imaging or surgical consult, plays an important factor in device programming. Electrodes outside of the cochlea should be identified and deactivated from any future programs. An abnormal course of the facial nerve, or need for increased current, may predispose a user to experience facial stimulation. Facial stimulation may be observed as a twitching of the eye, lip, neck, or side of face. The facial stimulation may occur with individual channel stimulation or when the microphone is activated. If the facial stimulation can be isolated to a specific channel or channels, the upper stimulation level of that channel can be reduced, clipped, or duration of the pulse (ie, pulsewidth) increased. If these attempts are made without resolution of the facial stimulation, or inability to achieve appropriate loudness growth on the channel, the channel itself may need to be deactivated from the active program. Frequencies previously allocated to that channel are then reallocated to adjacent channels in the electrode array.

The presence of cochlear malformations may impact performance outcomes.[13,14] Examples of these conditions are: a common cavity, postmeningitis ossified cochlea, or a small cochlear nerve. The presence of inner ear malformation can be related to other syndromic conditions that could also impact outcomes with a cochlear implant. These malformations may necessitate the surgeon to use a varied style of electrode arrays, such as a straight, compressed, or split array, to allow for the best electrode contact with surviving spiral ganglion cells. Families should have been counseled prior to surgery on the guarded performance expectations that may come with cochlear malformations. Exceptions always exist, but given their presence, the tonotopic organization of the significantly malformed cochlea or auditory nerve may not preserve the same frequency specificity afforded to a child with typical anatomy.

In these cases, more optimal language outcomes are associated with an earlier age of implantation.[15]

PROGRAMMING CHILDREN WITH OTHER DIAGNOSES

Many factors beyond age will impact programming methods, some of which may not be known at initial evaluation. Developmental, cognitive, sensory, or motor limitations may impair a child's ability to consistently show sound awareness. Children with developmental delays or deficits may need extended time to show a response to a sound, or require much longer conditioning time prior to being able to confidently respond to sound with independence. Some children will never be able to consistently respond to a sound. In these cases, a clinician must rely on objective testing, behavioral observation, parent and professional reports to optimize parameters.

Children with other sensory limitations such as vision impairment may need further accommodations. For example: moving a visual reinforcement toy into their reduced visual field, turning down lights in a room to increase visual contrast of a reinforcing toy, moving away other toys that may distract from the testing (eg, a child distracted by a certain color and disregarding the reinforcing toy). Parents and educators are an important resource, as they often know how to structure the child's environment to provide the greatest opportunity to provide consistent responses.

Head control and motor skills are important factors in showing behavioral responses. If a child is not able to turn his head to a certain degree needed, false negative responses may be obtained, confounding programming. Mobile VRA toys, on a pole with wheels, for example, are useful in positioning the reinforcing toy for optimal sight lines.

Other conditions, such as autism, or sensory integration issues not previously diagnosed preoperatively, may impact programming methods and possibly outcomes with cochlear implantation.[16,17] Some children present with aversion to certain aspects of programming: hand over hand instruction, wearing the processor without the microphone active, or even the feel of the programming cable of the back of their neck. It is the role of the clinician to accommodate the child given these aversions to maximize the probability of obtaining the desired measurements needed for accurate programming. There will be successes and failures in choosing programming techniques, but each challenging programming session can serve to better prepare the clinician for the next session.

a speech-language pathologist, a teacher of the deaf, a social worker, and an early interventionist. Other professionals can be included as necessary, such as a developmental psychologist.

Experienced professionals should weigh known expectations of listening and language development with factors of the child acclimating to new electrical stimulation and possible language, learning, and cognitive issues. Programming parameters should be kept current and consistently remapped at least every 6 to 12 months in long-term pediatric users with over 3 to 4 years of experience. Poor or slow progress with a cochlear implant is not necessarily related to inappropriate programming parameters, rather a multitude of factors as listed in the preoperative evaluation. Changes in program parameters will not necessarily address poor outcomes. A whole-child approach is best when managing this population, as the reason for poor progress may be more than just a "need for a mapping."

COLLABORATION WITH OTHER PROFESSIONALS

The short amount of time a clinician works with a child during a mapping session is not adequate to understand the scope of the child's progress with the cochlear implant. If not already available on the cochlear implant team, the audiologist should collaborate with other professionals working with the child. These professionals should be familiar with issues surrounding hearing loss, comfortable with providing habilitation services, and able to demonstrate understanding of the auditory hierarchy. They may include:

CONCLUSION

Working with children and their cochlear implants is a challenging and rewarding experience. Hopefully, this chapter has served as a general introduction to some of the important considerations in working with this population. Specific programming parameters and techniques are dependent on each cochlear implant manufacturer. Methods and protocols vary clinic to clinic as well. Several current texts provide a comprehensive review of cochlear implant programming beyond the scope of this chapter.[18–20] Please consult current texts, company Web sites, and company representatives for further information. Comprehensive understanding of all of these factors, as well as learned experiences, will help children maximize their communicative potential with their cochlear implants.

REFERENCES

1. Hellman SA, Chute PM, Kretschmer RE, Nevins ME, Parisier SC, Thurston LC. The development of a children's implant profile. *Am Ann Deaf.* 1991 Apr;136(2):77–81.
2. Daya H, Figueirido JC, Gordon KA, Twitchell K, Gysin C, Papsin BC. The role of a graded profile analysis in determining candidacy and outcome for cochlear implantation in children. *Int J Pediatr Otorhinolaryngol.* 1999 Aug 5;49(2):135–142.
3. Thomas F, Rajput K. Use of a revised children's implant profile (GOSHChIP) in candidacy for paediatric cochlear implantation and in predicting outcome. *Int J Audiol.* 2009 Aug;48(8):554–560.
4. Lazaridis E, Therres M, Marsh RR. How is the children's implant profile used in the cochlear implant candidacy process? *Int J Pediatr Otorhinolaryngol.* 2010 Apr;74(4): 412–415.
5. Houston DM, Miyamoto RT. Effects of early auditory experience on word learning and speech perception in deaf children with cochlear implants: implications for sensitive periods of language development. *Otol Neurotol.* 2010 Oct;31(8):1248–1253.
6. Hodges AV, Balkany TJ, Ruth RA, Lambert PR, Dolan-Ash S, Schloffman JJ. Electrical middle ear muscle reflex: use in cochlear implant programming. *Otolaryngol Head Neck Surg.* 1997;117:255–261.
7. Bresnihan M, Norman G, Scott F, Viani L. Measurement of comfort levels by means of electrical stapedial reflex in children. *Arch Otolaryngol Head Neck Surg.* 2001; 127:963–966.
8. Holstad BA, Sonneveldt VG, Fears BT, et al. Relation of electrically evoked compound action potential thresholds to behavioral T- and C-levels in children with cochlear implants. *Ear Hear.* 2009 Feb;30(1):115–127.
9. Ling D. The Six-Sound Test. In: Estabrooks W, Birkenshaw-Fleming L, eds, *Songs for Listening! Songs for Life!* Washington, DC, A. G. Bell Association for the Deaf and Hard of Hearing; 2003:227–229.
10. Erber, N. Evaluating speech perception ability in hearing-impaired children. Bess FH, ed. *Childhood Deafness: Causation, Assessment, and Management.* New York, NY: Grune & Stratton; 1977.
11. McClatchie A, Therres M. *AuSpLan: A Manual for Professionals Working with Children Who Have Cochlear Implants or Amplification.* Oakland, CA: Audiology Department, Children's Hospital & Research Center, (510-428-3344); 2003.
12. Moog, J, Biedenstein J, Davidson L. *Speech Perception Instructional Curriculum and Evaluation (SPICE).* St. Louis, MO: Central Institute for the Deaf; 1995.
13. Papsin BC. Cochlear implantation in children with anomalous cochleovestibular anatomy. *Laryngoscope.* 2005 Jan;115(1 pt 2 suppl 106):1–26.
14. Warren FM 3rd, Wiggins RH 3rd, Pitt C, Harnsberger HR, Shelton C. Apparent cochlear nerve aplasia: to implant or not to implant? *Otol Neurotol.* 2010 Sep;31(7): 1088–1094.
15. Dettman S, Sadeghi-Barzalighi A, Ambett R, Dowell R, Trotter M, Briggs R. Cochlear implants in forty-eight children with cochlear and/or vestibular abnormality. *Audiol Neurotol.* 2010;16(4):222–232.
16. Edwards LC. Children with cochlear implants and complex needs: a review of outcome research and psychological practice. *J Deaf Stud Deaf Educ.* 2007 Summer; 12(3):258–268.
17. Daneshi A, Hassanzadeh S. Cochlear implantation in prelingually deaf persons with additional disability. *J Laryngol Otol.* 2007 Jul;121(7):635–638.
18. Cullington H, ed. *Cochlear Implants Objective Measures.* London and Philadelphia: Whurr Publishers; 2003.

19. Niparko JK. *Cochlear Implants Principles and Practices*. 2nd ed. Philadelphia, PA: Wolters Kluwer/Lippincott Williams & Wilkins; 2009.

20. Wolfe J, Schafer EC. *Programming Cochlear Implants*. San Diego, CA: Plural Publishing; 2010.

Chapter 14

Measuring Auditory Outcomes of Cochlear Implant Use in Children with Behavioral and Electrophysiologic Tests

KAREN A. GORDON AND BLAKE C. PAPSIN

INTRODUCTION

Cochlear implants are designed to give children who are deaf access to sound. At the most basic level, this means that children should be able to detect at least some of the sounds in their environment. If we measure the outcome after cochlear implantation (CI) using sound detection alone, we find that the device is hugely successful. In our experience, only those children who have absent or significantly narrowed cochlear branches of the auditory nerve cannot detect any sound with a cochlear implant. Of course, our expectations of multichannel devices have increased well beyond simple sound detection and we now expect children using cochlear implants to accurately perceive speech sounds so that they can develop normal oral communication

skills. Although most children do hear and understand speech with their implants and many use oral speech and language as their primary mode of communication, there is considerable variability in performance.[1-5] In order to understand why this variability occurs and to improve hearing for children who are deaf, we need to accurately assess current outcomes of CI. In this chapter, we review behavioral and electrophysiologic measures that are being used to monitor auditory development after CI in children.

Because children who are deaf develop their hearing skills over time after CI, a number of different behavioral measures are used to track these changes. We therefore review outcome measures along a hierarchical ascension of auditory skills beginning from sound detection, discrimination between sounds, and finally perception of words and sentences. We should also realize that these behavioral changes reflect processes occurring along the auditory pathways. Consequently, electrophysiologic measures have been used to determine what parts of the auditory system respond to cochlear implant stimulation and to examine whether some areas are more resistant to change than others. Effects of cochlear implant stimulation on the auditory nerve, brainstem and thalamocortex are reviewed. Electrophysiologic measures are also helpful for ensuring that the cochlear implant is working properly and that stimulation is not causing unwanted nonauditory activity from areas such as the facial nerve (cranial nerve VII) or the vestibular component of the auditory nerve (cranial nerve VIII). Moreover, these recordings can be completed in most children regardless of age or developmental ability and thus may provide important information when behavioral outcome measures are not available. Together, behavioral and electrophysiologic outcome measures offer ways to assess the effectiveness of CI for auditory development in groups of children as well as for individual children.

TRADITIONAL BEHAVIORAL MEASURES OF AUDITORY DEVELOPMENT

Behavioral measures are often thought of as the "gold standard" for measuring outcome of a particular intervention. The advantage of these measures is that they reflect any improvements or decrements in function. We must remember, however, that there are many aspects of function and that specific abilities will be targeted by the tests used and behavioral responses

required. A variety of tests and tasks have been used in the clinic to assess functional changes in hearing after CI; these include simple tasks such as detecting the presence of a target sound to more complex tasks requiring speech understanding.

DETECTION OF SOUNDS

Sound detection is the most basic of auditory skills and is commonly used to assess hearing sensitivity. Adults are asked to press a button or raise a hand when they detect a sound whereas young children may respond by taking a turn in a game or looking toward a re-enforcer (often a dancing puppet). Tones or speech sounds are presented at progressively lower intensity levels; the softest level that elicits a reliable behavioral response is defined as the threshold for that auditory stimulus. Most children receiving cochlear implants can only detect loud sounds (ie, >70 dB HL) which means that, without auditory prostheses, they have little access to normal conversational speech (typically 40 to 60 dB HL) and miss environmental sounds that are softer than their hearing thresholds.

Cochlear implants can give children with severe to profound hearing loss access to moderate sounds and to speech at normal conversational levels by converting the acoustic information into electrical pulses that stimulate the auditory nerve. Figure 14–1 shows an x-ray of the internal components of two types of cochlear implant devices in a child implanted bilaterally. Depending on the device used, a number of stimulating electrodes are inserted into the scala tympani of the cochlea. Acoustic input is divided into separate frequency bands and each band is allocated to a single electrode. The

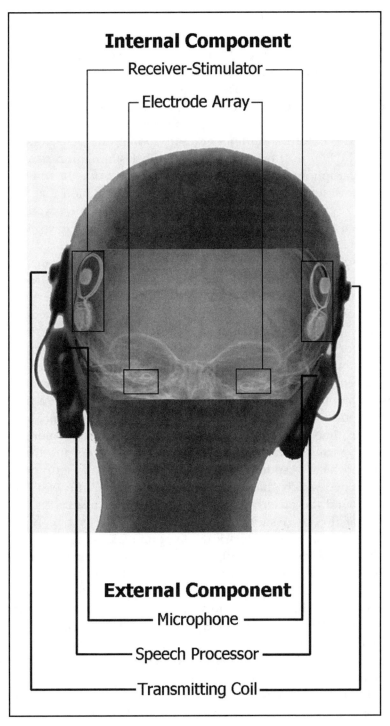

Internal Component

Receiver-Stimulator

Electrode Array

External Component

Microphone

Speech Processor

Transmitting Coil

Figure 14–1. *Two sets of cochlear implant components (external and internal) are shown. The x-ray of internal components has a smaller scale than the picture of external components on the head. The microphone picks up acoustic sound and the speech processor analyses it for frequency and intensity over time. Instructions are sent by the external transmitting coil to the internal receiver-stimulator. Electrical pulses are delivered by electrodes on the array implanted in the scala tympani of the cochlea.*

arrangement of frequencies to cochlear implant electrodes mimics the normal cochlea; high frequencies are allocated to basal electrodes with lower frequencies allocated to progressively more apical electrodes. The external equipment is also shown in Figure 14–1; in this example, the microphone (which picks up acoustic sound) and speech processor (which analyzes the sound) sit on the ear and the transmitting coil (which sends instructions to the internal device) sits on the head in close proximity to the internal receiver-stimulator. The current levels required to elicit hearing will depend on a number of factors including the size and integrity of the neural population that can be stimulated,[6] the distance between the electrode and the neurons,[7,8] and the focus of the electrical field as produced by monopolar, bipolar, tripolar or other modes of stimulation.[9,10] These levels can also change over time both in the short and long term.[11,12] Such changes might reflect an intracochlear response to the indwelling electrode which changes the environment around the electrode array (eg, formation of fibrous tissue) [13–15] or a physiologic adaption to the electrical stimulation.[16] Adaptation with implant use could also be a more cognitive learning process whereby children grow accustomed to the input and, for instance, find levels which were previously too loud becoming comfortable or too soft.

Clearly, we would like to provide a dynamic range of hearing with cochlear implants so that the adults and children who use these devices can comfortably perceive both the softness and loudness of sounds. The range of electrical current levels required to do this must be determined for the multiple cochlear implant electrodes in each cochlear implant user. Behavioral measures have long been considered to be the best way of ensuring optimal stimulation levels for cochlear implant users. However, the specific measurements have changed over the years. It was once considered necessary to measure behavioral thresholds to electrical stimulation delivered by each implant electrode. In addition, the upper levels of stimulation that remained comfortable for listening were measured for every stimulating electrode. The need to collect both measures for all implant electrodes reflected the sometimes large differences in stimulation requirements for individual electrodes even if they were in similar regions of the implanted array (sometimes side by side). Monopolar stimulation, now used in most cochlear implant devices, reduces the variability between electrodes for comfortable and audible stimulation.[10] As a result, behavioral measures may only be required at a number of electrodes along the array. The stimulation levels for the intermediate electrodes can be extrapolated with no known adverse effects on speech understanding. The need to use extrapolation and inference is become increasingly important as the age at implantation falls with routine implantation of infants.

Thresholds to electrical stimulation can be measured using the same techniques used to assess hearing sensitivity prior to CI. Typically, a bracketing approached proposed by Hughson and Westlake is used.[17] Both adults and children provide a reliable conditioned response to the input. This response is then tracked over a range of stimulus intensities. The lowest intensity that yields a consistent response across multiple presentations is considered to be the threshold. The test re-test reliability of these measures when usingacoustic pure tones that decrease by 10 dB and increase in

5 dB steps has been found to be less than 5 dB in adults.[18]

Upper limits of comfort tend to be measured in a variety of ways. Adults with prior hearing experience are asked to indicate when the sound becomes "too loud" and maximum levels are set below this. Children may be shown a visual scale of comfort. An example of such a scale is shown in Figure 14–2. Typically, the scale shows a series of simple cartoon faces which range from a happy smiling face to a sad frowning face. Intolerance to an electrical stimulation can be indicated by pointing to the latter face. Recent reports indicate that this type of categorical scaling of loudness is reliable in adults and significantly related to threshold measures at least for soft and moderately loud sounds.[19] However, there is high test-retest variability in children 7 to 12 years of age[20] which makes this a questionable technique for younger children. In addition, it can be argued that this is very difficult task for children with severe to profound hearing loss who have limited hearing even with hearing aids. Consequently, the upper limits of stimulation are often established in children by using a set dynamic range over the measured threshold levels.[12,21]

Some cochlear implant manufacturers no longer require that behavioral measures of threshold or upper limits of comfort be completed for individual electrodes. Manufacturers of these devices suggest that stimulation should be audible and comfortable for stimulation delivered by groups of electrodes. For children, a scale of comfort as described above has been used; levels at which the child indicates he or she heard the sound and that it was not uncomfortable are programmed into the cochlear implant. Soft sounds are not measured by behavioral thresholds but, rather, are set at a fixed percentage lower than the comfortably audible levels. This procedure appears to be a move away from the initial approach whereby the perception of electrical stimulation as soft or loud was carefully measured for all electrodes. Little is known about the effects of this type of approach in comparison to previously used programming methods but there are no reports that this adversely affects outcomes of speech perception. Nonetheless, as we discuss below, there may be subtle changes in stimulation required to best elicit auditory activity and development that might not be captured using these behavioral response-based techniques.

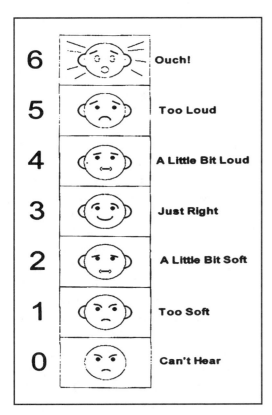

Figure 14–2. *Loudness rating categories used by Ellis and Wynne in their 1999 study (Figure 1, p. 44).[20]*

In general, we have always endeavored to provide audible and comfortable stimulation through a cochlear implant which gives the user access to hearing sounds as both soft and loud. There is less known about how stimulation levels should be increased in order to provide the most accurate growth of loudness between minimum and maximum levels or how this growth should be balanced between two cochlear implants for bilateral implant users. Pitch balancing between the implants might also be important but how this might be achieved in the pediatric population remains a question.

SPEECH PERCEPTION

Despite the multiple approaches for setting cochlear implant stimulation levels, most users are able to detect sounds including speech. This might be bewildering for a young child who heard very little with their hearing aids but with encouragement, consistent implant use, and therapy, it is hoped that he or she will begin to discriminate between different sounds and learn to understand what is heard. This process of hearing and associating consistent sounds with meaning forms the basis of oral communication.

There are multiple tests which can be used to examine the child's ability to perceive speech through their cochlear implants. Many of these tests were originally designed to be part of a hearing assessment battery and use vocabulary that should be familiar to preschool- and school-age children. Of course, this assumption is often not met for children who are acquiring language in parallel with their development of speech perception. In addition, young children may not be ready to respond as required by these tests (ie repeating a word or pointing to a picture). In these cases, the parents or caregivers can be asked about the child's listening behavior using structured questionnaires.

Questionnaires

There are several questionnaires which can be used to assess early hearing development in children using cochlear implants. The Meaningful Auditory Integration Scale (MAIS)[22] and Infant-Toddler Meaningful Auditory Integration Scale (IT-MAIS)[23] are sets of 10 questions each designed to measure the impact of cochlear implant use in the child's daily life.[22] In general, the targeted information is whether the child consistently uses the device, whether he or she alerts to sound, and whether he or she understands the sounds heard. The original intention was for parents or caregivers of children with profound hearing loss to be interviewed regarding these issues rather than questioned. Based on the responses obtained during the interview, the examiner rates the frequency of the child's experience on a scale of 0 through 4 (where 0 is never and 4 is frequent)[22] for each of the 10 questions. The developers of the MAIS used this tool to assess hearing in 4 groups of children: 2 groups used 2 different types of cochlear implant devices, another group used hearing aids, and the last group used a Tactaid (a device that converts acoustic input into vibrotactile information).[22] They found the best scores in children using hearing aids, the poorest scores in children using the Tactaid and intermediate scores in the cochlear implant users.

One of the strengths of these types of questionnaires is that they are not specific to one particular language. Indeed, the IT-MAIS has been used to assess outcomes of CI in children all over the world.[24-27] Data from normal-hearing infants and young children (5 to 36 months of age) have also been reported and compared with outcomes in children who were implanted at ages 12 to 18 months, 19 to 24 months, or between 24 and 36 months.[24] Although not specifically stated, most of the children using cochlear implants were likely to have been deaf since infancy. The youngest group of cochlear implant users achieved IT-MAIS scores similar to their normal hearing peers by 24 months of age. The children receiving cochlear implants between 24 and 36 months showed a slightly reduced rate of improvement during the first year of cochlear implant use compared to children receiving a cochlear implant at younger ages. Overall, these data demonstrated an advantage of early implantation on hearing outcomes. The authors suggested that the hearing skills assessed using the IT-MAIS and obtained rapidly by children receiving cochlear implants at young ages were an important foundation for spoken language competence. Tests of speech perception and language acquisition can be used to confirm this.

Open- and Closed-Set Tests

There are a number of tests which have been used to assess the development of speech perception in the pediatric cochlear implant population. These measures tend to be grouped into closed- and open-set tests. In closed-set tests, the child is provided with a set of words or pictures (the "set" of possible targets therefore is limited or "closed"). The child is then asked to choose the word, picture or object that most closely represents a given auditory target. The target sound

is often a word but may be a phrase or another type of verbal (eg, crying or laughing) or nonverbal sound (eg, car horn, telephone ring). The stimuli may be prerecorded or can be administered by an examiner who monitors the level of his or her voice to make sure that each stimulus is delivered at the targeted level.

Many closed-set tests ask the child to choose from 3 or more items requiring the child to hear and understand the word and then find the item (picture or toy) which most closely corresponds to it. By comparison, a simpler task is to ask the child to discriminate between 2 sounds. A typical response would be for the child to indicate whether the sounds are the same or different. In that situation, the child does not need to attach meaning to either sound but only has to listen for differences. This type of discrimination can also be assessed by teaching the child to respond only when there is a change from one sound to another.[28] This works well when one sound is presented frequently with an infrequent presentation of the other; responses to the infrequent sound can be head turns with visual reinforcement[29] or taking a turn in a game.[30] These methods have been used successfully to evaluate hearing skills in children of very young ages.[28,29,31]

In comparison to closed-set tests, open-set tests do not provide the child with any choices for responses (the "set" of possible targets therefore is "open"). Open-set testing is significantly more difficult as it relies exclusively on the correct perception of an auditory stimulus. Targets can be single speech sounds, words, sentences, or questions and the child is asked to either repeat what was spoken or to answer the question posed. Generally, multisyllabic words are considered easier to repeat accurately compared with monosyllabic words because the latter can be easily confused by the incorrect identification of a single phoneme (ie, cat rather than bat or phone rather than foam).

The accuracy of speech perception will depend upon the test being used. Closed-set tests allow a degree of accuracy based on chance alone. For example if the child has 4 pictures to choose from, chance dictates an accuracy of 25%; if there are 6 pictures, an accuracy of 17% could be due to chance alone. In addition, accuracy will depend on the level of the vocabulary used. Many of the tests used to monitor speech perception in children using cochlear implants were designed specifically to so that children tested would be familiar with the words they are asked to identify or repeat. This is particularly evident in closed-set tests that require the child to understand the word and choose a picture which best represents it. It is also important to con-

sider the ability of the child to perform the required task. Young children might not understand, for example, that they must choose the toy that the examiner asks for rather than the toy they would most like to play with.

Over the years, several closed-set and several open-set tests have been used to monitor development of speech perception in children using cochlear implants. Some of the tests in English that have been commonly used in the United States and Canada are listed in Table 14–1. Similar tests exist in many different languages around the world. Given the many different tests available and the need to use different tests depending on the age and abilities of the child, it can be difficult to gather speech perception data using a single test in a group of children using cochlear implants. Geers and Moog[32] suggested that speech perception tests might be ordered into a hierarchy based on the

Table 14–1. Speech Perception Tests

Speech Perception Tests	*Reference*
Closed-Set Tests	
Early Speech Perception (ESP) Test: Low Verbal Version	Moog and Geers[82]
Early Speech Perception (ESP) Test: Standard Version	Moog and Geers[82]
Test of Auditory Comprehension (TAC) for Hearing Impaired Pupils	Hoversten[83]
Northwestern University Children's Perception of Speech (NU-CHIPS) Test	Elliott and Katz[84]
Word Intelligibility by Picture Identification (WIPI) Test	Ross and Lerman[85]
Open-Set Tests	
Glendonald Auditory Screening Procedure (GASP)	Erber[86]
Multisyllabic Lexical Neighborhood Test (MLNT)	Kirk et al[87]
Lexical Neighborhood Test (LNT)	Kirk et al[87]
Phonetically Balanced Kindergarten Word List (PBK)	Haskins[88]
Bamford-Kowal-Bench (BKB) Sentences	Bench et al[89]

difficulty of the task and the vocabulary required. Based on their work, our group devised a Pediatric Ranked Order Speech Perception (PROSPER) score which ranks speech perception skills according to the test completed and the accuracy scored on that test.[33] The hierarchy of tests and corresponding PROSPER score are detailed in Table 14–2. We found that this was very helpful in analyzing speech perception results in a group of children who had multiple disabilities.

Predicting Speech Perception Outcomes in Children Using Cochlear Implants

Speech perception tests have been used to assess changes in hearing with cochlear implant use and to predict which children develop good hearing skills with their cochlear implants. There is typically a high degree of variability in speech perception test scores and no one factor has been found to explain this. Of the many factors studied, the clearest finding is that increasing age at implantation is associated with poorer speech perception scores.[2,24–36] Although not always stated, most children studied have been deaf from an early age. Some of these children were likely to have had little access to sound early in life and thus were deaf for durations equivalent to their age. A number of groups have tried to determine whether there is a critical or sensitive period for development of speech perception after which CI will have more limited effects. In general, implantation for children with early onset deafness has been shown to have the greatest advantages for development of speech perception when performed at ages younger than 3 years.[1,36,37] In past work, our research group used a statistical method (binary

partitioning analyses) to identify a "cutoff" age that best delineated speech perception scores in groups implanted at younger versus older ages.[38] We found that the "cutoff" age depended on the speech perception measure used, suggesting that there is no universal age or critical period for development of speech perception through cochlear implant use. These findings reflected the changing complexity in the language of the tests used and suggested that there is a hierarchy of language acquisition that can only proceed when auditory development occurs within sensitive periods. Recently, Tajudeen and colleagues[1] examined this issue in 117 children who received cochlear implants before 3 years of age. Testing was measured repeatedly with increasing durations of cochlear implant use. They found that children implanted as infants (<1 year of age) achieved higher scores than their peers implanted at later ages but that scores were not significantly different between these groups when considered over the duration of cochlear implant use or "hearing age." This means that children implanted early have an early start for hearing development, thereby minimizing potential delays relative to their normal-hearing peers but that they do not have enhanced rates of auditory development relative to their peers implanted at slightly older ages (up to 3 years). The authors concluded that there is no sensitive period for acquiring speech perception within the first 3 years of life. It should be noted that longer periods of deafness do result in decreased speech perception outcomes but this does not necessarily mean that all children implanted at older ages will fail to develop speech perception. Those children who develop auditory skills prior to implantation (with normal hearing or

Table 14–2. Pediatric Ranked Order Speech Perception (PROSPER) Score. A hierarchy of speech perception tests ranging from parent reports to closed-set phoneme and word recognition to open-set phoneme, sentence, and word recognition.

Rank	Speech Perception Test Score
0	Test could not be completed
1	MAIS or IT-MAIS <50%
2	MAIS or IT-MAIS ≥50%
3	ESP low verbal pattern perception <50%
4	ESP low verbal pattern perception ≥50%
5	ESP low verbal spondee <50%
6	ESP low verbal spondee ≥50%
7	ESP low verbal monosyllable <50%
8	ESP low verbal monosyllable ≥50%
9	ESP standard pattern perception <50%
10	ESP standard pattern perception ≥50%
11	ESP standard spondee <50%
12	ESP standard spondee ≥50%
13	ESP standard monosyllable <50%
14	ESP standard monosyllable ≥50%
15	WIPI <50%
16	WIPI ≥50%
17	GASP sentences <50%
18	GASP sentences ≥50%
19	GASP word <50%
20	GASP word ≥50%
21	MLNT phoneme <50%
22	MLNT phoneme ≥50%
23	MLNT word <50%
24	MLNT word ≥50%
25	BKB word <50%
26	BKB word ≥50%
27	LNT phoneme <50%
28	LNT phoneme ≥50%
29	LNT word <50%
30	LNT word ≥50%
31	PBK phoneme <50%
32	PBK phoneme ≥50%
33	PBK word <50%
34	PBK word ≥50%

through hearing aids) and then receive cochlear implants at older ages do have good potential to perceive speech accurately with their cochlear implants.[5,39]

Other factors can play a role in speech perception outcomes after CI. Children with particular cochlear abnormalities (common cavity deformity) and those in whom there was hypoplasia of the auditory or cochlear division of the vestibule-cochlear nerve achieve poorer speech perception skills than their peers with normal cochlear and primary nerve anatomy.[40] This reflects the need for the cochlear implant to effectively stimulate the auditory system. There has been recent interest in this area with a particular emphasis on where the cochlear implant electrode array sits in the cochlea[41] and the type of stimulation that might be most effective.[42] Also of great importance for speech perception is the type of therapy that the children receive after implantation and their mode of communication. Children involved in therapies that emphasize listening and who primarily use spoken communication show better hearing skills after implantation than children using manual communication or modes of therapy that combine oral and manual communication modes.[43]

BEHAVIORAL MEASURES TO MONITOR EFFECTS OF BILATERAL COCHLEAR IMPLANTATION

Bilateral cochlear implants are now being provided to children in order to improve hearing. It is clear that it is difficult to localize sounds when hearing is only available from one side[44] and that hearing in noise is impaired relative to binaural hearing.[45] These binaural hearing skills have been evaluated using behavioral measures to evaluate whether there are advantages of bilateral over unilateral cochlear implant use. A number of studies have shown improved speech perception scores in both quiet and noise when children are using bilateral rather than unilateral cochlear implants.[46–49] In our study, speech perception was measured repeatedly in children using the test that was most appropriate for the child's age, development, and language abilities.[49]

Sound localization appears to be a difficult task for children using bilateral cochlear implants when a large set of sound sources are used. A simpler discrimination task has been developed in which children listen to 2 sounds and are asked whether the first sound "moved."[50–52] The two sounds are delivered at a wide range of angles so that the "minimal audible angle" can be determined. This procedure has been very effective in demonstrating advantages of bilateral over unilateral CI in children ages 2 to 16 years.[50–52] Another group has showed improved sound localization in children with bilateral implants by providing a closed-set of 3 possible answers.[53] Children were ages 4 to 15 years at the time of testing and the authors found that this task was too difficult for younger children.[53]

Binaural processing has also been evaluated using behavioral tests. We assessed perception of interimplant level and timing cues (needed for binaural hearing) using a task with 4 possible responses[54] and van Deun and colleagues[55] asked children to identify a sound in noise in a set of 3. These data have provided interesting information on how children use interimplant level and timing differences carried by bilateral cochlear implant stimulation but has been limited to children who are at least 5 years of age. We have recently used play and visual reinforcement techniques to measure speech detection in noise in slightly younger children who received bilateral implants simultaneously.[56]

SUMMARY OF BEHAVIORAL MEASURES

Behavioral measures after CI are used both to program the cochlear implant and to monitor the development of speech perception. Reliable detection of sounds is evidence that the child is hearing through their cochlear implant(s). Accurate discrimination between 2 different sounds indicates that the child is able to hear specific cues in the sound, accurate responses on open-set speech perception tests indicate that the child hears and can reproduce speech sounds, and accurate responses in closed (and some open) set speech perception tests demonstrate that the speech sounds have meaning and are being understood. Overall, behavioral measures provide an indication of auditory function or how the child is using their cochlear implant(s) to hear. Speech perception results in groups of children using cochlear implants are typically highly variable and can change for different tests and response tasks. It is thus impossible to predict what these outcomes will be for any one child. Although age at implantation (likely reflecting the duration of deafness in early life) is clearly a very important factor, there are many other issues which also play a role in the development of hearing with a cochlear implant. Improvements of bilateral over unilateral cochlear implants have been assessed and found using both open- and closed-set speech perception tests. Other aspects of binaural hearing, including sound localization, have been measured using closed-set tasks and show improv-ed function over unilateral cochlear implant use but with considerable variability in accuracy.

ELECTROPHYSIOLOGIC MEASURES OF AUDITORY FUNCTION AND DEVELOPMENT

Behavioral measures have both the advantage and disadvantage of requiring responses from children. The advantage is that an accurate behavioral response provides confirmation that the cochlear implant is working, that the electrical pulses stimulated the auditory system, that there was cognitive processing and recognition of the sound, and that the child was able to formulate a response to the sound. The corollary, an inaccurate response or lack of response, could mean that there was a breakdown in any or all of these areas. This is a disadvantage of behavioral measures. Electrophysiologic measures can thus be useful tools in addition to behavioral measures to assess auditory function and development in children using cochlear implants. These measures do not require the child to respond and can provide information about auditory development from discrete areas along the auditory pathways. Moreover, they can be done repeatedly at any time postimplantation and can identify changes that occur rapidly with cochlear implant use.

RESPONSES FROM THE AUDITORY PATHWAYS

The cochlear implant is designed to stimulate the auditory nerve and relies on intact connections from this primary nerve to more central areas of the auditory system. These connections are largely present through the auditory brainstem and midbrain in children who are deaf.[57,58] This was found by recording clear responses from the auditory nerve and brainstem in the operating room immediately after the electrode array is inserted and at initial device use. The potential methods used to observe and record auditory activity in cochlear implant users is limited by the magnet in the receiver-stimulator that interferes with both functional magnetic resonance imaging and magnetoencephalography. It is possible, however, to measure electrical field potentials generated by groups of neurons responding to cochlear implant input. These potentials are measured in amplitude over time.

Figure 14–3 shows examples of the types of electrophysiologic responses that can be evoked in cochlear implant users. The earliest latency response (0 to 2 ms) is the compound action potential of the primary auditory nerve (ECAP). The next is the electrically evoked auditory brainstem response (EABR) which extends from 0 to 5 ms and includes activity from the auditory nerve, brainstem and midbrain. The first peak (eI) is obscured by stimulus artifact but the next (eII) can be seen; both these peaks reflect activity in the auditory nerve.[59] Wave eIII is generated at or near the cochlear nucleus and wave eV is from the lateral lemniscus.[59] Further on in latency is the electrically evoked middle latency response (EMLR) from the thalamocortex. This response has a negative peak (eNa) at approximately 10 ms followed by a positive peak (ePa) and a second negative peak (eNb).[60] Finally, there is an obligatory cortical response which, when mature, occurs between 50 and 300 ms and has three clear peaks (P1, N1 and P2). [61] Unlike the ECAP, EABR, and EMLR, which are often evoked by single electrical pulses, the cortical response is more typically evoked by trains of pulses or by sound which is picked up and processed by the cochlear implant and translated into electrical pulses. The cortical response shown is from a 9-year-old child with 7 years of cochlear implant experience and is dominated by a large positive peak at approximately 100 ms. This response is still immature in comparison to the cortical response from an adult.[61] Because it is not clear whether the large positive peak in the immature response is from the same neural population that later generates the mature P1, we have identified it as P1ci.

Most of the evoked potential responses recorded in cochlear implant users are measured using recording electrodes which sit on the surface of the head. The EABR and EMLR typically are collected from the midline center of the head and referenced to the ipsilateral and/or contralateral earlobes or mastoids. The later latency cortical response can be recorded using the same setup but stimulus artifact, when it occurs, can obscure the waveform of interest. This effect can be minimized by using short duration stimuli or by moving the reference electrode to other locations on the head.[62] Another suggestion has been to eliminate the auditory response using a forward-masking technique and then subtract this measure, which contains the stimulus artifact alone, from the original response.[63] If the response is recorded from multiple electrodes on the head, principal or independent component analyses can be used to isolate the artefact and remove it from the response.[62,64] We have reported the use of a novel beam-former that can be applied to cortical responses collected from 64 cephalic locations to re-move cochlear implant stimulus artifact.[65] This

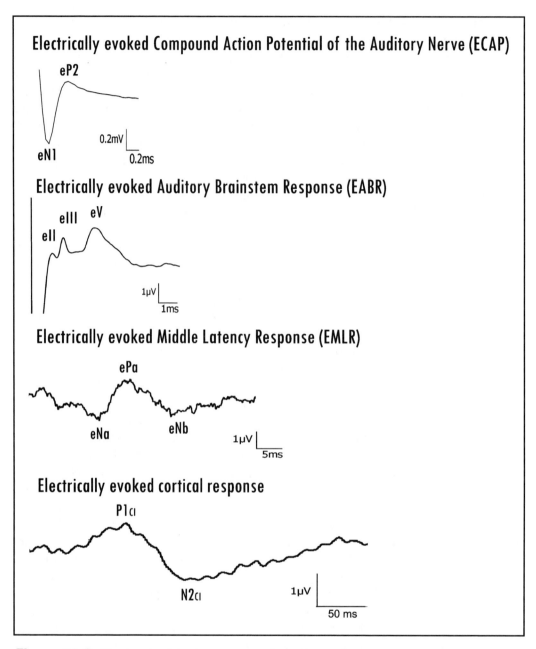

Figure 14–3. *Electrophysiologic responses from the auditory system.*

technique is also able to identify the locations in the brain which generate each amplitude peak in the cochlear implant-evoked response.

As shown in Figure 14-3, the early wave eI of the EABR is obscured by stimulus artefact. This response from the primary auditory nerve can be recorded using the telemetry system from the implant. The advantage of the telemetry system is that one of the electrodes on the implanted array is used to stimulate activity in the auditory nerve and a neighboring electrode records the response. The telemetry system then sends the information through the implant to a computer for analysis. The problem of stimulus artefact is solved by using a subtraction technique described previously.[66] This has provided a very effective way to measure primary auditory nerve activity in cochlear implant users without having to apply external recording electrodes. Moreover, the proximity of the recording electrode to the neurons being recorded provides a high amplitude response that is much better isolated from other neurologic responses or environmental noise than if recorded by external cephalic electrodes.

MONITORING EVOLUTION OF COCHLEAR IMPLANT DEVICES

The interface between the cochlear implant electrode array and the primary auditory neurons is critical for provision of efficient and effective auditory stimulation for children who are deaf. This interface can be affected by any deleterious changes in the auditory neurons occurring during the period of deafness or by how the cochlear implant delivers electrical pulses.[9] The latter issue has been addressed by modifying the shape of the cochlear implant electrodes and the array and by adjusting where in the cochlea the array will sit. Precurved electrodes have been designed to sit closer to the modiolus which is where the cell bodies of the auditory neurons are located (spiral ganglia). We would like to monitor effects of these implant design changes on the development of hearing in children but this has been difficult to do with behavioral speech perception measures. This is due, in part, because of the variability

in these measures across implant users. Using electrophysiologic measures have provided a means to do this and we have found that evolutions in cochlear implant design affect responses from the auditory nerves (monitored by changes in ECAP thresholds).[7] The EABR also appears to have some potential for monitoring the electrode-neuron interface as stimulated by monopolar versus a more focused tripolar stimulation.[67]

MONITORING EFFECTS OF DEAFNESS AND DEVELOPMENT OF THE AUDITORY SYSTEM

Evoked potential measures have been used effectively to assess the effects of deafness on the auditory pathways prior to implantation and to monitor developmental changes with implant use. Effects of deafness on the auditory pathways can be explored by stimulating the deprived auditory system with the cochlear implant prior to consistent cochlear implant use. The same measures can be repeated after regular intervals of cochlear implant use. Whereas the child may not be able to perform the tasks required by speech perception tests or might not have developed sufficient language to do these tests, we are able to use electrophysiologic measures to monitor auditory development several times during this same period.

Our group measures evoked potential responses in children immediately following the activation of the cochlear implant(s) in the clinic. By measuring ECAP and EABR latencies in a large group of children at initial cochlear implant use, we have shown that the auditory nerve does develop somewhat during the first year of life even when children are deaf and have little to no access to auditory input.[58] These changes are demonstrated by decreasing latencies in the EABR with the largest changes between eN1 and eII (from the auditory nerve). Because this is an asynaptic part of the pathway,[68] this diminution in latency (a positive developmental change) likely reflects myelination along the primary auditory nerve. After the first year of life, however, there are no significant changes in ECAP and EABR wave latencies or amplitudes when stimulated by a basal electrode.[57,59] This electrode provides stimulation in an area of the cochlea which was unlikely to have received acoustic input even with hearing aid use and thus we conclude that that further development of the auditory nerve and brainstem are arrested without auditory input.

Whereas ECAPs and EABR were clear in most children receiving cochlear implants at initial device activation, we found that EMLRs were difficult to measure at this time in young children.[60] Interestingly, EMLRs were more evident in older children who had longer periods of bilateral deafness than the younger cohort which means that the thalamocortical networks that generate the EMLR become more synchronous with age in the absence of hearing. It is possible then that these networks do not require auditory input to develop and/or that they are influenced by nonauditory input. If the latter is true, the increased ability to detect EMLRs after long periods of bilateral deafness could reflect an abnormal reorganization of the auditory thalamocortical generators.

We have also examined late latency cortical responses in children at initial cochlear implant use. In a recent paper,[69] we reported that cortical responses measured at initial device use in children are highly variable. In that study, 72 children were studied and all had received bilateral cochlear implants simultaneously; cortical responses were evoked by both the right and left implants yielding 144 responses. The most striking finding was the high degree of variability in the responses. We suggested that deafness in childhood does not produce uniform effects in the brain for all children. In support, we found that children whose deafness was associated with bilallelic mutations of the GJB-2 gene had more uniform cortical responses at this early stage of implant use than their peers whose deafness was due to other factors. This means that there are likely to be individual changes in the auditory system depending on the type of deafness in children. We are currently investigating jow this impacts auditory development with cochlear implants.

Auditory development after the initial stage of implant use can be evaluated by monitoring changes in the electrophysiologic responses once the child begins to use the cochlear implant(s) consistently. In general, the auditory pathways undergo rapid changes at many different levels once the implant is activated. ECAP and EABR latencies significantly decrease over the first 2 to 6 months of cochlear implant use even in children with long durations of deafness[57,70] and the EMLR becomes detectible by 6 months.[60] The cortical response also shows impressive change over the first 6 to 8 months of implant use in children implanted at young ages/short durations of deafness.[71] Changes in the cortical response are more limited in children implanted at older ages.[71] This finding indicates that the plasticity of the auditory system decreases with age and/or that is has been irreparably changed during the period of deafness in childhood. We have also found that some children show atypical cortical responses even after long-term cochlear implant use and these types of responses are associated with poor speech perception scores.[64,72] Although many of these children were implanted at older ages, some were implanted at ages as young as 4 years. This suggests that there may be additional factors that can restrict development of the auditory brain after CI. Certainly, age at implantation does not fully explain the variability in speech perception scores and thus this notion is consistent with the behavioral data.

CENTRAL AUDITORY DEVELOPMENT PROMOTED BY UNILATERAL VERSUS BILATERAL COCHLEAR IMPLANT USE

We have recently suggested that auditory development promoted by unilateral cochlear implant use could cause reorganization along the auditory pathways, potentially compromising development of bilateral auditory pathways and binaural auditory processing.[73] As discussed above, behavioral measures have been used to demonstrate that there are benefits of bilateral CI in children for binaural hearing measured by improved speech detection and perception in quiet and noise[46–49] and better sound localization.[50,51,53] However, there are some concerns that these children do not have the same access to timing and level cues between the ears (needed for binaural hearing) as their normal hearing peers. We are currently exploring binaural processing using electrophysiologic measures.[54,74–77] We have shown that unilateral cochlear implant use promotes auditory development preferentially in pathways innervated by the stimulated ear thus leaving asymmetries

in activity between these pathways and those from the opposite ear. These asymmetries are not found in children who received bilateral cochlear implants simultaneously or after a short period of delay after 9 to12 months of bilateral implant use. Moreover, we found that unilateral cochlear implant use allows an abnormal expansion of activity in the contralateral auditory cortex that can be limited by providing bilateral cochlear implants with short or no delays. This re-organization in the auditory brain with unilateral cochlear implant use was not reversed after a considerable period (3 to 4 years) of bilateral cochlear implant experience.[78] We now need to determine whether these unilaterally driven changes in the auditory system have implications for binaural processing and whether providing both implants at the same time or with minimal delays will promote bilateral auditory pathways that can make use of binaural cues.

PROGRAMMING COCHLEAR IMPLANT STIMULATION LEVELS

Once a child receives a cochlear implant, it is important to ensure that he or she is receiving audible and comfortable stimulation from the device. We have already described behavioral measures used to determine whether sound is detected and to program a range of stimulation levels so that the child hears sounds ranging from soft to loud. However, we have also noted that behavioral measures have been difficult to use to determine changes at the level of the electrode-neural interface. This means that there can be useful information provided by both behavioral and electrophysiologic measures for programming cochlear implants for individual children.

Currently, clinicians in our cochlear implant program use ECAP measures taken immediately following device activation in the operating room to set initial stimulation parameters in children. ECAP thresholds are determined for several electrodes along the array and these values are programmed into the implant. These levels are decreased by the same amount for all electrodes and then increased at small and equal levels until the child provides a behavioral reaction. We then ensure that these levels are comfortable. Using these levels in the cochlear implant achieves our primary objective which is to provide audible and comfortable levels. Once this is achieved, the child can be taught to respond consistently to cochlear implant input and the levels can be modified further. We have found that ECAP thresholds can depend on the position along the implanted array but that behavioral thresholds do not.[7] This discrepancy is consistent with findings that the relationship between ECAP and behavioral thresholds is significant but not strong enough to use one to predict the other for individual cases.[12,21,79] Because behavioral measures remain the "gold standard" for setting cochlear implant levels, we use these when available. However, it remains unclear what information we are missing by ignoring differences in electrical stimulation revealed by electrophysiologic measures including the ECAP threshold.

With the emergence of bilateral cochlear implants, we now need to consider whether the sound provided by the two independent devices is balanced. Imbalances in level could distort important interaural level cues and mismatches in pitch cues could impair the fusion of sound between the two devices. As discussed above, we have used behavioral measures in children who were at least 5 years of age to determine whether bilateral input is heard as coming from one side or the other.[54] Where there was no preference for side, we interpreted levels to be balanced. In the same study, we assessed differences in EABR wave eV amplitude evoked by the right versus left implant. We found that, as wave eV amplitudes in the two responses became more dissimilar, the perception of sound lateralized to one side. Thus, EABR wave amplitudes might help in providing balanced level cues in young bilateral cochlear implant users. To date, there are no proposed behavioral or electrophysiologic methods for ensuring matched pitches between bilateral cochlear implants in children.

AVOIDING UNWANTED NONAUDITORY STIMULATION FROM COCHLEAR IMPLANTS

Electrophysiologic measures have been helpful for isolating some nonauditory effects of CI. We have reported on one situation in which evoked responses were useful in identifying unwanted facial nerve stimulation. Cochlear implant stimulation can induce facial twitching in which case stimulation levels provided by the offending electrodes should be reduced. We discovered a myogenic response which obscured the EABR in some children.[80,81] As shown in Figure 14–4, this was confirmed in the operating room by suppressing the response with a muscle relaxant. The top panel of Figure 14–4 shows an electromyogenic response from the thenar muscle to ensure the effectiveness of the medication; the response is absent when the muscle relaxant is active and returns

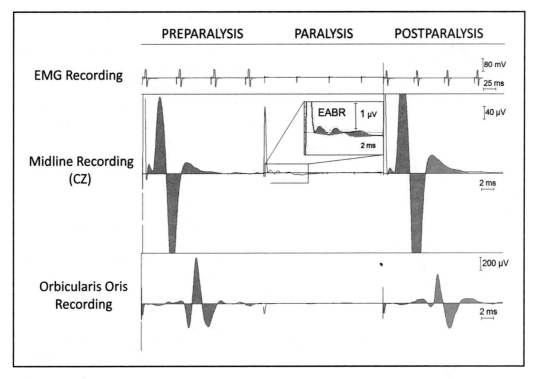

Figure 14–4. *Biphasic responses evoked by cochlear implant stimulation and recorded at midline of the head (CZ) were identified as myogenic by introducing a paralytic (rocuronium). The effectiveness of the paralytic was confirmed as shown in the top panel through an electromyogenic response from the thenar muscle (response was absent during paralysis). Paralysis eliminated the large midline response revealing an underlying EABR. Recordings from a branch of the facial nerve innervating the orbicularis orus (around the mouth) confirmed that the midline response was associated with facial nerve stimulation.*

upon reversal of the drug. The middle panel shows the large biphasic response recorded from midline which occurred at the same latency as the EABR. This was eliminated by paralysis revealing the underlying EABR. The lower panel shows responses recorded from the orbicularis orus (around the mouth) confirming facial nerve stimulation before and after paralysis. In a group of children, muscle activity evoked by cochlear implant stimulation was isolated to the eyes, mouth, and neck. This myogenic response could be elicited in most of the children using cochlear implants with high stimulation levels (independent of where the electrode was along the implanted array) without any noticeable facial twitching. The children felt nothing despite the presence of these responses but, with increased stimulation levels, reported sensations in the affected areas of the face and/or neck. Further increases in stimulation levels resulted in noticeable twitches on the face. The electrophysiologic response in this case was able to detect myogenic responses at lower levels than a clinician watching the face or a child reporting nonauditory sensations.

SUMMARY AND CONCLUSIONS

Over the past three decades, cochlear implants have restored the sense of audition to adults and children with severe to profound deafness allowing them to develop and/or maintain oral communication skills. Successful perception of speech and language through cochlear implants is the ultimate objective of the device and we are constantly trying to improve these skills; modifications to the internal array, stimulation modes, and speech processing strategies are ongoing, attempts to limit the period of deafness in both adults and children are made through early identification and intervention, and device programming continues to evolve to provide optimal stimulation parameters for each cochlear implant recipient. Although there are important limitations in measuring outcome after CI with speech detection and recognition tests, they arguably still provide an estimate of auditory function which is needed for successful educability, sociability and employability.

Behavioral and electrophysiologic indices of auditory development after CI provide evidence of device success. By contrast, deterioration in auditory activity or hearing skills measured by electrophysiologic and/or behavioral responses can be a sentinel of device failure. Successful cochlear implant teams therefore use these tests carefully and judiciously to monitor progress and identify problems.

It should be recognized that the battery of behavioral and electrophysiologic tests described in this chapter only tell a portion of the fascinating story about restoring hearing using electrical pulses for individuals who are deaf. We are becoming increasingly aware that perception of music and the perception of emotional content in speech and language are other important auditory abilities to be evaluated after CI so that these skills can be improved. Similarly, the optimal timing and programming of bilateral cochlear implants has yet to be maximally ascertained. Still, it is clear that, by employing the combination of behavioral and electrophysiologic tests outlined in this chapter, the phenomenal process of auditory development and function after deafness in humans can be accurately observed and measured.

REFERENCES

1. Tajudeen BA, Waltzman SB, Jethanamest D, Svirsky MA. Speech perception in congenitally deaf children receiving cochlear implants in the first year of life. *Otol Neurotol.* 2010;31(8):1254–1260.
2. Zwolan TA, Ashbaugh CM, Alarfaj A, et al. Pediatric cochlear implant patient performance as a function of age at implantation. *Otol Neurotol.* 2004;25(2):112–120.
3. Svirsky MA, Teoh SW, Neuburger H. Development of language and speech perception in congenitally, profoundly deaf children as a function of age at cochlear implantation. *Audiol Neurotol.* 2004;9(4):224–233.
4. Nikolopoulos TP, Gibbin KP, Dyar D. Predicting speech perception outcomes following cochlear implantation using Nottingham children's implant profile (NChIP). *Int J Pediatr Otorhinolaryngol.* 2004;68(2):137–141.
5. Geers AE. Speech, language, and reading skills after early cochlear implantation. *Arch Otolaryngol Head Neck Surg.* 2004;130(5):634–638.

6. Donaldson GS, Viemeister NF, Nelson DA. Psychometric functions and temporal integration in electric hearing. *J Acoust Soc Am.* 1997;101(6):3706–3721.

7. Gordin A, Papsin B, James A, Gordon K. Evolution of cochlear implant arrays result in changes in behavioral and physiological responses in children. *Otol Neurotol.* 2009;30(7):908–915.

8. Gordin A, Papsin B, Gordon K. Packing of the cochleostomy site affects auditory nerve response thresholds in precurved off-stylet cochlear implants. *Otol Neurotol.* 2010;31(2):204–209.

9. Goldwyn JH, Bierer SM, Bierer JA. Modeling the electrode-neuron interface of cochlear implants: effects of neural survival, electrode placement, and the partial tripolar configuration. *Hear Res.* 2010; 268(1–2):93–104.

10. Bierer JA. Threshold and channel interaction in cochlear implant users: evaluation of the tripolar electrode configuration. *J Acoust Soc Am.* 2007;121(3):1642–1653.

11. Zwolan TA, O'Sullivan MB, Fink NE, Niparko JK. Electric charge requirements of pediatric cochlear implant recipients enrolled in the Childhood Development After Cochlear Implantation study. *Otol Neurotol.* 2008;29(2):143–148.

12. Gordon KA, Papsin BC, Harrison RV. Toward a battery of behavioral and objective measures to achieve optimal cochlear implant stimulation levels in children. *Ear Hear.* 2004;25(5):447–463.

13. Charlet de Sauvage R, Lima da Costa D, Erre JP, Aran JM. Electrical and physiological changes during short-term and chronic electrical stimulation of the normal cochlea. *Hear Res.* 1997;110(1–2):119–134.

14. Paasche G, Tasche C, Stover T, Lesinski-Schiedat A, Lenarz T. The long-term effects of modified electrode surfaces and intracochlear corticosteroids on postoperative impedances in cochlear implant patients. *Otol Neurotol.* 2009;30(5):592–598.

15. Somdas MA, Li PM, Whiten DM, Eddington DK, Nadol JB Jr. Quantitative evaluation of new bone and fibrous tissue in the cochlea following cochlear implantation in the human. *Audiol Neurotol.* 2007; 12(5):277–284.

16. Heffer LF, Sly DJ, Fallon JB, White MW, Shepherd RK, O'Leary SJ. Examining the auditory nerve fiber response to high rate cochlear implant stimulation: chronic sensorineural hearing loss and facilitation. *J Neurophysiol.* 2010;104:3124–3135.

17. Carhart R, Jerger J. Preferred method for clinical determination of pure-tone thresholds. *J Speech Hear Disord.* 1959; 24:330–345.

18. Swanepoel de W, Mngemane S, Molemong S, Mkwanazi H, Tutshini S. Hearing assessment-reliability, accuracy, and efficiency of automated audiometry. *Telemed J E Health.* 2010;16(5):557–563.

19. Al-Salim SC, Kopun JG, Neely ST, Jesteadt W, Stiegemann B, Gorga MP. Reliability of categorical loudness scaling and its relation to threshold. *Ear Hear.* 2010;31(4): 567–578.

20. Ellis MR, Wynne MK. Measurements of loudness growth in 1/2-octave bands for children and adults with normal hearing. *Am J Audiol.* 1999;8(1):40–46.

21. Holstad BA, Sonneveldt VG, Fears BT, et al. Relation of electrically evoked compound action potential thresholds to behavioral T- and C-levels in children with cochlear implants. *Ear Hear.* 2009;30(1):115–127.

22. Robbins AM, Renshaw JJ, Berry SW. Evaluating meaningful auditory integration in profoundly hearing-impaired children. *Am J Otol.* 1991;12(suppl):144–150.

23. Zimmerman-Phillips S, Robbins AM, Osberger MJ. Assessing cochlear implant benefit in very young children. *Ann Otol Rhinol Laryngol* (suppl). 2000;109(12): 42–43.

24. McConkey Robbins A, Koch DB, Osberger MJ, Zimmerman-Phillips S, Kishon-Rabin L. Effect of age at cochlear implantation on auditory skill development in infants and toddlers. *Arch Otolaryngol Head Neck Surg.* 2004;130(5):570–574.

25. Chen X, Liu S, Liu B, et al. The effects of age at cochlear implantation and hearing aid trial on auditory performance of Chinese infants. *Acta Otolaryngol*. 2010; 130(2):263–270.

26. Kubo T, Iwaki T, Sasaki T. Auditory perception and speech production skills of children with cochlear implant assessed by means of questionnaire batteries. *ORL J Otorhinolaryngol Relat Spec*. 2008;70(4): 224–228.

27. Osberger MJ, Soli S, von der Haar-Heise S. Comparative study of English- and German-speaking children with the Clarion cochlear implant. *Am J Otol*. 1997;18(6 suppl):S164–S165.

28. Menary S, Trehub SE, McNutt J. Speech discrimination in preschool children: a comparison of two tasks. *J Speech Hear Res*. 1982;25(2):202–207.

29. Eilers RE, WilsonWR, Moore JM. Developmental changes in speech discrimination in infants. *J Speech Hear Res*. 1977;20(4): 766–780.

30. Dawson PW, Nott PE, Clark GM, Cowan RS. A modification of play audiometry to assess speech discrimination ability in severe-profoundly deaf 2- to 4-year-old children. *Ear Hear*. 1998;19(5):371–384.

31. Trehub S. The discrimination of foreign speech contrasts by infants and adults. *Child Dev*. 1976;47:466–472.

32. Geers AE, Moog JS. Predicting spoken language acquisition of profoundly hearing-impaired children. *J Speech Hear Disord*. 1987;52(1):84–94.

33. Trimble K, Rosella LC, Propst E, Gordon KA, Papaioannou V, Papsin BC. Speech perception outcome in multiply disabled children following cochlear implantation: investigating a predictive score. *J Am Acad Audiol*. 2008;19(8):602–611; quiz 651.

34. Uziel AS, Sillon M, Vieu A, et al. Ten-year follow-up of a consecutive series of children with multichannel cochlear implants. *Otol Neurotol*. 2007;28(5):615–628.

35. Manrique M, Cervera-Paz FJ, Huarte A, Molina M. Prospective long-term auditory results of cochlear implantation in prelinguistically deafened children: the importance of early implantation. *Acta Otolaryngol Suppl*. 2004;(552):55–63.

36. Hassanzadeh S, Farhadi M, Daneshi A, Emamdjomeh H. The effects of age on auditory speech perception development in cochlear-implanted prelingually deaf children. *Otolaryngol Head Neck Surg*. 2002;126(5):524–527.

37. Manrique M, Cervera-Paz FJ, Huarte A, Molina M. Advantages of cochlear implantation in prelingual deaf children before 2 years of age when compared with later implantation. *Laryngoscope*. 2004;114(8): 1462–1469.

38. Harrison RV, Gordon KA, Mount RJ. Is there a critical period for cochlear implantation in congenitally deaf children? Analyses of hearing and speech perception performance after implantation. *Dev Psychobiol*. 2005;46(3):252–261.

39. Dowell RC, Dettman SJ, Hill K, Winton E, Barker EJ, Clark GM. Speech perception outcomes in older children who use multichannel cochlear implants: older is not always poorer. *Ann Otol Rhinol Laryngol Suppl*. 2002;189:97–101.

40. Papsin BC. Cochlear implantation in children with anomalous cochleovestibular anatomy. *Laryngoscope*. 2005;115(1 pt 2 suppl 106):1–26.

41. Verbist BM, Skinner MW, Cohen LT, et al. Consensus panel on a cochlear coordinate system applicable in histologic, physiologic, and radiologic studies of the human cochlea. *Otol Neurotol*. 2010;31(5): 722–730.

42. Arenberg Bierer J. Probing the electrode-neuron interface with focused cochlear implant stimulation. *Trends Amplif*. 2010; 14(2):84–95.

43. Geers A, Brenner C, Davidson L. Factors associated with development of speech perception skills in children implanted by age five. *Ear Hear*. 2003;24(1 suppl): 24S–35S.

44. Johnstone PM, Nabelek AK, RobertsonVS. Sound localization acuity in children with unilateral hearing loss who wear a hear-

ing aid in the impaired ear. *J Am Acad Audiol.* 2010;21(8):522–534.

45. Ruscetta MN, Arjmand EM, Pratt SR. Speech recognition abilities in noise for children with severe-to-profound unilateral hearing impairment. *Int J Pediatr Otorhinolaryngol.* 2005;69(6):771–779.

46. Van Deun L, van Wieringen A, Wouters J. Spatial speech perception benefits in young children with normal hearing and cochlear implants. *Ear Hear.* 2010;31(5): 702–713.

47. Sparreboom M, Snik AF, Mylanus EA. Sequential bilateral cochlear implantation in children: development of the primary auditory abilities of bilateral stimulation. *Audiol Neurotol.* 2010;16(4):203–213.

48. Dunn CC, Noble W, Tyler RS, Kordus M, Gantz BJ, Ji H. Bilateral and unilateral cochlear implant users compared on speech perception in noise. *Ear Hear.* 2010;31(2):296–298.

49. Gordon KA, Papsin BC. Benefits of short interimplant delays in children receiving bilateral cochlear implants. *Otol Neurotol.* 2009;30(3):319–331.

50. Grieco-Calub TM, Litovsky RY. Sound localization skills in children who use bilateral cochlear implants and in children with normal acoustic hearing. *Ear Hear.* 2010;31(5):645–656.

51. Grieco-Calub TM, Litovsky RY, Werner LA. Using the observer-based psychophysical procedure to assess localization acuity in toddlers who use bilateral cochlear implants. *Otol Neurotol.* 2008;29(2):235–239.

52. Litovsky RY, Johnstone PM, Godar S, et al. Bilateral cochlear implants in children: localization acuity measured with minimum audible angle. *Ear Hear.* 2006;27(1): 43–59.

53. Van Deun L, van Wieringen A, Scherf F, et al. Earlier intervention leads to better sound localization in children with bilateral cochlear implants. *Audiol Neurotol.* 2010;15(1):7–17.

54. Salloum CA, Valero J, Wong DD, Papsin BC, van Hoesel R, Gordon KA. Lateralization of interimplant timing and level

differences in children who use bilateral cochlear implants. *Ear Hear.* 2010;31(4): 441–456.

55. Van Deun L, van Wieringen A, Francart T, et al. Bilateral cochlear implants in children: binaural unmasking. *Audiol Neurotol.* 2009;14(4):240–247.

56. Chadha NK, Papsin BC, Jiwani S, Gordon KA. Speech detection in noise and spatial unmasking in children with simultaneous versus sequential bilateral cochlear implants. *Otol Neurotol.* 2011;32(7):1057–1064.

57. Gordon KA, Papsin BC, Harrison RV. Activity-dependent developmental plasticity of the auditory brain stem in children who use cochlear implants. *Ear Hear.* 2003;24(6):485–500.

58. Gordon KA, Valero J, Jewell SF, Ahn J, Papsin BC. Auditory development in the absence of hearing in infancy. *Neuroreport.* 2010;21(3):163–167.

59. Gordon KA, Papsin BC, Harrison RV. An evoked potential study of the developmental time course of the auditory nerve and brainstem in children using cochlear implants. *Audiol Neurotol.* 2006;11(1):7–23.

60. Gordon KA, Papsin BC, Harrison RV. Effects of cochlear implant use on the electrically evoked middle latency response in children. *Hear Res.* 2005;204(1–2):78–89.

61. Ponton CW, Don M, Eggermont JJ, Waring MD, Masuda A. Maturation of human cortical auditory function: differences between normal-hearing children and children with cochlear implants. *Ear Hear.* 1996;17(5):430–437.

62. Gilley PM, Sharma A, Dorman M, Finley CC, Panch AS, Martin K. Minimization of cochlear implant stimulus artifact in cortical auditory evoked potentials. *Clin Neurophysiol.* 2006;117(8):1772–1782.

63. Friesen LM, Picton TW. A method for removing cochlear implant artifact. *Hear Res.* 2010;259(1–2):95–106.

64. Gordon KA, Tanaka S, Wong DD, Papsin BC. Characterizing responses from auditory cortex in young people with several years of cochlear implant experience. *Clin Neurophysiol.* 2008;119(10):2347–2362.

65. Wong DD, Gordon KA. Beamformer suppression of cochlear implant artifacts in an electroencephalography dataset. *IEEE Trans Biomed Eng.* 2009;56(12):2851–2857.

66. Abbas PJ, Brown CJ, Shallop JK, et al. Summary of results using the nucleus CI24M implant to record the electrically evoked compound action potential. *Ear Hear.* 1999;20(1):45–59.

67. Bierer JA, Faulkner KF, Tremblay KL. Identifying cochlear implant channels with poor electrode-neuron interfaces: electrically evoked auditory brain stem responses measured with the partial tripolar configuration. *Ear Hear.* 2010;32(4):436–444.

68. Moller AR, Jannetta PJ, Sekhar LN. Contributions from the auditory nerve to the brain-stem auditory evoked potentials (BAEPs): results of intracranial recording in man. *Electroencephalogr Clin Neurophysiol.* 1988;71(3):198–211.

69. Gordon KA, Tanaka S, Wong DD, et al. Multiple effects of childhood deafness on cortical activity in children receiving bilateral cochlear implants simultaneously. *Clin Neurophysiol.* 2010;122(4):823–833.

70. Gordon KA, Papsin BC, Harrison RV. Auditory brainstem activity and development evoked by apical versus basal cochlear implant electrode stimulation in children. *Clin Neurophysiol.* 2007;118(8):1671–1684.

71. Sharma A, Dorman MF, Kral A. The influence of a sensitive period on central auditory development in children with unilateral and bilateral cochlear implants. *Hear Res.* 2005;203(1–2):134–143.

72. Gordon KA, Tanaka S, Papsin BC. Atypical cortical responses underlie poor speech perception in children using cochlear implants. *NeuroReport.* 2005;16(18):2041–2045.

73. Papsin BC, Gordon KA. Bilateral cochlear implants should be the standard for children with bilateral sensorineural deafness. *Curr Opin Otolaryngol Head Neck Surg.* 2008;16(1):69–74.

74. Gordon KA, Valero J, Papsin BC. Auditory brainstem activity in children with 9–30 months of bilateral cochlear implant use. *Hear Res.* 2007;233(1–2):97–107.

75. Gordon KA, Valero J, Papsin BC. Binaural processing in children using bilateral cochlear implants. *NeuroReport.* 2007;18(6):613–617.

76. Gordon, KA, Valero J, van Hoesel R, Papsin BC. Abnormal timing delays in auditory brainstem responses evoked by bilateral cochlear implant use in children. *Otol Neurotol.* 2008;29(2):193–198.

77. Gordon KA, Wong DD, Papsin BC. Cortical function in children receiving bilateral cochlear implants simultaneously or after a period of interimplant delay. *Otol Neurotol.* 2010;31(8):293–299.

78. Wong, DDE, Gordon KA. Hemispheric lateralization of cortical responses in children using bilateral cochlear implants. In: *33rd Midwinter Research Meeting of the Association for Research in Otolaryngology*; 2010, Anaheim, CA.

79. Brown CJ. Clinical uses of electrically evoked auditory nerve and brainstem responses. *Curr Opin Otolaryngol Head Neck Surg.* 2003;11(5):383–387.

80. Cushing SL, Papsin BC, Gordon KA. Incidence and characteristics of facial nerve stimulation in children with cochlear implants. *Laryngoscope.* 2006;116(10):1787–1791.

81. Cushing SL, Papsin BC, Strantzas S, Gordon KA. Facial nerve electromyography: a useful tool in detecting nonauditory side effects of cochlear implantation. *J Otolaryngol Head Neck Surg.* 2009;38(2):157–165.

82. Moog JS, Geers AE. *Early Speech Perception Test for Profoundly Hearing-impaired Children.* St. Louis, MO: Central Institute for the Deaf; 1990.

83. Hoversten GH. *Test of Auditory Comprehension (TAC) for Hearing Impaired Pupils: Reliability and Validity Study.* Washington DC: ERIC Clearinghouse; 1997.

84. Elliott LL, Katz D. *Development of a New Children's Test of Speech Discrimination*

[Technical manual]. St. Louis, MO: Auditec; 1980.

85. Ross M, Lerman J. A picture identification test for hearing-impaired children. *J Speech Hear Res*. 1979;13:44–53.

86. Erber NP. *Auditory Training*. Washington DC: AG Bell Association for the Deaf; 1982.

87. Kirk KI, Pisoni DB, Osberger MJ. Lexical effects on spoken word recognition by pediatric cochlear implant users. *Ear Hear*. 1995;16:470–481.

88. Haskins HA. A phonetically balanced test of speech discrimination for children [Unpublished master's thesis]. Northwestern University, Evanston, IL; 1949.

89. Bench J, Kowal A, Bamford J. The BKB (Bamford-Kowal-Bench) sentence lists for partially-hearing children. *Br J Audiol*. 1979; 13:108–112.

Chapter 15

Treatment Outcomes of Adult Cochlear Implantation

PAUL T. MICK, LENDRA M. FRIESEN, DAVID B. SHIPP, AND JOSEPH M. CHEN

INTRODUCTION

Cochlear implantation is, arguably, the single most important therapeutic intervention in Otology. Its impact is underscored by the transformative experience we routinely observe in an ever-increasing segment of the hearing impaired that is often taken for granted. Cochlear implantation has generated a tremendous amount of publicity and health care resources for our specialty and we often pay tribute to the pioneers who led us here, whereas the unsung heroes are the engineers and programmers from an industry that is committed to research and development. Improvement in outcomes among cochlear implant (CI) recipients appeared to have kept pace with technology, while successive expansion in candidacy criteria also gave rise to high performance. David et al[1] compared different generations of implant systems and coding strategies in the context of functional outcomes to illustrate that the improvement in performance over time were due to technologic improvement in similar cohorts. In well-matched, profoundly hearing-impaired subjects, newer implant technology and speech coding strategies allowed subjects to perform better in word and sentence recognition tests (Figs 15–1A and 15–1B).

Although it is difficult to quantify any one particular feature in hardware design that had the biggest impact on performance, some of the more notable changes are: body to ear-level devices, microphone, electrode design, battery life, and the size of receiver-stimulator. Some led to improvement in efficiency, others focused on convenience and cosmetics.

It is generally agreed that the most important aspects of a cochlear implant system that contributed to performance were improvement in signal processing and speech coding strategies. In the late 1980s and early 1990s, speech coding evolved from frequency extraction to "envelope-based" strategies such as:

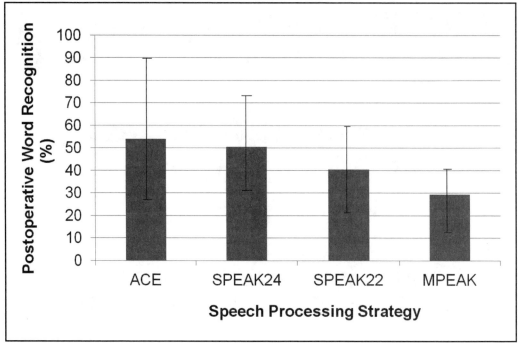

A

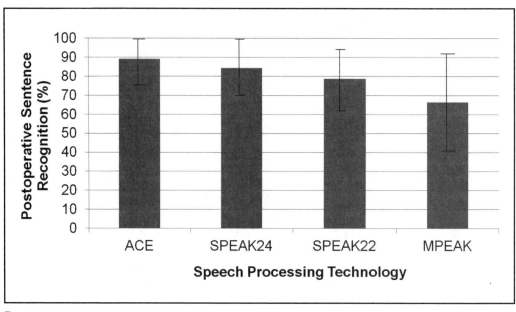

B

Figure 15–1. A. *CNC word recognition scores in 4 groups of Nucleus CI users (across 4 generations of speech coding strategies) who had profound hearing loss prior to surgery, showing improved outcomes (n = 105).* **B.** *HINT sentence recognition scores in 4 groups of Nucleus CI users (across 4 generations of speech coding strategies) who had profound hearing loss prior to surgery, showing improved outcomes (n = 105). Adapted from David, Ostroff, Shipp, Chen, and Nedzelski.[1]*

continuous interleaved sampling –CIS,[2] n-of-m,[3] and spectral peak-SPEAK[4] strategies. Two of these are still in widespread use today (CIS and n-of m). The currently used HiResolution[5] strategy is a variation of CIS that uses high rates of stimulation, while ACE[6] evolved from n-of-m.

During the past several years, increasing attention has been devoted to "fine structure" representation or fine frequency information.[7-12] This relates to frequency variations within band-pass channels that may not be represented well with CIS and other "envelope-based' strategies. Such a loss could degrade the representation of speech sounds[7] and tone patterns in tonal languages,[13] and greatly diminish the representation of musical sounds. Some fine structure information is transmitted via envelope-based strategies, but it has yet to be revealed how much. It is generally believed that true fine structure representation of sound is not possible due to the lack of neural integrity and as a result, implantees, by and large, perform poorly in the context of noise, multiple speakers, and in music perception.

Although both relaxed candidacy criteria and technologic advances have occurred concurrently with improved CI performance, it was the latter that defined the real impact we see today. In this chapter, we discuss modern multichannel implants and their performance outcomes.

OUTCOMES MEASURES

TESTS OF SPEECH RECOGNITION

Improved speech understanding is the primary goal of cochlear implantation in adults, and tests of speech discrimination help set the standards for determining candidacy and benefit. These tests are also used to track the progress of aural rehabilitation, optimize speech processor strategies, and serve as research outcome measures.

Several tests of speech perception have been developed (Table 15–1). In 2001, the American Academy of Otolaryngology-Head and Neck Surgery, in conjunction with the American Academy of Audiology and CI manufacturers, published a Minimum Speech Test Battery (MSTB) for postlingually deafened English-speaking adults with cochlear implants.[14] The group recommended that Hearing-in-Noise Test (HINT) sentences[15] and Consonant/Nucleus/Consonant (CNC) words[16] be included as part of a standardized set-list in any audiologic evaluation of CI patients to facilitate comparison of outcomes. The group also recommended that during each preoperative and postoperative evaluation, one 50-word CNC list and two 10-sentence HINT lists should be presented in quiet at 70 dB (SPL). Nevertheless, a wide variety of outcome measures continue to be used in clinical settings, often making intertrial comparisons difficult[17]; understanding how they differ with the standard test battery is important when reviewing outcomes.

Several internal and external methodological factors may affect the results of the various tests. Internal factors include whether they are objective or subjective, the type of response format employed (open- versus closed-set) and/or the number and equivalence of test lists. External factors include the use of recorded versus live voices, the stimulus presentation level, the use of competing noise, and whether or not visual cues are used.

Table 15–1. Common Tests of Speech Recognition

Test	Sentences or Words	Visual Cues	Background Noise	Live vs Recorded Voice	Equivalency of Lists	Number of Lists	Open vs Closed Set	Comment
HINT	Sentences	No	Yes	Recorded	Yes	25 lists of 10 sentences	Open	Commonly tested in quiet or with a fixed SNR, but originally described with an adaptive SNR technique
CID Everyday Sentences	Sentences	No	Yes	Recorded or live	No	10 lists of 10 sentences	Open	Scoring based on the number of correct key words
BKB	Sentences	No	No	Recorded	Yes	20 lists of 16 sentences	Open	
BKB-SIN	Sentences	No	Yes	Recorded	Yes	18 list pairs	Open	Scoring by adaptive SNR technique
Quick-SIN	Sentences	No	Yes	Recorded	Yes	12 lists of 6 sentences	Open	Scoring by adaptive SNR technique, using key words. Test takes approximately one minute to administer.
AzBio	Sentences	No	Yes	Recorded	Yes	33 lists of 20 sentences	Open	Sentences spoken by untrained speakers in casual style with background babble

Test	Sentences or Words	Visual Cues	Background Noise	Live vs Recorded Voice	Equivalency of Lists	Number of Lists	Open vs Closed Set	Comment
CUNY sentences	Sentences	Yes	Yes	Recorded	Yes	72 lists of 12 sentences	Open	Test can be performed with or without visual cues
CNC	Words	No	No	Recorded	Yes	10 lists of 50 words each	Open	Monosyllabic words with equal phonemic distribution across lists, with approximately the same phonemic distribution as the English language.
Words in Noise (WIN)	Words	No	Yes	Recorded	Yes	CNC words used with background noise	Open	
Arthur Boothroyd words	Words	No	No	Recorded or live	Yes	15 lists of 10 words	Open	Scoring based on the number of correct phonemes (3 phonemes per word)

HINT = Hearing in Noise Test (Nilsson et al[15]; CID = Central Institute for the Deaf (Silverman[153]; BKB = Bamford-Kowal-Bench (Bench et al[33]; BKB-SIN = Bamford-Kowal-Bench—Speech in Noise[33]; Quick-SIN = Quick Speech in Noise (Killion[34]); CUNY = City University of New York (Boothroyd[20]; CNC = Consonant/Nucleus/Consonant (Peterson and Lehiste[154]); Words in Noise (Wilson[155]); Arthur Boothroyd words (Boothroyd[156]).

Objective tests require listeners to repeat presented syllables, phonemes, words, or sentences. In contrast, subjective tests ask the listener or someone else to report on listening behaviors, often in the form of questionnaires. Subjective tests are used almost exclusively for children.[18,19]

Open-set tests are those in which the listener is given a test stimulus (eg, a phoneme, word, or sentence) and is asked to respond with what he or she believes was said. In contrast, in closed-set tests, the listener chooses a response from a list of potential answers, one of which is correct. Open-set testing is more lifelike and difficult. It requires cognitive processing, which is influenced by an individual's vocabulary and linguistic knowledge. Closed-set testing is rarely used for adults in the modern clinical setting, as more difficult tests are required to avoid ceiling effects. Researchers still use closed-set tests in adults to determine which speech features are well conveyed by a particular CI system, or to evaluate an individual's capabilities without the influence of cognitive factors.[20,21]

It was noted that recorded voice (as opposed to live voice) may increase consistency in speech perception testing between listeners.[22] Significantly different speech recognition results are often obtained for the same test materials when they are administered by different talkers,[23,24] and even when using different recordings made over time by the same speaker.[25] Clinicians may differ with regard to how they say test words, with some using a conversational manner and others attempting to enunciate. This can be a significant factor because intelligibility is affected by the use of conversational versus clear speech.[26] The AzBio test, developed at the Cochlear Implant Laboratory

at Arizona State University, is a new test in which the speakers are untrained persons speaking in conversational style. It consists of 33 equivalent lists of 20 sentences recorded by untrained speakers using a conversational speaking style.[27] This test is now a routine part of the test battery at our center to circumvent the issues of the ceiling effect commonly observed with the HINT test. Live voice testing may be used when the examiner requires more flexibility, such as when testing children.

Postoperative speech perception testing is performed repeatedly to assess progress and aid in processor fitting. So that patients do not memorize responses over time, each test should include multiple lists of stimuli. The number of lists provided by each speech perception test varies (see Table 15–1). List equivalency and test-retest reliability has been established for most, but not all, tests of speech discrimination.

In the past, as described for the MSTB, speech perception outcomes were usually tested at 70 dB SPL.[28,29] Conversational speech typically occurs at 50 to 60 dB SPL. Some authors have advocated lowering testing levels to better reflect conversational speech and thus provide more meaningful results.[30] Speech recognition scores may drop significantly with decreased presentation levels.[31]

In addition, although there is background noise in most regular conversations, testing has generally been performed in quiet sound-booths. Testing in quiet may produce "ceiling effects," in which top performers all achieve near-perfect scores. In other words, the independent variable (ability to discriminate speech) no longer has an effect on the dependent variable (test score). Conversely, if patients are tested with a large amount of background noise, the test may become so difficult as to produce "floor effects," in which poor performers all score near zero. Testing in noise can be presented at a fixed signal-to-noise ratio (SNR) to measure the percent of words or sentences correctly identified.[31,32] However, it is difficult to find a SNR that avoids ceiling and floor effects in all participants. A second method avoids ceiling and floor effects by keeping the speech signal constant while noise levels are varied until the listener scores a certain target score (typically 50% correct). The dependent measure is the SNR that yields the target score.[32,15] The Bamford-Kowal-Bench Speech-in-Noise (BKB-SIN)[33] and Quick-SIN[34] tests are performed this way. The HINT was also originally described using this technique, but for cochlear implant patients it is often administered in quiet, at +10, +5, or even 0 dB SNR.[35]

Speech discrimination is usually tested without visual cues. Normal speech, however, usually occurs in the presence of visible articulatory gestures that give information as to what is being said (eg, lip reading). Visual cues may significantly improve speech recognition scores, especially in challenging acoustic environments.[36–38] Auditory-only tests, therefore, may not adequately characterize the performance of patients with cochlear implants. Ideally, performance should be assessed using auditory only, visual only, and auditory plus visual modalities. The City University of New York (CUNY) sentence test is one of the few tests of speech discrimination that can be presented in all three modalities.[20]

With continued improvements in CI outcomes, many previously used measures are no longer rigorous enough to adequately assess speech perception. New, more difficult tests have been developed. Tests may be made more difficult by

increasing the SNR,[15,36] using background multitalker babble[27] or controlling lexical characteristics of stimulus items.[39,40] Word tests (such as the CNC test) are being used more frequently as they are more difficult than sentence tests.

Tests in which speech can be presented with background noise include the HINT, BKB-SIN, and the Quick-SIN test. The HINT test consists of 25 lists of 10 sentences selected from the BKB test for their uniformity in length and their representation of natural speech. Speech is presented at a fixed level and noise is adaptively varied. The BKB-SIN and Quick-SIN tests both contain multiple sentence lists. Four-talker babble background noise, designed to simulate a typical social gathering, can be varied. The dependent measure in both tests is the signal-to-babble ratio that yields 50% correct.

PERFORMANCE LEVELS

The evidence for cochlear implantation is unequivocal as it relates to improved speech perception abilities in appropriately selected candidates. At our institution, 1,128 adult patients have been managed and tracked through an extensive prospective database since inception in 1985. In Figure 15–1, performance outcomes were significantly improved over time, through newer generations of implant systems to suggest that technology and new programming strategies are driving the performance curves in comparable cohorts.[1] In 2005, Bodmer reviewed 455 late-deafened adults over a 10-year period who were implanted and fitted with contemporary speech processors.[41] The average one-year postoperative HINT score was 82% in quiet, and 68% in noise compared to a preoperative score of 19% in quiet. The average one-year postoperative CNC word score was 53.5%, compared to the average preoperative score of 9.9%. In this cohort, 44% were deemed high CI performers (HINT scores >90%) whereas 13% were poor CI performers (HINT scores <10%); it was clear that preoperative speech recognition function and prelingual deafness were major predictors of outcome, whereas the use of hearing aid, vestibular function, and device types were not statistically significant. Interestingly, a subset of perilingually deafened subjects was able to achieve high performance status with a strong auditory-verbal background. A most recent review of 417 postlingually deafened adult implant users from 2001 to 2011 revealed a similar trend in performance with the most recent iterations of implant technology (unpublished data, Fig 15–2).

As candidacy criteria became more relaxed, patients who had pre-operative hearing function better than the conventional threshold (<60% HINT score) but struggled with hearing aids were considered for implantation. In a group of 27 subjects with preoperative HINT scores >60%, Amoodi et al[42] reported the mean HINT score improvement from 69% to 95%, with one-third of the patients reached the ceiling effect of 100%. CNC Word scores improved from 29 to 65% on average. Six subjects who reached the ceiling effect of 100% were tested with the AzBio Sentences to further define the degree of performance; scores ranged from 90 to 100% (in quiet) to 32 to 92% (in noise) (Fig 15–3). The Hearing Handicap Inventory (HHI) further supported their performance and satisfaction in this group of higher functioning participants who previously struggled with hearing aids, but were considered as nonconforming candidates.[42] It is exciting to see that patients continue to derive benefit beyond the conventional thresholds established to date, notwithstanding the move toward electroacoustic stimulation, and implanting those with single-sided deafness and tinnitus as some of the newer, albeit more controversial, indications for implantation.

Our clinical results mirror published data from other centers that use different test batteries. One large study from the United Kingdom Cochlear Implant Study Group[43] with over 300 subjects used the BKB sentence test. Participants were divided into "traditional candidates" (TC: PTA = 117.1 dB) or "marginal hearing aid users (MHU: PTA =108.7 dB) on the basis of preoperative speech intelligibility tests. The mean scores for both groups improved by 9 months compared with preimplantation, with the TC group showing significantly more improvement than the MHU group. Parkinson and colleagues[44] studied 216 subjects using CUNY sentences and words. They found significant benefits at 3 months postimplantation as the average improvement ranged from 35% for CUNY words in quiet to 67% for CUNY sentences in quiet.[44]

Speech understanding in the context of telephone use is a subjective measure of performance outcome without a standardized method. Telephone use challenges the implant user both in terms of lacking visual cueing, and reduced audibility from decreased frequency transmission.[45,46] Surveys of implant users indicated that most (66 to 87%) were able to use the telephone at least some of the time.[47-50] Telephone use has been found to be significantly associated with post-implantation sentence scores and possibly education level.[50,51] Telephone conversations are easier to understand for implant users if they are familiar with the topic of conversation and with the

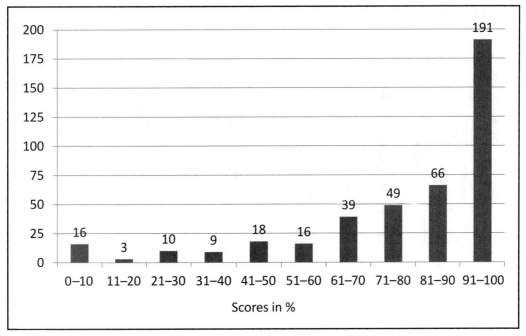

A

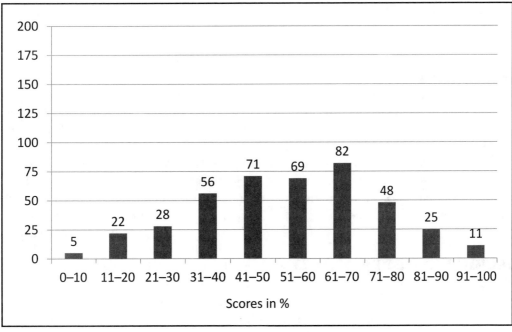

B

Figure 15–2. **A.** *Postlingually deafened adults open-set sentence (HINT-in-quiet) recognition scores 2000–2011 1-year postactivation (*N = 417*).* **B.** *Postlingually deafened adults open-set word (CNC) recognition scores 2000–2011 1-year postactivation (*N = 417*).*

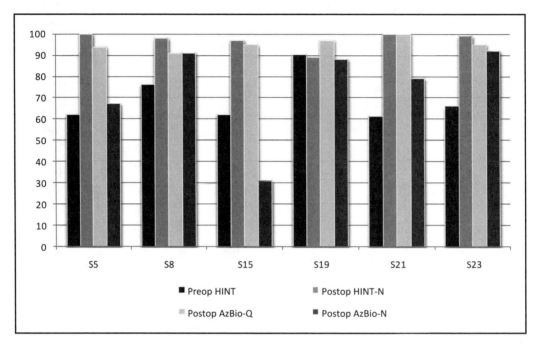

Figure 15–3. *Audiometric testing for high performers who reached the ceiling effect of 100% on HINT-in-quiet test. HINT-in- noise, and AzBio sentence (in quiet and noise with +5 dB SNR) tests were performed to further differentiate outcomes.*

person on the other end of the line. The ability to use a telephone has been significantly associated with increased quality of life.[50]

Performance levels for nontraditional indications such as hearing preservation technique, electroacoustic stimulation, bilateral implantation, and single-sided deafness are discussed elsewhere.

MUSIC PERCEPTION AND ENJOYMENT

Presently, one of the most challenging areas in CI functionality relates to music enjoyment and perception. Patients who may have a high degree of speech understanding in the quiet often feel frustrated as their speech performance may not translate into a high degree of music enjoyment and listening.

There are several variables that determine enjoyment, such as preferences in types of music, familiarity, and listener characteristics. For instance, CI listeners, in general appear to prefer pop and country western music that typically contains short simple melodies, repetitive rhythms, and harmonic changes compared to classical music which often consists of complex rhythmic structures, harmonic changes, and organization.[52-55] However, a recent study has found stronger preference of CI listener in classical music over jazz, country, and pop music.[56] The reasons for the inconsistent results are not clear, and may be related to the choice of musical excerpts of the same musical style being presented at varying complexities across studies.

Structural features associated with a musical excerpt (lyrics, voice quality, rhythm) assist the CI recipient in recognition of familiar musical excerpts.[54,57,58] In fact, CI recipients tend to perform at a level close to chance in identifying familiar melodies presented without their lyrics, either as instrumental or melody-line versions. This is likely due to the implant being better at transmitting speech than pitch.

Several studies pertaining to CI listeners have found individual characteristics influential to the quality of music listening.[57,59–61] Specifically, age of adult CI listeners is negatively correlated with self-reported enjoyment, appraisal, and perceptual accuracy for rhythm, pitch, pitch sequences, melody recognition, and timbre recognition in music listening.[55,62,63] Commitment to listening is another issue as older adults report spending less time listening to music.[55]

Through a qualitative report, Bartel et al[64] demonstrated that when it comes to music enjoyment, prior experience of musical skills, critical listening, and one's expectations are important determinants of outcome. Furthermore, focus and attention skills during a period of self-rehabilitation may prove to be a critical piece in both enjoyment and performance in music with a CI.

A number of researcher groups have attempted to qualify and quantify music perception in small samples of CI users by breaking down various components of music as independent variables, namely pitch,[65–67] timbre,[66,67] and rhythm.[65,67–68] It is generally accepted that the lack of neural integrity and the inability for the implant system to deliver sufficient fine structure cues prevents CI users from accurately perceiving music. Studies have shown that pitch and timbre perception can be improved in implantees following auditory rehabilitation. After 12 weeks of training, Gfeller et al [63] reported that post-lingually deafened cochlear implant recipients showed significant improve-

ment in timbre recognition and appraisal compared with a control group. It has been shown that pitch perception performance correlated significantly with a longer duration of musical training in children with cochlear implants. Esra Yucel et al[69] studied 18 profoundly hearing-impaired children with unilateral CIs. The participants were separated into a control group where no training was completed, and a training group, where participants were given 12 months of rhythm and pitch training. The participants in the training group were more interested in listening to music in cars, at school and during music lessons after 12 months of rhythm and pitch training compared to the control group. In addition, by the end of 24 months, the training group showed remarkable improvement in all developmental areas of musical perception.

Overall, there is less auditory training and related research performed in adult CI recipients than in children, whether due to financial reasons or lack of compelling evidence for the usefulness of such training. However, Galvin et al[66] found that the CI participants' mean melodic contour identification performance significantly improved with targeted melodic contour training. The authors also suggested that CI participants' music perception and appreciation may improve after melodic contour identification training.

Although auditory training generally improved performance in the targeted listening task, the improvement often generalized to auditory tasks that were not explicitly trained (eg, improved sentence recognition after training with phonetic contrasts, or improved familiar melody identification after training with simple melodic sequences).[70] It has been also documented that musical exposure and training have transfer effects on the non-musical skills of children with cochlear implants, similar to normal-hearing children. In a Japanese study, including 17 congenitally deaf children, music-listening initiators (those who, based on parent questionnaires, initiated music listening) had significantly higher word-recognition scores than non-initiators. The authors related the finding that music listening, especially focused music listening, may involve the training of auditory attention. In other words, learning that occurs in the context of music listening may transfer to other auditory but nonmusical contexts.[71] Pitch is important in speech for prosodic cues in most languages and semantic or grammatical cues in tonal languages. As most music training protocols are focused on improving pitch perception, which is known to be very poor in CI users compared to NH subjects, it therefore is logical that an improvement in pitch perception will lead to an improvement in speech perception.

Numerous challenges are facing researchers in designing effective auditory training programs for CI users. One of the major difficulties is creating a training protocol that mimics the real life CI users' daily encounters. It is also essential to develop a protocol that will provide quick improvement over a relatively short time period; otherwise, the participants will lose interest and motivation during training sessions. Ideal duration of training has also been investigated. Longitudinal studies showed that most gains in performance occurred in the first 3 to 6 months of use. Improvements continue, however, but at a much slower rate up to 24 months following implantation. [72–74]

Evidence has shown that a significant variable in a listener's potential to enjoy music is the ability to maintain focus and to employ selective, alternating, and divided attentions in the context of pitch processing, an area that had been overlooked in the past. Rather than focusing only on perceptual skills in the basic elements of music (pitch, timbre, and rhythm),[63,75,76] a more holistic approach should be adopted by adding tasks with increasing levels of complexity, involving pattern and melody recognition. A novel study to develop a diagnostic software as a first step toward an expanded rehabilitation tool by Alexander et al, called Music-EAR,[56] compared the music perception and enjoyment of CI users, normal-hearing musicians and normal-hearing nonmusicians, revealed that CI users performed significantly worse than normal hearing subjects in all of the perceptual tasks. They performed most poorly, however, on pitch and timbre perception tasks. Additionally, overall CI user scores were lowest in those tasks that required the recipient to differentiate multiple lines of concurrent music, to divide attention between different melodies, or to distinguish variations in pitch and timbre simultaneously.

Their findings were concurrent with Galvin et al[66] who showed that CI users performed poorly on listening tasks requiring differentiation between multiple instruments being played simultaneously. Galvin et al also concluded that CI users have limited access to the fundamental frequency and timbre cues necessary to isolate competing voices or musical instruments. In a qualitative report, Bartel and colleagues[64] studied "high-performing" CI users with varied musical training and functional perceptual abilities who demonstrated a high ability to focus their attention and to sustain their practice in the form of rehabilitation. The results are a reflection on the increased complexity of the given tasks in regard to perception, memory, and concentration with some implant users capable of processing complex melodies and harmonies. Additionally, these findings also confirmed that subjects with similar musical backgrounds, education, and duration of hearing loss, can achieve radically different post-implant musical ability depending on persistence in listening training. These case studies provide real-world examples of the benefits that can be achieved through consistent attention-based learning pointing to the fundamental need for more standardized and customized rehabilitation training.[64]

Although many question the ability of the CI technology to provide the necessary spectral information needed to accurately perceive music, particularly in the context of a damaged cochlea, many enjoy listening to music whereas others have very high music perceptual skills to suggest that these are achievable goals even with current technology. The advent of training programs designed to improve auditory processing, and especially those incorporating attention-based tasks may prove important in the future.

QUALITY OF LIFE AND COST EFFECTIVENESS

It is clear that cochlear implantation confers audiologic benefits. How these benefits translate into health related quality-of-life (HRQL) improvements in other domains are the focus of many clinical studies in recent years. Quality of life can be defined as an individual's contentment or satisfaction. Contributing factors include health and nonmedical factors such as living conditions, relationships, finances, and other individual and environmental characteristics.[77]

Specific instruments have been designed to measure the impact of otologic illness on HRQL and include the Tinnitus Handicap Inventory (THI),[78] the Hearing Handicap Inventory (HHI),[79] and, more recently, the Nijmegen Cochlear Implant Questionnaire (NCIQ).[80]

In a more comprehensive fashion, quality of life may be assessed through validated instruments, such as the Short Form 36 Questionnaire (SF-36),[81] Health Utilities Index (HUI),[82] and European Quality of Life.[83] The SF-36 is popular as it is one of the oldest HRQL tool with proven robustness and is well standardized. The HUI is appropriate for use in otology and CI research because it contains statement items relating to functional limitations due to impaired hearing or speech. The utility weights were based on Canadian and U.S. populations.[82]

Chung et al[84] administered the SF-36 to 283 adult subjects pre- and postoperatively and reported a significant improvement in 5 of the 8 domains, including: role functioning (physical), role functioning (emotional), vitality, social functioning, and mental health. When age stratification was applied to those under the age of 45, and over 65 years, the same patterns were observed; the entire group performed better than the Canadian norm (Fig 15–4). Similar results of improved HRQL were seen with smaller cohorts.[85–88] Klop administered HUI and the NCIQ to postlingually deafened adult implant users. When clinical significance was assessed by minimal significant difference (MID) and effective size(ES), he found important clinical improvements on 6 health domains of the NCIQ and on the sensation domain of the HUI in most patients.[87]

The importance and relevance of HRQL research in cochlear implantation are reinforced by the challenges we face in the era of limited resources. To compete for healthcare dollars, it is critical to

HRQoL Improvements
Overall Results

N = 283   Mean age = 52.88 +/- 15.05

Domain	Pre-CI Mean	Post-CI Mean	Mean Difference	*p*-value
Physical functioning	80.55 (21.74)	82.74 (20.12)	2.19 (18.64)	0.214
Role functioning (physical)	74.65 (36.83)	85.6 (29.06)	10.95 (36.82)	<0.001
Bodily Pain	74.1(23.84)	76.48 (21.74)	2.38 (24.6)	0.216
General health perception	71.99 (20.48)	75.06 (20.02)	3.07 (17.45)	0.072
Vitality	62.95 (21.1)	68.94 (18.36)	5.99 (19.03)	<0.001
Social functioning	72.89 (27.6)	86.60 (20.26)	13.71 (24.75)	<0.001
Role functioning (emotional)	72.42 (38.35)	87.65 (26.94)	15.22 (39.48)	<0.001
Mental Health	70.49 (19.75)	79.38 (15.32)	8.89 (16.33)	<0.001

Figure 15–4. *Health-related quality of life measures (SF36) in 283 adult cochlear implant users demonstrating improvement in 5 of 8 domains at 1-year postimplantation.*

set outcomes standards not just by performance metrics, but also through the lens of health economics. Health economics research is what public and private providers look to when evaluating new drugs and technology that are responsible for a significant part of the cost increases in health care delivery[89]; the goal, of course, is to establish the net effect of an intervention compared to its cost relative to other types of therapy. The cost-effectiveness of a therapy is often established by what is known as the Cost-Utility Index, and the incremental cost effectiveness ratio (ICER). They are used interchangeably to define the net cost of a treatment to the net effects in quality-adjusted life years (QALYs). A QALY is a unit that incorpo-

rates both mortality and HRQL. It is calculated by multiplying an intervention's effect on life expectancy (in years) by a "health utility" conversion factor valued between 0 and 1; 0 represents death and 1 represents perfect health, with the continuum in between representing the spectrum of HRQL. Health utility can be determined directly or indirectly[90]; direct methods include the visual analog scale (VAS),[91] time tradeoff (TTO),[92] or Standard Gamble techniques.[82] Indirect methods include the use of "utility metrics" such as the validated questionnaires described above for measuring HRQL.

The cost-utility benefit of unilateral cochlear implantation in postlingually deafened adults is well established.[93–97]

The largest study was published by the United Kingdom Cochlear Implant Study Group (UKCISG) in 2004 that involved 13 centers.[98] It documented the preoperative and 9-month postoperative HUI (Mark III) results of 311 postlinguistically deafened adults, from 18 to 82 years of age, divided into 4 performance groups within the definition of severe to profound hearing loss. For the entire group, average utility score increased from 0.433 to 0.630, an increase of 0.197. Averaged over the entire cohort, the cost of gaining a QALY was €27,142; cost/QALY varied with age at implantation from €19,223 for subjects who were younger than 30 yr of age to €45,411 for subjects who were older than 70 yr of age. The study concluded that cochlear implantation was a cost-effective intervention for the majority of subjects, including the older group, although relaxation of candidacy criteria will reduce cost-effectiveness. In the event of resource prioritization, the authors contended that the provision of care in cochlear implantation should take into account "duration of profound deafness," and "preoperative word recognition" as predictors of success and benefit.[98]

The methodology with which QALY or "utility" is determined remains a very contentious issue as the cost side (numerator) of the equation is relatively fixed but the denominator is subject to great interpretation and how the utility tools are presented to the stakeholder. Significant degrees of conflict of interest exist depending on who is involved in the assessment. Notwithstanding this variability, the most comprehensive review cost-effectiveness was published by Bond et al[17] in 2009, who used published data to create an economic model to assign incremental cost-effectiveness ratio (ICER). For postlingually profoundly deaf adults, the corresponding ICERs were £14,163 (unilateral implant), £49,559 (simultaneous bilateral implants) and £60,301 (sequential bilateral implants) per QALY respectively. Probabilistic threshold analyses estimated that, when measured on a lifetime horizon and compared with nontechnologic support or acoustic hearing aids, cochlear implants were highly likely to be considered cost-effective for adults at willingness-to-pay thresholds of £20,000 and £30,000 per QALY. At those same thresholds, for simultaneous bilateral implantation to become cost-effective, a discount of approximately 75% on the cost of the second implant system was required. Of course, this type of modeling can be misleading due to the highly uncertain utility gain estimates contained within a large pool of studies, as well as the uncertainty related to discount pricing.

So far, most cost utility or effectiveness studies have not focused on socioeconomic benefit to the individual and to society. Monteiro et al[99] used known Canadian economic surrogates and income groups to indirectly determine the personal economic impact of both deafness and unilateral cochlear implantation in 637 subjects. The main outcome measures included employment rates and personal income estimates prior to and following cochlear implantation. 36.7% suffered a negative economic impact as a result of their deafness. Cochlear implantation was associated with a significant increase in estimated median annual income, compared to pre-implantation ($42,672 vs $30,432; $p = 0.007$). The ideal method of calculating economic impact would entail the use of personal income tax information, which presents enormous challenges to researchers, not the least of which include privacy and enrollment, but would offer a perspective to utility gain that has not been accessible to date.

Individual Variability in Outcome

Multivariate analysis has identified predictors of improved speech discrimination after cochlear implantation. The two most significant predictors are duration of deafness and preoperative speech discrimination. Combined, these factors account for approximately 80% of the variance in postimplant word recognition.[100] Factors that have been associated with better outcomes include postlingual deafness, education level, lip-reading ability, and higher promontory thresholds.[1,101–104] Parameters such as sex, age, caloric response, and the side of implantation are not predictive. Hearing aid use, and etiologies of hearing loss may be relevant to specific groups. Knowledge of salient predictive factors supports the decision process and helps establish expectations and the needs related to auditory rehabilitation.

Duration of Deafness

Duration of deafness is a well established predictor of speech recognition with a cochlear implant.[41,100,104] Each additional year of profound deafness has been found to result in a 0.7 to 0.8% decrease in the expected postoperative CNC word recognition score. The rate may be less in older patients, who have a more established auditory foundation than younger ones.[106]

It is theorized that over time, there would be a gradual reduction of the hair cell population in most implant subjects leading to the loss of their trophic support, and the secondary degeneration of the spiral ganglion.[107] Of course, there is

a tremendous amount of individual and disease variability in the degenerative effect within the end-organ. Variation in residual speech discrimination may also reflect the viability of central auditory pathways, whereby the trophic effects are not as clearly defined as they are at the periphery. This explains why patients with higher preoperative sentence scores can be expected to perform better than those with lower scores, even if they have had hearing loss for the same length of time.[100]

Preoperative Speech Discrimination

Speech discrimination is in itself an independent predictor of postoperative outcome.[41,100,103–104] Rubinstein and colleagues[100] found that for each 2% increase in Central Institute for the Deaf (CID) sentence scores preoperatively there was an approximate 1% increase in CNC word scores postoperatively. Thus, for a given duration of deafness, a patient with a preoperative sentence score of 40% would be expected to have a postoperative CNC word score that was 20% higher than a patient with no open-set speech recognition. In a large case-control study at our institution, in which implantees were divided into excellent and poor performers based on their postoperative speech discrimination scores ($n = 445$), excellent performers had significantly higher preoperative sentence scores than did poor performers (14%:7%, $p = 0.004$).[41] It has been found that even a small amount of preoperative speech discrimination is associated with higher than average performance and less variance in results.[100] In spite of the above, patients with no preoperative speech reception may still do very well, suggesting the clinical-pathologic correlation to hair cell and spiral ganglion survival is not clearly understood.

Amoodi et al[42] showed that as a whole, implant recipients who were functioning at a preoperative level that exceeded the conventional criteria of <60% HINT in quiet, performed better than the historical controls; the mean postoperative score was 94% as compared to approximately 80%,[1,41,50,97,102,103] whereas 30% of the recipients reached the ceiling effect on HINT sentence tests. Clearly, we are no longer married to a fixed threshold in terms of candidacy. Those with hearing loss at levels that are previously considered non-forming, but struggle with hearing aids, should undergo a broader audiometric assessment and counseling in light of this finding.

Prelingual Versus Postlingual Deafness

Speech discrimination outcomes are poorer in adult patients with pre- or perilingual deafness. Deafness at an early age results in deficiencies in both auditory-receptive and spoken-expressive language centers. Adult patients who have experienced prolonged sensory deprivation or distortion since a very young age lack the brain plasticity to achieve adequate neural integration and their implant performance is expectedly poorer. However, it has been shown that exposure to the oral environment in various degrees will have a differentiating impact on outcomes. Kaplan et al[108] demonstrated that those who received auditory-verbal therapy (AV) performed better than those who were defined as oral deaf (OD), whereas the group that included those educated through total communication (TC), or reared primarily through American Sign Language (ASL) with little oral communi-

cation performed the poorest. The mean postimplant composite scores (using open-set words, phoneme, and sentence recognition) were significantly different amongst the three groups.[108]

Clinical studies have repeatedly shown that prelingually deafened adult implantees score poorly on speech discrimination measures. There are also higher rates of sporadic use or nonuse in these patients, who are more likely to require more extensive rehabilitation than their postlingually deafened counterparts.[109,110] Nevertheless, this group of patients can still benefit from cochlear implantation, and can achieve some degree of open-set speech discrimination.[108] Auditory-verbal therapy (AVT) was found to be a significant predictor when comparing performance levels in this group of subjects, whereby 21% of the poor performers and 75% of the high performers received AVT.[41] Chee et al[111] showed that 77% of the early deafened adults were employed, 96.7% were satisfied with their implants and use them for most of their waking hours. Family support and a positive attitude were thought to be important factors other than AVT in maximizing benefit.

Aging

How aging affects cochlear implantation performance remains a topic of debate based on an assumption by some that elderly patients do not derive as much benefit from CI as younger patients due to both age-related degenerative changes in auditory systems and cognitive factors. Speech recognition as measured by phoneme score in patients above 70 years of age did not improve as much as younger age groups following cochlear implant.[112] Similarly, elderly patients over 70 years of age did not perform as well on consonant words, Central Institute for the Deaf sentences, and HINT sentences as younger patients postimplant.[113] One might suspect that elderly individuals may have poorer rehabilitation outcomes than their younger peers evidenced by animal and human studies demonstrating age-related degeneration of spiral ganglion cells crucial to the success of implantation.[114,115]

Notwithstanding the potential age-related effects on speech understanding, the improvement in performance with implantation in the elderly remains significant. Park and colleagues[97] demonstrated that the improvement in HINT scores (in quiet) following implantation in the oldest age group (66 years of age or older) was comparable to those of younger age groups. When the age cutoff for the "elderly" group was adjusted to 70 years of age or older, speech recognition still improved to a similar extent as younger patients following CI (4.7-fold increase in patients ≥ age 70 versus 4.1-fold increase in patients < age 70). These findings are in agreement with those of others,[106,116,117] and lend support to the notion that a candidate's age is not an important factor in audiometric benefits of CI and should not play a primary role in determination of candidacy. In our study,[97] we did find significant differences between the two age groups when HINT sentences were presented in noise with a +5 dB S/N ratio (Fig 15–5). It might be that age-related effects on speech understanding begin to emerge more robustly in complex listening environments such as with noise or when listening to music, and when more difficult speech tasks are presented. This may be one of the reasons for the discrepancy in results across studies.

For a given duration of deafness, some older patients may have better speech recognition outcomes than younger patients, an observation that led to the concept of "Durage," in reference to the ratio of "duration of deafness" to "age," that is, the percentage of life lived in deafness.[102] Patients with a lower "Durage" have better outcomes after cochlear implantation to suggest that older patients may have a more developed foundation of central auditory processing than younger patients, accounting for improved outcomes when duration of deafness is equal. An auditory foundation is a form of cognition reflecting an internalized memory of sounds and the ability to process acoustic inputs. However, one must keep in mind that this does not stop the aging process. Even with the benefits of an auditory foundation, age-related effects are being observed in elderly individuals' speech understanding as the underlying physiology relevant to their auditory systems changes over time.

Age at implantation does not seem to impact on quality of life improvement. There was no significant difference in pre- or postimplant Hearing Handicap Index (HHI) scores between different age groups.[97] In addition, the United Kingdom Cochlear Implant Study Group found no significant differences in quality of life outcomes between age groups as measured by the HUI-3, Glasgow Health Status Inventory (GHSI), or Glasgow Benefit Inventory (GBI).[98]

Etiologies of Hearing Loss

The largest group of patients within an adult cochlear implant program consists of those diagnosed with "bilateral progressive idiopathic sensorineural hearing loss," a category that has no real etiological meaning. When combined with those who suffered rapid onset bilateral SNHL, and those with early idiopathic hearing loss, more than 50% of the adult implant recipients did not have a clear diagnosis.

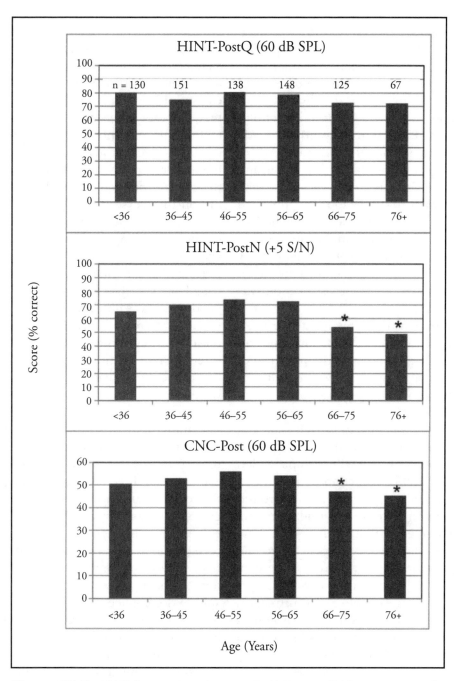

Figure 15–5. *HINT Scores in quiet, +5 dB SNR, and CNC word scores for CI patients of different age groups. Repeated measures ANOVAs indicated significant main effects for the two older age groups on the HINT +5 dB SNR and on the CNC word test. Asterisks indicate the scores that were significantly different at the .05 significance level. The number of patients is the same for each condition (listed above the top columns).*

Table 15–2 includes other possible diagnoses based on our experience with 908 unilateral cochlear implant recipients.[1,41,50,97–99,110] It seems, with all other variables being equal, cochlear implant outcomes are similar for most etiologies.[104,118] Exceptions should be made for autoimmune inner ear disease (AIED), for which outcomes have been better, and meningitis, for which outcomes have been poorer. Wang and colleagues[119] published results in 25 patients with AIED who had average one-year postimplantation open-set sentence scores of 97%, significantly higher than age- and sex-matched controls, although cochlear ossification was not identified.

Patients with postmeningitic deafness had, by and large, significantly poorer speech discrimination in the presence of labyrinthitis ossificans.[120,121] Results for patients with partial ossification, in which only the basal turn required a drill-out, better approximated those who did not suffer postmenigitic ossification.[120] When the cochlea is totally ossified, implantation with a radical drill-out can be performed by skeletonizing the modiolus around which an electrode was then draped. Gantz contends that such a technique rarely results in open-set speech discrimination either due to poor electrode contact and reduced neuronal substrate,[121] based on histopathologic confirmation of decreased spiral ganglion cells counts and new bone formation observed in human temporal bone studies.[122,123]

Side of Implantation

Many factors come into play when determining which ear should receive a patient's first implant. Each ear is compared to the other with respect to residual hearing ability, length of deafness, radiographic appearance, hearing aid use, vestibular function, and the presence of associated otologic disease. Controversy exists as to whether a better or worse hearing ear should be implanted. Some theorize that, all other things being equal, the better hearing ear should be used to take advantage of healthier neural elements in the auditory pathway.[100] Others feel that the general otologic principle of operating on the worse hearing ear should be observed, so that if complications arise, the better hearing ear has not been damaged. Several studies have revealed no significant difference in implant performance based on whether the better or worse hearing ear was implanted,[124] when other variables were well matched. A primary reason for selecting the worse ear was often related to the caloric asymmetry that drove the decision to implant the ear with reduced function.

There is no proven advantage to implanting either the left or the right ear with regards to perceived dominance with regards to the auditory system. Research over the past three decades has suggested that central auditory pathways may process speech asymmetrically, with the left cerebral hemisphere supporting speech recognition and production, and the right hemisphere supporting emotional and tonal aspects of speech.[125] Left hemisphere dominance is found in 95 to 98% of right handed people and 70 to 80% of left-handed people.[126,127] Despite these findings, if all other factors are equal, the side of implantation has not been shown to influence postoperative speech recognition.[97,128]

Cognitive and Linguistic Skills

There are theoretical advantages to having higher cognitive and linguistic skills

Table 15–2. Etiologies of Hearing Loss in Patients Who Received Single-Sided Implants Between 1987 and 2010

Sunnybrook CI Program	
Etiologies	Numbers Affected
acute temporal bone infections	1
auditory neuropathy	5
autoimmune	9
bilateral fistulae	1
B-O-R syndrome	1
cochlear hydrops	1
Cogan syndrome	8
congenital syphilis	2
CSOM	16
CSOM/Ménière's	1
DFNA36	3
diphtheria	1
early idiopathic	139 (15.4%)
encephalitis	1
Fabry	2
GJB2/Connexin 26	28
hereditary progressive	103 (11.4%)
Kallman syndrome	1
Kearns-Sayre syndrome	2
measles	5
MELAS	4
Ménière's	25
meningitis	37
mitochondrial cytopathy	1
NF2	1
otosclerosis	66 (7.3%)
ototoxicity	15
Pendred syndrome	12
pertussis	2
progressive idiopathic	263 (29.2%)
Radio/Chemo Tx	8
rapidly progressive idiopathic	69 (7.6%)
rubella	21
scarlet fever	3
sudden idiopathic	20
trauma	13
Turner syndrome	2
Usher syndrome	10
Total	**902**

for an implantee with regards to better speech recognition. To understand speech, individuals must match variable acoustic signals with abstract linguistic units, phonemes and syllables, which are then used to identify words in the context of sentences. During the rapid matching process, individuals must hold acoustic signals in their working memory, and use their long-term memory to access words and their acoustic representations.[130]

Waltzman et al,[131] in a multivariate analysis, showed that intelligence quotient along with lip-reading skills and age of implantation were independent variables to better speech recognition. Lyxell contended that verbal cognitive abilities (internal speech functions, speed of verbal information processing, and working memory capacity) are somewhat predictive of outcomes at 6 to 8 months post-implantation.[132] In another study, attention, memory span and working memory were found to be significantly related to word recognition, communication mode, and speech rate.[133] Speed of processing as well as focused, sustained and selective attention have been found to affect vowel and consonant recognition.[134]

In contrast, Collison[130] did not find any correlation between post-implantation performance with a battery of cognitive tests that included the Expressive Vocabulary Test, the Test of Nonverbal Intelligence-3, and the Woodcock-Johnson III Tests of Cognitive Abilities (verbal comprehension section) in a study of 15 patients. Additionally, in a group of 37 patients, a preoperative psychological questionnaire was not predictive of postoperative speech discrimination.[135]

It may be that language and cognition are subtle predictors of performance in certain groups of patients. In patients with poor psychophysical skills, in those with poor representation of the speech signal from their implants, the pervasiveness of unfamiliar speech sounds might result in high demands on their cognitive and linguistic capacities in order for the limited signals to be contextualized. This may be the group that could benefit from a robust linguistic knowledge base and superior cognition.[130] Neurodegenerative processes such as dementia is obviously toward the extreme of the cognitive spectrum. Gates et al[136] theorized that in dementia, the neurodegenerative process leads to reduced executive functioning which is part and parcel of central auditory processing and not a primary auditory function. The role and impact of cochlear implantation in this group of individuals are not at all clear.

Tinnitus

There is now sufficient clinical evidence that cochlear implantation does, by and large, have a positive effect on the perception of tinnitus in those with symptoms prior to surgery; up to 75% of implant users in large database cohorts will report complete tinnitus suppression or reduction with implant activation. A relatively small percentage of implant users will report worsening of tinnitus or a new onset of the same. When compared to hearing aid users, cochlear implant subjects appear to have higher prevalence of tinnitus while declaring better tinnitus suppression or reduction with their devices as compared with hearing aid users.[137] The mechanisms by which a cochlear implant suppresses or exacerbates tinnitus are not well understood, and likely to be multivariate as is the origin of the symptom itself. Masking and distraction through improved sound awareness likely play an important role. A more complex explanation may involve changes in areas of the central auditory system. The effect of tinnitus suppression goes beyond tinnitus reduction or abolition during device activation, as many will report residual inhibition and even contralateral residual inhibition to suggest a cortical effect.[138] Osaki[139] used positron-emission tomography to investigate residual inhibition in three cochlear implantees with tinnitus in whom the right cerebellum was activated during tinnitus while the right anterior, middle and superior temporal gyri were activated during a period of tinnitus suppression and residual inhibition. The authors theorized that the effect was related to cortical networks of auditory higher order processing, also involving memory and attention.

The rate of electrical stimulation has been a subject of studies to determine the optimal range of effect. A high rate pulse train in the range of 5000 pps was proposed as a paradigm for promontory or cochlear implant stimulation with its intensity scalable by patients to achieve tinnitus suppression.[140] More recently, Zheng[141] proposed a low rate of stimulation (<100 Hz) delivered at an intensity lower than the tinnitus to the cochlear apex; this technique appeared to reduce the cortical N100 potentials while increasing the spontaneous alpha power in the auditory cortex. There is some indication in the literature that the more complex the speech-coding strategy the more effective is tinnitus management.[142]

As candidacy expansion creeps into the very controversial area of unilateral deafness, the functional disability of this population of patients including those with severe tinnitus are being put forward as a legitimate reason for implantation. Buechner[143] reported on 5 subjects, 3 had significant tinnitus suppression as well as reported speech recognition benefits. Arndt[144] showed similar outcomes in 11 subjects who "failed" conventional CROS or Baha® aids, the authors suggested that cochlear implantation in this group of patients was superior to those conventional techniques.

Tinnitus management in cochlear implant users through electrical suppression will remain a topic of significant interest to many as it potentially could translate into a viable therapy for those sufferers with less severe hearing loss.

Dizziness

Patients who undergo cochlear implantation have variable degrees of peripheral vestibular function as determined by preoperative clinical examination and caloric-electronystagmography (ENG) responses; yet, the majority will have little or no symptoms. It is recognized, however, that following implantation, many will have transient symptoms and a small proportion will experience long-term dizziness. Dizziness and imbalance are thought to be related to surgical trauma leading to hypofunction of the vestibular end-organ and incomplete adaptation. Reports of benign positional vertigo[145] and delayed dizziness suggestive of endolymphatic hydrops[146] are less commonly identified sequelae.

Self-administered Dizziness Handicap Inventory (DHI), usually performed within the first year, suggests that up to 30% of implant users report a deterioration following surgery; 20 to 40% will have some degree of caloric hypofunction, yet, they are not necessarily predictive of each other.[145-151] Age, preoperative ENG function, electrode placement were not predicative of vestibular outcome, whereas advanced age (>70 yrs) is predictive of postoperative caloric hypofunction.[151] A customized approach was recommended by Melvin[152] to quantify semicircular canal and saccular functions spanning the entire range of stimuli encoded by the labyrinth to address difficult clinical scenarios. Clinical head impulse test (cHIT) remains a simple but a highly specific method of determining high-frequency peripheral vestibular dysfunction that should be part of the preoperative assessment, whereas tests such as quantitative head impulse test (qHIT), ENG, VEMP, and posturography yielded variable responses that had less clinical and diagnostic impact.

The above suggests that vestibular redundancy and compensation are likely responsible for clinical masking of peripheral vestibular injuries. However, when faced with the scenario of severe caloric asymmetry, the default position in choosing which side to implant tends to favor the ear with the weaker response, to avoid causing bilateral peripheral vestibular loss and chronic oscillopsia; there is some evidence to suggest that this risk may be exaggerated. When the ear with the only measurable ENG function is implanted due to audiometric advantage in unilateral implantation, or, in the context of sequential bilateral implantation, permanent bilateral vestibular dysfunctions are rare.[152] Of course, a patient who is not symptomatic following implantation in the above scenario would be less vestibular tolerant in the event of another vestibular injury at a later time. The vestibular risks continue to weigh heavily on the decision process in a select group of patients and they must be fully apprised.

the expectations of even the most ardent early supporter of this technology. As clinical outcomes of adult cochlear implantation continue to improve in stride with technology, it is exciting to see the expansion of candidacy criteria, pointing to future possibilities. The next immediate frontier of performance improvement will likely be measured by how implant users perform in noise and with music perception. To truly optimize the capabilities of a cochlear implant, regardless of performance levels or technology, clinicians must devote and develop more resources for aural rehabilitation.

The challenges down the road for many adult programs are the expected influx of pediatric graduates who will enter adulthood with aging implant systems; it is not at all clear how onerous this might be from a provision of care standpoint. Additionally, we will see increased demands for more resources due to expansion and relaxation of candidacy criteria in the adult population. The above scenario will severely challenge both public and private health care providers as a matter of course; health economic studies will become more relevant in the context of prioritization in many jurisdictions around the world. How to do that in a fair and equitable manner will be a decision each implant program will have to determine vis-à-vis a regional or national policy based on quality evidence related to the real costs and benefits of this treatment.

CONCLUSION

The transformative effect of cochlear implantation on the deaf population has been the single most important therapeutic modality in Otology and has far exceeded

REFERENCES

1. David EE, Ostroff JM, Shipp D, Chen J, Nedzelski J. Speech coding strategies and revised cochlear implant candidacy:

an analysis of post-implant performance. *Otol Neurotol.* 2003;24:228–233.

2. Wilson BS, Finley CC, Lawson DT, Wolford RD, Eddington DK, Rabinowitz WM. Better speech recognition with cochlear implants. *Nature.* 1991;352(6332):236–238.

3. Wilson BS, Finley CC, Farmer JC Jr, et al. Comparative studies of speech processing strategies for cochlear implants. *Laryngoscope.* 1988;98(10):1069–1077.

4. Skinner MW, Clark GM, Whitford LA, et al. Evaluation of a new spectral peak coding strategy for the Nucleus 22 Channel Cochlear Implant System. *Am J Otol.* 1994;suppl 2:15–27.

5. Koch DB, Osberger MJ, Segel P, Kessler D. HiResolution and conventional sound processing in the HiResolution bionic ear: using appropriate outcome measures to assess speech recognition ability. *Audiol Neurotol.* 2004;9(4):214–223.

6. Kiefer J, Hohl S, Sturzebecher E, Pfennigdorff T, Gstoettner W. Comparison of speech recognition with different speech coding strategies (SPEAK, CIS, and ACE) and their relationship to telemetric measures of compound action potentials in the nucleus CI 24M cochlear implant system. *Audiology.* 2001;40(1):32–42.

7. Smith ZM, Delgutte B, Oxenham AJ. Chimaeric sounds reveal dichotomies in auditory perception. *Nature.* 2002;416(6876): 87–90.

8. Nie K, Stickney G, Zeng FG. Encoding frequency modulation to improve cochlear implant performance in noise. *IEEE Trans Biomed Eng.* 2005;52(1):64–73.

9. Zeng, FG. Trends in cochlear implants. *Trends Amplif.* 2004;8:1–34.

10. Hochmair I, Nopp P, Jolly C, et al. MED-EL Cochlear implants: state of the art and a glimpse into the future. *Trends Amplif.* 2006;10(4):201–219.

11. Arnoldner C, Riss D, Brunner M, Durisin M, Baumgartner WD, Hamzavi JS. Speech and music perception with the new fine structure speech coding strategy: preliminary results. *Acta Otolaryngol.* 2007 Dec;127(12):1298–1303.

12. Litvak LM, Krubsack DA, Overstreet EH. Method and system to convey the within-channel fine structure with a cochlear implant. US Patent 7317945 (2008).

13. Xu L, Pfingst BE. Relative importance of temporal envelope and fine structure in lexical-tone perception. *J Acoust Soc Am.* 2003;114(6 pt 1):3024–3027.

14. Luxford W and the ad hoc Subcommittee of the Committee on Hearing and Equilibrium of the American Academy of Otolaryngology-Head and Neck Surgery. Minimum speech test battery for postlingually deafened adult cochlear implant patients. *Otolaryngol Head Neck Surg.* 2001;124:125–126.

15. Nilsson M, Soli SD, Sullivan JA. Development of the Hearing-in-Noise Test for the measurement of speech reception thresholds in quiet and in noise. *J Acoust Soc Am.* 1994;95(2):1085–1099.

16. Lehiste I, Peterson GE. Vowel amplitude and phonemic stress in American English. *J Acoust Soc Am.* 1959;31:428–435.

17. Bond M, Mealing S, Anderson R, et al. The effectiveness and cost-effectiveness of cochlear implants for severe to profound deafness in children and adults: a systematic review and economic model (Review). *Health Technol Assess.* 2009; 13(44):1–330.

18. Archbold S, Lutman ME, Nikolopoulos T. Categories of auditory performance: inter-user reliability. *Br J Audiol.* 1998; 32(1):7–12.

19. Lin FR, Ceh K, Bervinchak D, et al. Development of a communicative performance scale for pediatric cochlear implantation. *Ear Hear.* 2007;28(5):703–712.

20. Boothroyd A. Evaluation of speech production of the hearing impaired: some benefits of forced-choice testing. *J Speech Hear Res.* 1985;28:185–196.

21. Mackersie CL. Tests of speech perception abilities. *Curr Opin Otolaryngol Head Neck Surg.* 2002;10:392–397.

22. Mendel LL, Danhauer JD, eds. *Test Administration and Interpretation.* San Diego, CA: Singular Publishing Group; 1997.

23. Penrod JP. Talker effects on word discrimination scores of adults with sensorineural hearing impairment. *J Speech Hearing Disorders.* 1979;44:340–349.

24. Gengel RW, Kupperman GL. Word discrimination in noise: effect of different speakers. *Ear Hear.* 1980;1:156–160.

25. Hood JD, Poole JP. Influence of the speaker and other factors affecting speech intelligibility. *Audiology.* 1980; 19:434–455.

26. Picheny MA, Durlach N, Braida L. Speaking clearly for the hard of hearing: I. Intelligibility differences between clear and conversational speech. *J Speech Hear Res.* 1985;28:96–103.

27. Gifford KH, Shallop JR, Peterson AM. Speech recognition materials and ceiling effects-considerations for cochlear implant programs. *Audiol Neurotol.* 2008; 13(3):193–205.

28. Gantz B, Tyler R, Knutson J, et al. Evaluation of five different cochlear implant designs: audiologic assessment and predictors of performance. *Laryngoscope.* 1988;98:1100–1106.

29. Tyler RS, Lowder M, Parkinson AJ, et al. Performance of adult Ineraid and Nucleus cochlear implant patients after 3.5 years of use. *Audiology.* 1995;34(3):135–144.

30. Skinner MW, Holden LK, Holden TA, et al. Speech recognition at simulated soft, conversational and raised to loud vocal efforts by adults with cochlear implants. *J Acoust Soc Am.* 1997;101:3766–3782.

31. Firszt JB, Holden LD, Skinner MW, et al. Recognition of speech presented at soft to loud levels by adult cochlear implant recipients of three cochlear implant systems. *Ear Hear.* 2004;25(4):375–387.

32. Holt RF, Kirk KI, Eisenberg LS, et al. Spoken word recognition development in children with residual hearing using cochlear implants and hearing aids in opposite ears. *Ear Hear.* 2005;26:82S–91S.

33. Bench J, Kowal A, Bamford J. The BKB (Bamford-Kowal-Bench) Sentence Lists for partially-hearing children. *Br J Audiol.* 1997;13:108–112.

34. Killion MC, Niquette PA, Gudmundsen GI, Revit LJ, Banerjee S. Development of a quick speech-in-noise test for measuring signal-to-noise ratio loss in normal-hearing and hearing-impaired listeners. *J Acoust Soc Am.* 2004;116:2395–2405.

35. Nilsson MJ, McCawVM, Soli SD. *Minimum Speech Test Battery for Adult Cochlear Implant Users: User Manual.* Los Angeles, House Ear Institues; 1996.

36. Erber NP. Auditory, visual and auditory-visual recognition of consonants by children with normal and impaired hearing. *J Speech Hear Dis.* 1972;15:413–422.

37. MacLeod A, Summerfield AQ. Quantifying the contribution of vision to speech perception in noise. *Br J Audiol.* 1987;21: 131–141.

38. Massaro DW, Cohen MM. Perceiving talking faces. *Curr Direct Psychol Sci.* 1995; 4:104–109.

39. Bell TS, Wilson RH. Sentence recognition materials based on frequency of word use and lexical confusability. *J Am Acad Audiol.* 2001;12(10):514–522.

40. Dirks DD, Takayana S, Moshfegh A. Effects of lexical factors on word recognition among normal-hearing and hearing-impaired listeners. *J Am Acad Audiol.* 2001;12(5):233–244.

41. Bodmer D, Shipp DB, Ostroff J, et al. A comparison of postcochlear implantation speech scores in an adult population. *Laryngoscope.* 2007;117:1408–1411.

42. Amoodi H, Mick P, Shipp D, J Nedzelski, Chen J, Lin V. *Outcomes of cochlear implantation in individuals whose hearing loss exceeded conventional candidacy criteria.* (Abstract-COSM, Chicago, May 1, 2011)

43. UK Cochlear Implant Study Group. Criteria of candidacy for unilateral cochlear implantation in postlingually deafened adults. I: theory and measures of effectiveness. *Ear Hear.* 2004;25:310–335.

44. Parkinson AJ, Arcaroli J, Staller SJ, et al. The nucleus 24 contour cochlear implant system: adult clinical trial results. *Ear Hear.* 2002;23(1 suppl):41S–48S.

45. Cray JW, Allen RL, Stuart A, Hudson S, Layman E, Givens GD. An investigation of telephone use among cochlear implant recipients. *Am J Audiol.* 2004 Dec;13(2):200–212.

46. Başkent D, Shannon RV. Combined effects of frequency compression-expansion and shift on speech recognition. *Ear Hear.* 2007 Jun;28(3):277–289.

47. Dorman MF, Dove H, Parkin J, Zacharchuk S, Dankowski K. Telephone use by patients fitted with the Ineraid cochlear implant. *Ear Hear.* 1991 Oct;12(5): 368–369.

48. Adams JS, Hasenstab MS, Pippin GW, Sismanis A. Telephone use and understanding in patients with cochlear implants. *Ear Nose Throat J.* 2004 Feb;83(2):96, 99–100, 102–103.

49. Anderson I, Baumgartner WD, Böheim K, Nahler A, Arnoldner C, D'Haese P. Telephone use: what benefit do cochlear implant users receive? *Int J Audiol.* 2006 Aug;45(8):446–453.

50. Clinkard, D, Shipp, D, Friesen, L, et al. Telephone use and the factors that affect it among cochlear implant patients. *Cochlear Implants International.* In press.

51. Heydebrand G, Hale S, Potts L, Gotter B, Skinner M. Cognitive predictors of improvement in adults' spoken word recognition six months after cochlear implant activation. *Audiol Neurotol.* 2007;12(4):254–264.

52. Gfeller K, Knutson J F, Woodworth G, Witt S, & DeBus B. Timbral recognition and appraisal by adult cochlear implant users and normal-hearing adults. *J Am Acad Audio.* 1998;9:1–19.

53. Gfeller K, Christ A, Knutson J, Witt S, Mehr M. The effects of familiarity and complexity on appraisal of complex songs by cochlear implant recipients and normal hearing adults. *J Music Ther.* 2003;40(2), 78–112.

54. Gfeller K, Olszewski C, Rychener M, et al. Recognition of "real-world" musical excerpts by cochlear implant recipients and normal-hearing adults. *Ear Hear.* 2005;26(3), 237–250.

55. Looi V, She J. Music perception of cochlear implant users: a questionnaire, and its implications for a music training program. *Int J Audiol.* 2010;49(2):116–128.

56. Alexander AJ, Bartel L, Friesen L, Shipp D, Chen J. From fragments to the whole: a comparison between cochlear implant users and normal-hearing listeners in music perception and enjoyment. *J Otolaryngol Head Neck Surg.* 2011;40(1):1–7.

57. Nakata T, Trehub SE, Mitani C, Kanda Y, Shibasaki A, Schellenberg EG. Music recognition by Japanese children with cochlear implants. *J Physiol Anthropol Appl Human Sci.* 2005;24(1):29–32.

58. Vongpaisal T, Trehub SE, Schellenberg EG, Papsin B. Music recognition by children with implants. *International Congress Series.* 2004;1273:193–196.

59. Chen JK, Chuang AY, McMahon C, Hsieh JC, Tung TH, Li LP. Music training improves pitch perception in prelingually deafened children with cochlear implants. *Pediatrics.* 2010;125:e793–e800.

60. Mirza S, Douglas SA, Lindsey P, Hildreth T, Hawthorne M. Appreciation of music in adult patients with cochlear implants: a patient questionnaire. *Coch Implants Int.* 2003;4(2):85–95.

61. Nicholas JG, Geers AE. Effects of early auditory experience on the spoken language of deaf children at 3 years of age. *Ear Hear.* 2006;27(3):286–298.

62. Gfeller K, Christ A, Knutson JF, Witt S, Murray KT, Tyler RS. Musical backgrounds, listening habits, and aesthetic enjoyment of adult cochlear implant recipients. *J. Am. Acad. Audio.* 2000;11:390–406.

63. Gfeller K, Olszewski C, Rychener M, Sena K, Knutsson JF, Witt S, Mapherson B. Recognition of familiar melodies by adult cochlear implant recipients and normal-hearing adults. *Coch Implants Int.* 2002; 3:29–53.

64. Bartel LR, Greenberg S, Friesen LM, et al. Qualitative case studies of five cochlear implant recipients' experience

with music. *Coch Implants Int*. 2011; 12(1):27–33.

65. Cooper WB, Tobey E, Loizou PC. Music perception by cochlear implant and normal hearing listeners as measured by the Montreal Battery for Evaluation of Amusia. *Ear Hear*. 2008;29(4):618–626.

66. Galvin JJ 3rd, Fu QJ, Oba SI. Effect of a competing instrument on melodic contour identification by cochlear implant users. *J Acoust Soc Am*. 2009;125:98–103.

67. Kong YY, Cruz R, Jones JA, Zeng FG. Music perception with temporal cues in acoustic and electric hearing. *Ear Hear*. 2004;25:173–185.

68. Gfeller K, Oleson, J, Knutson JF, Breheny P, Driscoll V, Olszewski C. Multivariate predictors of music perception and appraisal by adult cochlear implant users. *J Am Acad Audiol*. 2008;19:120–134.

69. Yucel E, Sennaroglu G, Belgin E. The family oriented musical training for children with cochlear implants: speech and musical perception results of two-year follow-up. *Int J Pediatr Otorhinolaryngol*. 2009;73:1043–1052.

70. Fu QJ, Galvin JJ 3rd. Maximizing cochlear implant patients' performance with advanced speech training procedures. *Hear Res*. 2008;242:198–208.

71. Mitani C, Nakata T, TRehub SE, Kanda Y, Kumagami H, Takasaki K, Miyamoto I, Takashi H. Music recognition, music listening, and word recognition by deaf children with cochlear implants. *Ear Hear*. 2007;28:29S–33S.

72. Loeb GE, Kessler DK. Speech recognition performance over time with the Clarion cochlear prosthesis. *Ann Otol Rhinol Laryngol Suppl*. 1995;166:290–292.

73. Gray RF, Quinn SJ, Court I, Vanat Z, Baguley DM. Patient performance over eighteen months with the Ineraid intracochlear implant. *Ann Otol Rhinol Laryngol Suppl*. 1995;166:275–277.

74. George CR, Cafarelli Dees D, Sheridan C, Haacke N. Preliminary findings of the new Spectra 22 speech processor with first-time cochlear implant users. *Ann*

Otol Rhinol Laryngol Suppl. 1995;166: 272–275.

75. McDermott HJ. Music perception with cochlear implants: a review. *Trends Amplif*. 2004;8:49–82.

76. Fujita S, Ito J. Ability of nucleus cochlear implantees to recognize music. *Ann Otol Rhinol Laryngol*. 1999;108:634–640.

77. Lin FR, Niparko JK. Measuring health-related quality of life after pediatric cochlear implantation: a systematic review. *Int J Pediatr Otorhinolaryngol*. 2006 Oct; 70(10):1695–1706.

78. Newman CW, Jacobson GP, Spitzer JB. Development of the tinnitus handicap inventory. *Arch Otolaryngol Head Neck Surg*. 1996 Feb;122(2):143–148.

79. Ventry IM, Weinstein BE. The hearing handicap inventory for the elderly: a new tool. *Ear Hear*. 1982;3(3):128–134.

80. Hinderink JB, Krabbe PF, Van Den Broek P. Development and application of a health-related quality-of-life instrument for adults with cochlear implants: the Nijmegen cochlear implant questionnaire. *Otolaryngol Head Neck Surg*. 2000;123(6):756–765.

81. Ware JE, Snow KK, Kosinski M. *Health Survey: Manual and Interpretation Guide*. Lincoln, RI: Quality Metric; 2000.

82. Torrance GW. Measurement of health state utilities for economic appraisal. *J Health Econ*. 1986;5:1–30.

83. Nord E. EuroQol: health-related quality of life measurement. Valuations of health states by the general public in Norway. *Health Policy*. 1991;18(1):25–36.

84. Chung J, Chueng K, Shipp D, et al. *Unilateral multi-channel cochlear implantation results in significant improvement in quality of life*. (Abstract: COSM, Chicago, April 29, 2011)

85. Hirschfelder A, Gräbel S, Olze H. The impact of cochlear implantation on quality of life: the role of audiologic performance and variables. *Otolaryngol Head Neck Surg*. 2008;138(3):357–362.

86. Klop WM, Briaire JJ, Stiggelbout AM, Frijns JH. Cochlear implant outcomes

and quality of life in adults with prelingual deafness. *Laryngoscope.* 2007 Nov; 117(11):1982–1987.

87. Klop WM, Boermans PP, Ferrier MB, van den Hout WB, Stiggelbout AM, Frijns JH. Clinical relevance of quality of life outcome in cochlear implantation in postlingually deafened adults. *Otol Neurotol.* 2008;29(5):615–621.

88. Hogan A, Hawthorne G, Kethel L, et al. Health-related quality-of-life outcomes from adult cochlear implantation: a cross-sectional survey. *Coch Implants Int.* 2001;2(2):115–128.

89. Samuel F. Technology and costs: complex relationship. *Hospitals.* 1988;62:72.

90. Froberg DG, Kane RL. Methodology for measuring healthstate preferences—II: scaling methods. *J Clin Epidemiol.* 1989; 42:459–471.

91. Dolan P, Gudex C, Kind P, Williams A. *A social tariff for the EuroQol: results from a UK general population survey.* Discussion paper No. 38. York: University of York, Centre for Health Economics; 1995.

92. Burstrom, Johannesson M, Diderichsen F. A comparison of individual and social time-trade-off values for health states in the general population. *Health Policy.* 2006;76(3):359–370.

93. Palmer CS, Niparko JK, Wyatt JR, et al. A prospective study of the cost-utility of the multichannel cochlear implant. *Arch Otolaryngol Head Neck Surg.* 1999; 125(11):1221–1228.

94. Fugain C, et al. Abstract from the 1998 International Pediatric Cochlear Implantation Symposium, Netherlands, 1998.

95. Summerfield AQ, Marshall DH, Davis AC. Cochlear implantation: demands, costs, and utility. *Ann Otol Rhinol Laryngol Suppl.* 1995;104(suppl 166, pt 2): S245–S248.

96. Cheng AK, Niparko JK. Cost-utility of the cochlear implant in adults: a meta-analysis. *Arch Otolaryngol Head Neck Surg.* 1999 Nov;125(11):1214–1218.

97. Park E, Ship D, Chen J, Nedzelski J, Lin V. Assessment of speech recognition and quality of life in post-lingually deafened adults before and after cochlear implantation. *J Am Acad Audiol.* In press.

98. UK Cochlear Implant Study Group. Criteria of candidacy for unilateral cochlear implantation in postlingually deafened adults. II: cost-effectiveness analysis. *Ear Hear.* 2004;25:336–360.

99. Monteiro E, Shipp D, Chen J, Nedzelski J, Lin V. *Cochlear implantation: a personal and societal economic perspective.* (Abstract-Canadian Society of otolaryngology May 31, 2011)

100. Rubinstein JT, Parkinson WS, Tyler RS, et al. Residual speech recognition and cochlear implant performance: effects of implantation criteria. *Am J Otol.* 1999;20: 445–452.

101. Skinner MW, Arndt PL, Staller S. Nucleus 24 advanced encoder conversion study: Performance versus preference. *Ear Hearing Suppl.* 2002;23:2–17.

102. Shipp DB, Nedzelski JM. Prognostic indicators of speech recognition performace in adults cochlear implant users: a prospective analysis. *Ann Otol Rhinol Laryngol Suppl.* 1995;166:194–196.

103. Shipp DB, Nedzelski JM, Chen JM, et al. Prognostic indicators of speech recognition performance in post linguistically deafened adult cochlear implant users. *Adv Otorhinolaryngol.* 1997;52:74–77.

104. Waltzman SB, Niparko JK, Fisher SG, et al. Predictors of postoperative performance with cochlear implants. *Ann Otol Rhinol Laryngol.* 1995;104(suppl 165):15–18.

105. Gantz BJ, Woodworth GG, Abbas PJ, et al. Multivariate predictors of success with multichannel cochlear implants. *Ann Otol Rhinol Laryngol.* 1993;102:909–916.

106. Leung J, Wang N, Yeagle JD et al. Predictive models for cochlear implantation in elderly candidates. *Arch Otolaryngol Head Neck Surg.* 2005;131:1049–1054.

107. Nadol JB Jr, Young YS, Glynn RJ. Survival of spiral ganglion cells in profound sensorineural hearing loss: implications for cochlear implantation. *Ann Otol Rhinol Laryngol.* 1989 Jun;98(6):411–416.

108. Kaplan DM, Shipp DB, Chen JM, Ng AHC, Nedzelski JM. Early-deafened adult cochlear implant users: assessment of outcomes. *J Otolaryngol.* 2003;32:245–249.

109. Brimacombe J, Beiter, Barker M, et al. *Cochlear implant results in pre-perilingual deafened adults.* Presented at the American Academy of Otolaryngology-Head and Neck Surgery; 1989 Sept 24–28, New Orleans LA.

110. Waltzman SB, Cohen NL, Shapiro WH. Use of multichannel cochlear implant in the congenitally and prelingually deaf population. *Laryngoscope.* 1992;102:395–399.

111. Chee GH., Goldring JE, Shipp DB, Ng AHC, Chen JM, Nedzelski JM. Benefits of cochlear implantation in early-deafened adults: the Toronto experience. *J Otolaryngol.* 2004;33:26-31.

112. Vermeire K, Brokx JP, Wuyts FL, Cochet E, Hofkens A, Van de Heyning PH. Quality-of-life benefit from cochlear implantation in the elderly. *Otol Neurotol.* 2005 Mar;26(2):188–195.

113. Chatelin V, Kim EJ, Driscoll C, et al. Cochlear implant outcomes in the elderly. *Otol Neurotol.* 2004;25:298–301.

114. Bao J, Ohlemiller KK. Age-related loss of spiral ganglion neurons. *Hear Res.* 2010 Jun 1;264(1–2):93–97.

115. Nadol JB Jr, Young Y-S, Glynn RJ. Survival of spiral ganglion cells in profound SNHL: implications for cochlear implantation. *Ann Otol Rhinol Laryngol.* 1989;98:411–416.

116. Herzog M, Mueller J, Milewski C, Schoen F, Helms J. Cochlear implantation in the elderly. *Adv Otorhinolaryngol.* 2000;57:393–396.

117. Pasanisi E, Bacciu A, Vincenti V, et al. Speech recognition in elderly cochlear implant recipients. *Clin Otolaryngol Allied Sci.* 2003 Apr;28(2):154–157.

118. Marshall AH, Fanning N, Symons S, et al. Cochlear implantation in cochlear otosclerosis. *Laryngoscope.* 2005;115:1728–1733.

119. Wang JR, Yuen HW, Shipp DB, Lin V, Chen J, Nedzelski J. Cochlear implantation in patients with autoimmune inner ear disease including Cogan syndrome: a comparison with age- and sex-matched controls. *Laryngoscope.* 2010;120(12):2478–2483.

120. Rauch S, Herrmann BS, David LA, Nadol JB Jr. Nucleus 22 cochlear implantation results in postmeningitic deafness. *Laryngoscope.* 1997;107(12):1606–1609.

121. Gantz BJ, McCabe BF, Tyler RS. Use of multichannel cochlear implants in obstructed and obliterated cochleas. *Otolaryngol Head Neck Surg.* 1988;98:72–81.

122. Nadol JB Jr, Hsu W. Histopathologic correlation of spiral ganglion cell count and new bone formation in the cochlea following meningogenic labyrinthitis and deafness. *Ann Otol Rhinol Laryngol.* 1991;100:712–716.

123. Merchant SN, Gopen Q. A human temporal bone study of acute bacterial meningogenic labyrinthitis. *Am J Otol.* 1996;17:375–385.

124. Al-Abidi A, Ng A, Shipp D, Nedzelski J. Does choosing the "worse ear" impact on functional outcome of cochlear implantation? *Otol Neurotol.* 2001;2:335–339.

125. Boemio A, Fromm S, Braun A, et al. Hierarchical and asymmetric temporal sensitivity in human auditory cortices. *Nat Neurosci.* 2005;8:389–395.

126. Newcombe F, Ratcliffe G. Handedness, speech lateralization and ability. *Neuropsychologia.* 1973;11:399–407.

127. Rasmussen T, Milner B. The role of early left-brain injury in determining lateralization of cerebral speech functions. *Ann N Y Acad Sci.* 1977;299:355–369.

128. Budenz CL, Cosetti MK, Coelho DH, et al. The effects of cochlear implantation on speech perception in older adults. *J Am Geriatr Soc.* 2011;59(3):446–453.

129. Morris LG, Mallur PS, Roland T, Waltzmann SB, Lalwani AK. Implication of central asymmetry in speech processing on selecting the ear for cochlear implantation. *Otol Neurotol.* 2007;28(1):25–30.

130. Collison EA, Munson B, Carney AE. Relations among linguistic and cognitive

skills and spoken word recognition in adults with cochlear implants. *J Speech Lang Hear Res.* 2004;47:496–508.

131. Waltzman SB, Fisher SG, Niparko JK, Cohen NL. Predictors of postoperative performance with cochlear implants. *Ann Otol Rhinol Laryngol Suppl.* 1995 Apr;165:15–18.

132. Lyxell B, Andersson U, Borg E, Ohlsson IS. Working-memory capacity and phonological processing in deafened adults and individuals with a severe hearing impairment. *Int J Audiol.* 2003 Jul;42 suppl 1:S86–S89.

133. Pisoni DB, Cleary M. Measures of working memory span and verbal rehearsal speed in deaf children after cochlear implantation. *Ear Hear.* 2003;24(1 suppl): 106S–120S.

134. Schvartz KC, Chatterjee M, Gordon-Salant S. Recognition of spectrally degraded phonemes by younger, middle-aged, and older normal-hearing listeners. *J Acoust Soc Amer.* 2008;124(6):3972–3988.

135. van Dijk JE, van Olphen AF, Langereis MC, Mean LHM, Brokx JPL, Smoorenburg GF. Predictors of cochlear implant performance. *Audiology.* 1999;38:109–116.

136. Gates GA, Gibbons LE, McCusrry SM, Crane PK, Feeney MP, Larson EB. Executive dysfunction and presbycusis in older persons with and without memory loss and dementia. *Cogn Behav Neurol.* 2010 Dec;23(4):218–223.

137. Mo B, Harris S, Lindbaek M. Tinnitus in cochlear implant patients—a comparison with other hearing-impaired patients. *Int J Audiol.* 2002 Dec;41(8):527–534.

138. Souliere CR Jr, Kileny PR, Zwolan TA, Kemink JL. Tinnitus suppression following cochlear implantation. A multifactorial investigation. *Arch Otolaryngol Head Neck Surg.* 1992 Dec;118(12):1291–1297.

139. Osaki Y, Nishimura H, Takasawa M, et al.Neural mechanism of residual inhibition of tinnitus in cochlear implant users. *NeuroReport.* 2005 Oct 17;16(15): 1625–1628.

140. Rubinstein JT, Tyler RS, Johnson A, Brown CJ. Electrical suppression of tinnitus with high-rate pulse trains. *Otol Neurotol.* 2003 May;24(3):478–485.

141. Zeng FG, Tang Q, Dimitrijevic A, Starr A, Larky J, Blevins NH. Tinnitus suppression by low-rate electric stimulation and its electrophysiological mechanisms. *Hear Res.* 2011 Apr 5. [Epub ahead of print]

142. Quaranta N, Wagstaff S, Baguley DM. Tinnitus and cochlear implantation. *Int J Audiol.* 2004 May;43(5):245–251.

143. Buechner A, Brendel M, Lesinski-Schiedat A, et al. Cochlear implantation in unilateral deaf subjects associated with ipsilateral tinnitus. *Otol Neurotol.* 2010 Dec;31(9):1381–1385.

144. Arndt S, Aschendorff A, Laszig R, et al. Comparison of pseudobinaural hearing to real binaural hearing rehabilitation after cochlear implantation in patients with unilateral deafness and tinnitus. *Otol Neurotol.* 2011 Jan;32(1):39–47.

145. Limb CJ, Francis HF, Lustig LR, Niparko JK, Jammal H. Benign positional vertigo after cochlear implantation. *Otolaryngol Head Neck Surg.* 2005 May;132(5):741–745.

146. Fina M, Skinner M, Goebel JA, Piccirillo JF, Neely JG, Black O. Vestibular dysfunction after cochlear implantation. *Otol Neurotol.* 2003 Mar;24(2):234–242.

147. Pan T, Tyler RS, Ji H, Coelho C, Gehringer AK, Gogel SA. Changes in the tinnitus handicap questionnaire after cochlear implantation. *Am J Audiol.* 2009 Dec; 18(2):144–151.

148. Higgins KM, Chen JM, Nedzelski JM, Shipp DB, McIlmoyl LD. A matched-pair comparison of two cochlear implant systems. *J Otolaryngol.* 2002 Apr;31(2):97–105.

149. Chiong CM, Nedzelski JM, McIlmoyl LD, Shipp DB. Electro-oculographic findings pre- and post-cochlear implantation. *J Otolaryngol.* 1994 Dec;23(6):447–449.

150. Melvin TA, Della Santina CC, Carey JP, Migliaccio AA. The effects of cochlear implantation on vestibular function. *Otol Neurotol.* 2009 Jan;30(1):87–94.

151. Enticott JC, Tari S, Koh SM, Dowell RC, O'Leary SJ. Cochlear implant and vestibular function. *Otol Neurotol.* 2006 Sep; 27(6):824–830.

152. Chen J, Oh A, Shipp D, Nedzelski J, et al. *Does implanting the only ear with vestibular function lead to oscillopsia.* (Abstract-Canadian Society of Otolaryngology Annual Meeting. Vancouver, 2001).

153. Silverman SR, Hirsch IJ. Problems related to the use of speech in clinical audiometry. *Ann Otol Rhinol Laryngol.* 1955;64:1234–1245.

154. Peterson GE, Lehiste I. Revised CNC lists for audiotory tests. *J Speach Hear Dis.* 1962;27:62–70.

155. Wilson RH. Development of a speech in multitalker babble paradigm to assess word-recognition performance. *J Am Acad Audiol.* 2003;14:453–470.

156. Boothroyd A. Developments in speech audiomctry. *Br J Audiol.* 1968;2:3–10.

Chapter 16

Cochlear Implant-Mediated Perception of Environmental Sounds and Music

YELL INVERSO

INTRODUCTION

Nonlinguistic sounds allow individuals to feel safe in, as well as connected to, the environment that surrounds them.[1] Comprehending information about the sounds around us has practical and aesthetic significance for the listener. Listeners can alter their behavior depending on the sound-producing objects in their immediate environment. For example, knowing that a bus or train is approaching, or hearing the honk of a car horn or the growl of a nearby dog can help the listener avoid danger or respond to an immediate threat. Even in nonemergency situations, being able to identify the source of a sound allows an individual to respond appropriately. Identifying the sources of nonspeech sounds is a perceptual task that is routinely performed by individuals with hearing that is within normal limits. Nonlinguistic sounds (NLS), such as enjoying your favorite song or listening to your child laugh, also add plea-

sure to our lives that many of us take for granted. NLS perception goes beyond safety considerations and the esthetic ways in which nonlinguistic sound recognition enriches the acoustical environment; accurate recognition of familiar environmental sounds, and our ability to dismiss them as periphery, is suggested to lead to improved speech perception.[2]

The early goals of cochlear implantation were modest in that the focus was on rudimentary environmental sound perception; however, the great success of the modern multichannel cochlear implant (CI) and modern signal processing have led to a focus on the perception of complex speech stimuli. This focus on the perception of speech as the primary goal of CIs is exhibited by how the majority of the research and clinical progress with CIs is measured. Speech perception measures comprise the bulk of test methods used to assess patient candidacy, postimplant performance, and rehabilitation progress. Implant technology has been optimized and specially designed for speech perception such that modern multichannel CIs are essentially speech processing devices, with nonlinguistic stimuli processing achieved through algorithms geared toward the processing of speech. As a result of this emphasis on speech information, high-level speech performance is now consistently achieved in both postlingually deafened adults and early-implanted prelingually deafened children. Many implantees consider language perception to be significantly easier than the recognition and enjoyment of environmental, musical, and other nonlinguistic sounds.[3,4] Since the advent of the cochlear implant, the clinical utility of the device has increased dramatically as there have been numerous advancements in cochlear implant technology. Speech and language perception is now consistently achieved in the majority of implanted individuals. The perception and enjoyment of environmental sounds and music is a growing expectation of implantees and an area of increased research investigation.

If one only examines the number of articles published on nonlinguistic sound perception by CI users, it may not be apparent that hearing and recognizing this type of stimuli is very important to individuals with hearing loss. In fact, the perception of general nonlinguistic sounds, including environmental and music stimuli, is of great interest for patients.[4-6] Anecdotal reports from audiologists, aural rehabilitationists, and patients are that the new or renewed ability to hear and understand speech is amazing; however, as success becomes increasingly possible, the expectations for recognizing environmental sounds and enjoying music are growing. Although the perception of environmental sounds may seem to be a quite low expectation of success; however, it is important to consider the patient's ability to not only *hear*

nonlinguistic sounds but to *understand* them and identify their meaning.

Frequency coding by cochlear implants relies primarily on place cues that transmit envelope information. The majority of CI processing extracts the envelope of the incoming sound waveforms and discards the fine structure (FS) information.[7] Many patients perform very well on measures of speech perception; therefore, CI users are able to comprehend speech using only the envelope information from the incoming signal.[8] Although the envelope method has been shown to be effective for speech perception in quiet situations,[9,10] the lack of FS information has been shown to negatively affect speech recognition in background noise and music perception.[11] These negative effects of CI processing could also reduce a CI user's ability to identify the sources of other nonlinguistic sounds in addition to music. Several researchers are examining whether performance on speech measures can be further improved and if the perception of nonspeech (eg, music) materials can be improved by including FS information in the processing of the signal.[11-14]

ACOUSTIC STRUCTURE OF SPEECH VERSUS NONSPEECH

There has been a limited amount of research done on the acoustical characteristics of NLS when compared with the number of studies examining the acoustics of speech. Therefore, it is not uncommon for a specific speech sound to be recognizable to professionals based on a spectrogram or other spectral representations of that sound. In contrast, researchers have done comparatively little to identify the acoustical markers or to identify characteristics of nonlinguistic sounds. It is not the intention of the preceding statement to suggest that nonlinguistic sounds are never used as part of research test batteries. However, one possible explanation for why a systematic acoustical characterization of this classification of sounds is not available is that a number of the studies using NLS as stimuli have not been particularly concerned with the acoustical characteristics of the NLS used. Hearing science studies have used nonspeech sounds as stimuli[15,16] for evoked potential research or studies involving autistic or special-needs populations. However, the studies did not discuss the selected sounds; instead, they were simply described as a "set of environmental sounds." A large-scale study completed by Miller and Tanis[17] used nonlinguistic or "common" sounds as the stimuli; however, the focus of the research was on auditory memory and did not focus on or provide information regarding neither the acoustical characteristics of the sounds nor the general perception of the NLS stimuli.

Acoustically, speech and nonlinguistic sounds are not entirely different in their structure. In fact, they share some of the same attributes. They are both complex signals with waveforms that change over time.[18] Additionally, both speech and most environmental sounds have meaning derived from their acoustic properties. Finally, the meaning associated with every acoustic sound is based on the experience of the listener, which is the case for both speech and NLS alike. As nonlinguistic sounds come from a variety of sources, the range of spectral and temporal variation among nonspeech environmental sounds greatly exceeds that of speech, for which the source is always the human vocal tract.[19] In Table 16–1[18] some of the structural features of environmental sounds, speech, and music are presented. The table calls attention to the lack of information that is available. For instance, what unit of analysis is used to describe nonlinguistic environmental sounds? For speech, the syllable is widely known and used, as is the note for music. When Gygi compiled his comparison table, he needed to use a "?" symbol to denote his uncertainty about whether the unit of analysis for environmental sounds was an event. The term event is used by Gygi to describe the occurrence that caused the sound and as a way to describe the sound itself. The single bark of a dog, for example, would be described as an event.

Gygi[18] attempts to summarize speech, music, and environmental sounds by their temporal and spectral structural characteristics. Speech has well-documented characteristics, and the structural features of speech have been researched and documented for years. Music is more variable than speech. For example, Gygi's analysis indicates that the spectral structure for music is harmonic for the most part; however, percussion instruments are inharmonic. Table 16–1 also highlights some factors explaining why research using nonlinguistic sounds can be problematic. Gygi explains that this difficulty is due to the high level of variability across NLS. A similar sentiment has also been noted in recent literature.[20–22] Unlike the characteristics of speech (and to a lesser extent, music), the acoustical characteristics of NLS are not often defined.

ACOUSTIC CHARACTERISTICS OF MUSIC

This chapter focuses on the perception and identification of a range of nonlinguistic sounds, both "musical" and "nonmusical"; therefore, a brief description of

Table 16–1. Structural Features of Speech, Music, and Environmental Sounds

	Units of Analysis	Possible Sources
Speech	Phonemes	Finite: Human vocal tract
Music	Notes	Finite: Instruments (crafted or designated)
Environmental Sounds	Events	Possibly finite: Any naturally occurring sound-producing event
	Spectral Structure	**Temporal Structure**
Speech	Largely harmonic (vowels, voiced consonants); tend to group in formants. Some inharmonic (stops, fricatives).	Short (40–200 ms). More steady-state than dynamic. Timing constrained but variable. Amplitude modulation rate for sentences is slow (~ 4 Hz)
Music	Largely harmonic, some inharmonic (percussion)	Longer (600–1200 ms; Fraisse, 1956). Mix of steady-state (strings, winds) and transient (percussion). Strong periodicity.
Environmental Sounds	Proportion of harmonic vs inharmonic not known, although both exist.	Longer (500 ms–3 s). Proportion of steady-state to dynamic not known. Variable periodicity.
	Syntactic/Semantic Structure	
Speech	Symbolic, productive, can be combined in grammar.	
Music	Symbolic, productive, combined in a grammar.	
Environmental Sounds	Nomic, not productive, no known grammar, although meaningful sequences exist.	

Used with permission, from Gygi.[18]

the elements of music and its perception by humans is offered here. The acoustical features of music have been described; however, the literature often focuses on the characteristics of a specific type or Instrument such as the human voice.[23] Studies evaluating the perception of musical cues are less frequent than those of speech but more readily available than those of other nonlinguistic sounds.[20]

Music and speech share many acoustic characteristics: periodic as well as aperiodic structure, spectral shaping by resonant cavities, longer and shorter intervals of approximately steady-state sounds, intermittent abrupt temporal events, and others. Limb[24] explains that the ultimate goals of both speech and music are communication and expression, be it concrete or abstract.

Language and music are similar; they both contain rhythmic and prosodic features that are fundamental to their perception. For the majority of its duration, the signal generated by speech or music (of simple, monophonic melody type) is made up of quasiperiodic signals, which have period and amplitude variations. In music these are the sustained part of the musical notes; in speech, there are vowel sounds, nasals, approximants (eg, /l/, /r/, etc), and parts of some plosives. The spectral envelope usually has "large-scale features" such as formants. Musical formants are produced by the resonances of the bridge or the air in the body of a wind Instrument, or the tone-hole lattices in woodwinds. Speech formants are produced by resonances in the vocal tract. For both speech and music, the spectrum of the signal, as well as its envelope, changes over time. The sustained signals, such as the vowels for speech and the longer notes for music, usually occur when the spectra are mostly harmonic in nature. Although speech and music are both complex signals with many similarities, there are also differences. Limb[24] suggested that the differences between speech and music might be more distinctive. He proposes that the features that make music different from speech aid the listener's identification of both speech and musical sounds. One such difference is that in most speech, the pitch varies constantly, whereas the pitch of music notes is stable over intervals of time (notes). It is true that formants are present in both speech and music; however, the stability of these formants varies over time in speech compared to music. In speech, the formants of the different phonemes are distinctly different and change as a speaker produces one phoneme and then the next. In music, the formants are instrument dependent and usually determined by a factor that is nonvariable, such as the resonance of a violin bridge.[25]

The musical elements of rhythm, pitch, timbre and melody require a high level of discrimination in order to be identified.[24] The first and most basic element of music is rhythm. Rhythm is related to the timing, or temporal features, of musical sounds. The fidelity of the temporal information that is received is crucial to rhythmic perception. Limb[24] also points out that music is "by definition presented over time and cannot be perceived without its temporal dimension" (p. 338). The next fundamental component of music is pitch. Frequency describes a physical phenomenon, whereas pitch describes a perceptual one. Pitch is the psychoacoustic correlate to the acoustical term fundamental frequency.[26] Pitch "relates to the frequency of a given sound, perceived as a note within a musical scale" (p. 338).[24] Differences in pitch gain relative significance to other pitches within a musical context, and thus allow the listener to detect melody. Harmony is defined as the relationship between pitches presented in conjunction, unlike a melody, which is presented as a series of pitches. The quality of a sound, independent of its pitch, is described as timbre. Timbre allows us to differentiate the sound of a piano from that of a violin, flute, or guitar, even if all are playing the same note or melody. Timbre perception is typically studied as the ability to discriminate between musical instruments. Although there are numerous other aspects of music that are crucial to a deeper understanding, in its basic essence, music is the presentation of multitimbral sounds organized by principles of rhythm, pitch, and harmony. Also, although it is possible to deconstruct a piece of music into its basic elements, music is generally presented and perceived as whole. All of the elements of music hold value in the understanding of cochlear implant-mediated perception of music.

ACOUSTIC CHARACTERISTICS OF ENVIRONMENTAL SOUNDS

Although the area of environmental sound perception has not been studied to the same extent that speech perception has, it is apparent that NLS are a complex and diverse group of stimuli. Researchers identify other variables, in addition to the acoustic properties, that contribute to the perception of NLS. Additionally, research[27–31] showed that other factors also contribute to environmental sound perception such as the visibility and movement of a sound source, the frequency of a source's occurrence in the environment, and the amount of contextual information provided.

Environmental sounds, by our definition, include a wide variety of acoustic stimuli, we use the term environmental sounds here to include any acoustic stimulus with a real-world analog that is not a type of spoken language, excluding music (discussed separately in this chapter). Acoustically, speech and nonspeech sounds have important similarities and differences. They are both complex signals with waveforms that change over time,[18] often having perceptual implications derived from their acoustic properties that are semantic (for language) or contextual (eg, nonlinguistic sounds, such as a car honking). However, as nonlinguistic sounds come from a variety of sources, the range of spectral and temporal variation among nonspeech sounds greatly exceeds that of speech, for which the source is always the human vocal tract, referred to as "harmonic" in nature.[19] Some of the nonspeech sounds in our everyday environment are similar in structure to speech. Consider how many sounds are produced by the human speech mechanism that do not carry linguistic meaning.

COCHLEAR IMPLANT USERS' PERCEPTION OF ENVIRONMENTAL SOUNDS

The literature suggests that individuals with normal hearing can accurately identify a large number of environmental nonlinguistic sounds with minimal errors.[22,28,30,32] In contrast, nonlinguistic sound identification may present difficulty for cochlear implant users who have a reduced auditory memory for what specific NLS should sound like, and also who receive distorted input.[20,33,34]

In a study spearheading the revived interest in environmental sound perception by CI users, Reed and Delhorne[34] studied environmental sound perception in 11 postlingually deafened CI users (9 Ineraid and 2 Clarion). The sound tokens used consisted of 40 sound sources. The researchers chose to group the stimuli by 10 "everyday" settings in which these sounds could occur (ie, kitchen, home, office, and outside). The testing paradigm employed was closed-set, in that, for each presented sound, the study participant picked one of 10 options associated with a specific environmental setting. The average performance across each of the environments was 79.2% with little variation across the settings. The range was 87.2% for office sounds to 77.6% for kitchen sounds. There was a greater degree of variability noted for individual CI user performance, ranging from 45.3% to 93.8% correct. Reed and Delhorne's conclusions were though some of the users had difficulty; overall many of the study participants seemed to have generally satisfactory environmental sound perception abilities in quiet.[34]

In a more recent study of CI mediated perception of environmental sounds results show generally poor performance among CI patients. Twenty-two experienced cochlear implant users, all of whom were postlingually deafened, were presented with a beta version of the NonLinguistic Sound test (NLST) developed by the authors for clinical testing. Each of the study participants were users of Cochlear Corporation (12) and Advanced Bionics (10) devices, with 22 and 16 electrodes respectively. The NLST, in contrast with the study described above,[34] employs an open-set testing paradigm. The test includes 50 sound tokens drawn from five different sound categories (Human nonlinguistic, Animal Mechanical/Alerting, Nature, and Musical instrument). The test sounds were arranged in three 50-item lists chosen randomly for each patient. The CI user is instructed to respond to the sound heard by giving the source as well as a descriptor of the sound. As an example, if the participant hears a "bark bark" they were asked to respond as "dog barking." The scoring of the test allows for two scores to be calculated; if the CI user correctly identified the sound source, but also if the source identified was within the same category of sound. As an example, if the token played was that of a phone ringing, and the CI user's response was that they heard an alarm clock buzzing. The participant would not receive a point for correct identification; however, as the

response given was a mechanical source, they would receive a point for correct categorization. Alternatively, if the sound played was thunder clapping, and the CI user reported hearing a car engine running, they would have neither identified the sound correctly, nor guessed within the correct sound category. The results of this study showed that participants, although performing well on measures of speech perception, perform poorly in identifying the NLS (mean 48.3%, range 18% to 70%).

Acoustical analysis of the sound tokens used in this study show that environmental sounds that carry speech-like harmonic structure and temporal cues are easier for cochlear implant users to recognize. Specifically, human nonspeech and animal sounds were categorized with levels of accuracy that were similar to each other. These two categories had a mixture of both temporally distinct and not distinct sounds. Interestingly, when sounds from the animal or human nonspeech categories were miscategorized, they were frequently confused for one another. The sounds in the category with the lowest categorization scores were that of nature sounds. A possible explanation for the difficulty is that these sounds (eg, rain, thunder, moving water) had the least distinct temporal patterning, thereby forcing individuals to rely on spectral qualities. Often, subjects mistook these sounds for those of car engines or running motors, which are also sounds with a relatively lower degree of temporal patterning. Figure 16–1 shows the spectrograms for two such sounds (rain and an airplane engine); these sounds are similar in their spectral qualities (high quotient of broadband noise) and they both lack distinct temporal patterning. Neither sound has acoustic characteristics similar to speech.

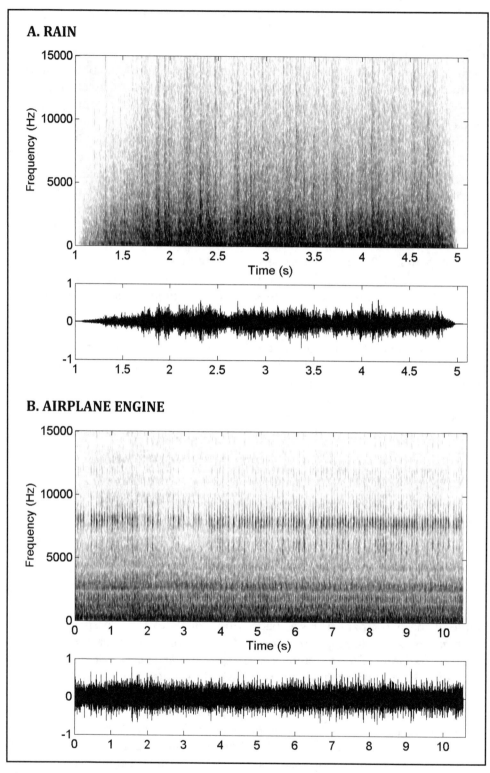

Figure 16–1. Spectrograms of rain falling and an airplane engine running illustrate the lack of distinct temporal patterning in many of the easily confused sound tokens (from Inverso and Limb[20]).

The nonlinguistic sounds that were identified most accurately, such as the human cough, dog bark, and bird chirp, were analyzed acoustically to determine why they might be easily recognized by CI users. Acoustical measurements revealed that these sounds all had distinct temporal events with spacing similar to speech syllables, as well as speechlike variations in amplitude, with abrupt interspersed onsets and broad spectral components. These acoustical characteristics are often used to describe speech[35] and can be seen in Figure 16–2.

The wide heterogeneity in the acoustic properties of nonlinguistic sound is likely partially responsible for the great difficulties that CI users display in identifying nonlinguistic stimuli, many of which are "inharmonic" in nature (eg, wind blowing). Identification of NLS declines significantly when the spectral features of the stimuli are smeared, a common result of CI signal processing algorithms.[30,36,37]

COCHLEAR IMPLANT USERS' PERCEPTION OF MUSIC

Postlingually deafened implantees and those who were implanted very young who often have excellent open set speech discrimination skills are motivated to improve their perception of complex acoustic sounds, including music.[38,39] Implant users rank music second only to speech in importance in their lives,[40] and many cochlear implant users find that music does not sound pleasing on their device. Anecdotal explanations for why CI users do not perceive music well are varied. First, implant users often have limited exposure to music prior to implantation due to their hearing loss. Second, individuals who are implanted often do not spend time in therapy learning how to hear music as they do with speech. There are other, more scientific reasons why music and other nonspeech sounds are not processed effectively by modern cochlear implants. Cochlear implants are primarily designed to transmit speech information and thus current technology remains limited when applied to musical stimuli.

CI-MEDIATED PITCH PERCEPTION

Pitch perception in cochlear implant users has been examined by several studies and is imperative in the enjoyment of music. The perception of pitch is directly tied to an individual's perception of melody. This is because melody is created when a series of pitches are temporally organized into patterns of varying musical contour and interval.[24] The ability to perceive melody requires the user to discriminate fine changes in pitch. Research has shown that CI users can listen to temporal changes in a stimulus and discriminate between pitches, hear musical intervals, and differentiate between melodies.[41,42] In implant users, the temporal pitch mechanism is only functional at low rates up to about 300 pps.[43] Modern processors use higher pulse rates (greater than 600 pps) in response to better speech perception; this results in CI processing that is not able to employ this temporal-pitch sensitivity using pulse rates. It is possible for listeners to discriminate complex tones produced by a musical instrument or the human voice. Doing so is very challenging for individuals with CIs because the place of excitation is masked because the complex and multiple sinusoidal components of

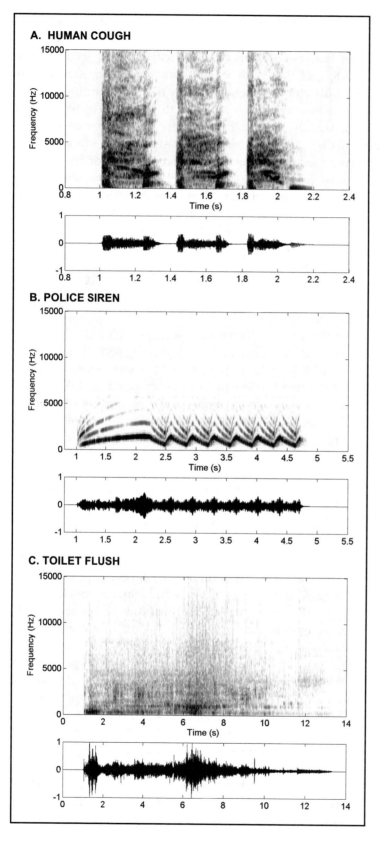

Figure 16–2. *Spectrograms of a human cough, a police siren, and a toilet flush are shown as representative examples of tokens with distinct temporal pattering (human cough and police siren) versus a token without distinct temporal pattering (toilet flush) (from Inverso and Limb[20]).*

musical sounds cause a spread of excitation across a range of electrodes. Additionally, due to the constant pulse rate of most CI processors, the periodicity of the stimulus is obscured.[44] In another study that was investigating the perception of melodic contour,[45] nine normal-hearing and eleven cochlear implant users were tested. The study participants listened to five-note melodic contours and were tasked to identify the contour shape from nine visual choices. The individuals with normal hearing did very well, achieving a mean performance of about 95% accuracy. However, the cochlear Implant study participants had dramatically varying results with a range from 14 to 90%.

CI-MEDIATED RHYTHM PERCEPTION

In comparison to other aspects of music (ie, timbre, pitch, etc), rhythm is the easiest for cochlear implant users to perceive; however, their perceptual abilities are less than normal hearing listeners.[46,47] Pitch and timbre rely on temporal features that occur rapidly, on the order of milliseconds. Comparatively, rhythm generally describes the temporal features of music that occur slower, on the order of seconds. For cochlear implant users, this translates to rhythmic patterns being perceived despite a skewed perception of other musical characteristics.[48] In a study evaluating recognition of familiar songs 49 CI receipients were tested. The investigators found that two-thirds of the correctly identified melodies had a highly memorable rhythm.[49]

Somewhat in contrast, an earlier study evaluated eight adult CI users' ability to recognize music.[50] Some of the participants tested showed a good ability to recognize songs that were sung with instrumental accompaniment; however, a poor ability to recognize songs played on an electronic keyboard without verbal cues. This result implicated that the users were using the verbal cues rather than recognizing the musical qualities such as tones and melodic intervals. The researchers reported that the subjects were barely able to distinguish between songs with the same rhythm and pitch range, and they showed poor ability to discriminate musical intervals. Gfeller and colleagues[51] evaluated rhythmic pattern discrimination using the Adapted Primary Measures of Musical Audiation (PMMA) test. In the PMMA test, listeners discriminate between two patterns that differ in their rhythmic pattern by note duration. In the 6-pulse task, study participants had to identify a change in the temporal location or short interval among four long intervals. The results for the PMMA test did not reveal a significant difference in performance between the normal hearing and CI users (~ 84%), however; there was a significant difference in performance on the 6-pulse task. The participants with normal hearing could hear the changes at a significantly shorter duration of 607 ms, whereas the CI group took longer to perceive the changes at an average duration of about 1,070 ms. Rhythm, as it relates to tempo discrimination, has also been shown to be near normal for CI users as compared to their normally hearing counterparts. Kong and colleagues (2004)[52] investigated tempo discrimination ability and complex rhythm discrimination ability using four listeners. They found that tempo discrimination was near normal in implant users. As in the study above, the researchers found that the CI users could not discriminate complex rhythm discrimination as well as normal-hearing listeners.

CI-MEDIATED TIMBRE PERCEPTION

Timbre perception is typically studied in order to determine the ability to discriminate between musical instruments. Several studies[46,50,53–56] have researched CI users' ability to differentiate between musical instruments. Upon review of these studies, it appears that the average percent correct identification score ranges from 35 to 46.6% for the CI users, whereas the normally hearing participants range in scores from 90 to 97%. Another key finding is that although normally hearing research participants also make errors, the errors are of a different nature, such as mistaking one wind instrument for another wind instrument, whereas errors made by the CI users are often not related to a specific type of instrument.[57] Additionally, CI users more often identify percussive instruments such as the piano correctly than brass or woodwind instruments.[54,57] Donnelly and Limb[58] denoted that such results would imply that it is the temporal cue of the attack that is distinctively associated with percussive instruments, such as the piano.

It is because of these subtle acoustic cues that timbre is so difficult for CI users to perceive. Additionally, this task is compounded as CI users must interpret these cues using a processor that is designed to code speech information. These issues in combination make the identification of musical instruments very challenging for CI users. In a study by Grasmeder and Lutman,[59] CI users and normally hearing adults were asked to report on a questionnaire about their ability to recognize musical instruments. The study reports that the self-reported ability of the CI users to recognize some musical instruments is poor. The instruments in particular that result in the poorest scores are the

saxophone, tuba, and clarinet. Additionally, the researchers created and analyzed both spectrograms and electrodograms for samples of music played on 10 different musical instruments. The electrodograms for the musical instrument sounds show that the more problematic instruments (saxophone, tuba, and clarinet) can only be identified using distorted spectral information or reduced temporal information. The findings agreed with the previously mentioned studies[54,57]; the more easily identifiable instruments, such as the drum and piano, can be identified using their salient temporal information.

A test of music perception called the Clinical Assessment of Music Perception (CAMP)[60] was used in a study by Nimmons and colleagues.[61] The researchers examined CI user recognition of eight live-recorded musical instruments. The mean timbre recognition for the eight CI users that participated was 49% correct, with a range of 21 to 54% correct. These results are not dissimilar to the mean 30.5% identification scores reported on the musical instrument section of the NLST by Inverso and Limb.[20] The cumulative results of this body of literature support that limited spectral resolution, as is the case with cochlear implants, makes the recognition of musical instruments difficult, especially when the instrument is not rich in temporal content.

IMPROVING CI-MEDIATED PERCEPTION OF NONLINGUISTIC AND MUSIC STIMULI

Nonlinguistic sounds continue to pose a challenge for cochlear implant users; however, the growing expectation for CI users to perceive and enjoy environmental sounds and music has prompted the cochlear implant developers to improve their designs and signal processing strategies. The changes being investigated and employed currently are varied and there is little consensus on which method provides the best signal. Some of the recent changes include the use of current steering, the combination of acoustic and electric stimulation, and signal processing designed to deliver more fine structure. One consideration that must be taken with any signal processing improvements or modifications is avoiding detrimental effects on speech processing. Although it may be possible for an adult cochlear implant user to change a program or their implant's settings to enjoy music; the remainder of nonlinguistic sounds happen spontaneously and naturally in an otherwise speech-filled environment. A listener cannot be expected to anticipate environmental sounds and make processor changes accordingly.

Current steering employs the simultaneous activation of adjacent electrodes that are weighted appropriately to match a spectral shape. Research has shown that the use of current steering increases the number of pitch percepts in cochlear implant users.[62,63] The primary suggested benefit of current steering is improved spectral resolution. Also, the increased number of pitch percepts available with current steering should be sufficiently high enough to enable improved music and nonlinguistic sound perception. Advanced Bionics newest design employs current steering in their processing called HiRes Fidelity 120™, which has the potential to aid in music and NLS perception. Although more independent studies need to be completed, the published literature that is currently available on HiRes Fidelity 120™ is promising.[64,65]

Cochlear Corporation recently created a processing strategy[66] that has nonlinguistic sound perception as well as speech in noise perception, in mind. The MP3000 coding strategy[66] attempts to eliminate some of the redundancies often found in the popular commercial Advanced Combination Encoder (ACE) strategy, resulting in fewer channels m ($<n$) being used to transmit the same amount of information. MP3000 is a coding strategy that is meant to increase the effective amount of spectral information presented if a similar number of selected maxima is specified.[67] Psychophysical masking I used to the transfer of masked acoustical information. MP3000 is a modification of the ACE strategy commonly used with Cochlear Corporation implants. ACE is a peak picking/"n of m" strategy that picks the maximum n spectral peaks of m channels to be delivered to the implantee. MP3000, which was once named Psychoacoustic Advanced Combination Encoder (PACE), similarly picks the largest amplitude component for transmission but chooses the masking pattern of this component and then selects the next largest acoustic component of the stimulus. This process accounts for the masking and nonlinear summation of excitation that would be produced in a normal-hearing auditory system.[44] The result of this processing scheme is that only the most perceptually salient components of the incoming signal will be delivered to the implantee. This differs from ACE which delivers the components based on amplitude alone. If successful, this processing scheme will improve spectral resolution and thereby enhance the perception of music and possible other nonlinguistic sounds.

A pilot study by Lai and Dillier[67] investigates music perception using the MP3000 coding strategy as compared to ACE. The researchers conducted instrument identification (timbre) and pitch ranking tests as well as a questionnaire to judge the sound quality of various music pieces. The study revealed that the CI users had greater difficulty using pitch cues versus timbre cues for instrument identification. Ultimately, the study did not reveal a significant advantage to using MP3000 over ACE in terms of music perception; however, the researchers mentioned that the subjects' familiarity with their own ACE maps might have been an important factor. Nogueira and colleagues[66] evaluated MP3000 with eight CI users. They found that a four-channel PACE (now MP3000) algorithm with 4 equaling the n in "n of m", surpassed the performance of ACE by 17%. Testing using eight channels yielded less significant results; however, the researchers did report a trend that would suggest better performance with MP3000 versus ACE. Although these results are preliminary they hold promise that this type of processing may result in better perception of nonspeech stimuli.

Another signal processing strategy that has been employed commercially is called Fine Structure Processing (FSP) by MED-EL in their newest generation implants. The FSP strategy is designed to attain better frequency coding in the low to mid-frequencies. The design's goal is to allow the neural structures in the inner ear to better phase-lock to the sound signal, similarly to how individuals with normal hearing would in this frequency range. In 2009, 22 children wearing MED-EL cochlear implants were evaluated for the development of music listening skills and also to assess the efficacy of a new training program called "Musical Ears."[68] The children were studied over an 18-month period. The first finding was that all the children showed statistically significant improvement over time. The study results suggest that these congenitally

deafened children were able to learn to sing as well as dance. These results were conducted through an internal study; therefore, further evaluation is needed into this topic of pediatric musical skills development. In a study of adult cochlear implant users, conducted by Arnolder and colleagues,[12] measures of speech and music perception yielded improved test scores following conversion from Continuous Interleaved Sampling (CIS) to the new FSP strategy. Following the study, the researchers reported that 12 of the 14 CI users that participated preferred the new FSP speech processing strategy over their CIS strategy. However, there is contrary data from another study that suggests this preference is user specific and offers a counteropinion on FSP for music perception.[69] Magnusson's work[69] indicates that users should be allowed to try both strategies and determine which one works best for them based on Audiologic testing as well as qualitative preference. The paired-comparison between the two strategies (FSP and HDCIS) did not reveal a statistically significant difference in performance; however, the total numbers of significant individual preferences broke down to: 11 FSP versus 12 HDCIS for speech perception, and 4 FSP versus 15 HDCIS for music perception. Finally, in testing speech perception in the users over time, the average speech recognition score significantly decreased at the one-month interval for the participants using FSP.

CONCLUSION

What is the definition of success with a cochlear implant? This question may never be answered, as success depends on the individual goals and expectations of the recipient. Consider though that the majority of individuals who choose to receive a cochlear implant optimistically anticipate that the device will restore the gestalt of their auditory environment, whereas music and other nonlinguistic sounds remain tremendously challenging for implant users. The sum total of our daily auditory experiences consists of much more than just speech stimuli; therefore, the clinical and research communities need to keep working to deliver as much of these sounds as possible. Continual developments in signal processing strategies and CI design, together with an increased appreciation of the importance of nonlinguistic sounds for safety and aesthetic pleasure should ultimately lead to substantial improvements in the ability of cochlear implants to transmit environmental and musical information.

REFERENCES

1. Ramsdell DA. The psychology of the hard-of-hearing and the deafened adult. In: Silverman HDSR, ed, *Hearing and Deafness*. New York, NY: Holt, Rinehart & Winston; 1978:499–510.
2. Oh EL, Lutfi RA. Informational masking by everyday sounds. *J Acoust Soc Am*. 1999; 106:3521–3528.
3. Parkinson AJ, Parkinson WS, Tyler RS, Lowder MW, Gantz BJ. Speech perception performance in experienced cochlear-implant patients receiving the SPEAK processing strategy in the Nucleus Spectra-22 cochlear implant. *J Speech Lang Hear Res*. 1998;41(5):1073–1087.
4. Gfeller K, Christ A, Knutson JF, Witt S, Murray KT, Tyler RS. Musical backgrounds, listening habits, and aesthetic enjoyment of adult cochlear implant recipients. *J Am Acad Audiol*. 2000;11(7):390–406.
5. Zhao F, Stephens SD, Sim SW, Meredith R. The use of qualitative questionnaires in patients having and being considered for cochlear implants. *Clin Otolaryngol Allied Sci*. 1997;22(3):254–259.
6. Tyler RS. Advantages and disadvantages expected and reported by cochlear implant patients. *Amer J Otolaryngol*. 1994; 15:523–531.
7. Wilson BS, Finley CC, Lawson DT, Wolford RD, Eddington DK, Rabinowitz WM. Better speech recognition with cochlear implants. *Nature*. 1991;352(6332):236–238.
8. Shannon RV, Zeng FG, Kamath V, Wygonski J, Ekelid M. Speech recognition with primarily temporal cues. *Science*. 1995; 270:303–304.
9. Loizou PC. Mimicking the human ear. *IEEE Signal Processing Magazine*. 1998; 15:101–130.
10. Rubinstein JT. How cochlear implants encode speech. *Curr Opin Otolaryngol Head Neck Surg*. 2004;12(5):444–448.
11. Smith ZM, Delgutte B, Oxenham AJ. Chimaeric sounds reveal dichotomies in auditory perception. *Nature*. 2002;416(6876): 87–90.
12. Arnoldner C, Riss D, Brunner M, Durisin M, Baumgartner WD, Hamzavi JS. Speech and music perception with the new fine structure speech coding strategy: preliminary results. *Acta Otolaryngol*. 2007 Dec; 127(12):1298–303.
13. Stickney GS, Nje K, Zeng, FG. Realistic listening improved by adding fine structure. *J Acoust Soci Amer*. 2002;112:2355.
14. Wilson B, Sun X, Schatzer R, Wolford R. Representation of fine structure or fine frequency information with cochlear implants. *Inter Congr Ser*. 2004;1273:3–6.
15. Cycowicz YM, Friedman D. A developmental study of the effect of temporal order on the ERPs elicited by novel environmental sounds. *Electroencephalog Clin Neurophysiol*. 1997;103(2):304–318.
16. Stuart GP, Jones DM. Priming the identification of environmental sounds. *J Exper Psychol*. 1995;48(3):741–761.

17. Miller JD, Tanis DC. Recognition memory for common sounds. *Psych Sci.* 1973;23: 307–308.

18. Gygi B. *Factors in the Identification of Environmental Sounds.* Unpublished doctoral dissertation, Indiana University, Bloomington; 2001.

19. Attias H, Schreiner CE. Temporal low-order statistics of natural sounds. In: Moxer M, ed. *Advances in Neural Info Processing Systems.* Cambridge, MA: MIT Press; 1997:27–33.

20. Inverso Y, Limb CJ. Cochlear implant-mediated perception of nonlinguistic sounds. *Ear Hear.* 2010;31(4):505–514.

21. Gygi B, Shafiro V. Development of the database for environmental sound research and application (DESRA): design, functionality, and retrieval considerations. *EURASIP J Audio, Speech, Music Processing.* 2010;2010. doi: 10.1155/2010/654914

22. Shafiro V. Development of a large-item environmental sound test and the effects of short- term training with spectrally-degraded stimuli. *Ear Hear.* 2008;29(5): 775–790.

23. Gobl C, Ní Chasaide A. Acoustic characteristics of voice quality. *Speech Comm.* 1992; 11:481–490.

24. Limb CJ. Cochlear implant-mediated perception of music. *Curr Opin Otolaryngol Head Neck Surg.* 2006;14(5):337–340.

25. Wolfe J. *Speech and Music, Acoustics, and Coding, and What Music Might Be For.* Adelaide, Australia: Causal Productions; 2002.

26. Howard DM, Angus JA. *Music Technology: Acoustics and Psychoacoustics.* 3rd ed. Oxford, UK: Focal Press; 2006.

27. Abe K, Ozawa K, Suzuki Y, Sone T. Comparison of the effects of verbal versus visual information about sound sources on the perception of environmental sounds. *Acta Acustica.* 2006;92:51–60.

28. Ballas JA. Common factors in the identification of an assortment of brief everyday sounds. *J Exp Psychol: Hum Percep Performance.* 1993;19(2):250–267.

29. Ballas JA, Mullins T. Effects of context on the identification of everyday sounds. *Hum Performance.* 1991;4(3):199–219.

30. Gygi B, Kidd GR, Watson CS. Spectral-temporal factors in the identification of environmental sounds. *J Acoust Soc Amer.* 2004;115(3):1252–1265.

31. Gygi BS, Shafiro V. Effect of context on the identification of environmental sounds. *J Acoust Soc Amer.* 2006;119:3334.

32. Marcell MM, Borella D, Greene M, Kerr E, Rogers S. Confrontation naming of environmental sounds. *J Clin Exper Neuropsychol.* 2000;22(6):830–864.

33. Tye-Murray N, Tyler RS, Woodworth GG, Gantz BJ. Performance over time with a nucleus or Ineraid cochlear implant. *Ear Hear.* 1992;13(3):200–209.

34. Reed CM, Delhorne LA. Reception of environmental sounds through cochlear implants. *Ear Hear.* 2005;26(1):48–61.

35. Bickley C, Lindblom B, Roug L. (1986). Acoustic measures of rhythm in infants' babbling, or "All God's children got rhythm." In: *Proceedings of the 12th International Congress on Acoustics*, Toronto; A6–A4.

36. Loebach J, Pisoni D. Perceptual learning of spectrally degraded speech and environmental sounds. *J Acoust Soc Amer.* 2008; 123(2):1126–1139.

37. Shafiro V. Identification of environmental sounds with varying spectral resolution. *Ear Hear.* 2008b;29(3):401–420.

38. Wendt-Harris B, Pollack P, Lassere A. What SHHH members say about hearing aids and audiological services. *J Self-Help Hard Hear People.* 2001;22(4):25–29.

39. Zhao F, Stephens SD, Sim SW, Meredith R. The use of qualitative questionnaires in patients having and being considered for cochlear implants. *Clin Otolaryngol All Sci.* 1997;22(3):254–259.

40. Gfeller K, Christ A, Knutson JF, Witt S, Murray KT, Tyler RS. Musical backgrounds, listening habits, and aesthetic enjoyment of adult cochlear implant recipients. *J Am Acad Audiol.* 2000;11(7):390–406.

41. Pijl S, Schwarz DW. Melody recognition and musical interval perception by deaf subjects stimulated with electrical pulse trains through single cochlear implant electrodes. *J Acoust Soc Am*. 1995;98(2 pt 1):886–895.

42. McDermott HJ, McKay CM. Musical pitch perception with electrical stimulation of the cochlea. *J Acoust Soc Am*. 1997;101(3):1622–1631.

43. Zeng FG. Trends in cochlear implants. *Trends Amplif*. 2004;8(1):1–34.

44. Drennan WR, Rubinstein J. Music perception in cochlear implant users and its relationship with psychophysical capabilities. *J Rehab Res Dev*. 2008;45(5):779–790.

45. Galvin JJ, Fu QJ, Nogaki G. Melodic contour identification by cochlear implant listeners. *Ear Hear*. 2007; 28: 302–319.

46. Leal MC, Shin YJ, Laborde M-L, Calmels MNL, Verges S, Lugardon S, et al. Music perception in adult cochlear implant recipients. *Acta Oto-Laryngol*. 2003;123(7):826–835.

47. McDermott HJ. Music perception with cochlear implants: a review. *Trends Amplif*. 2004;8(2):49–82.

48. Gfeller K, Christ A, Knutson J, Witt S, Mehr M. The effects of familiarity and complexity on appraisal of complex songs by cochlear implant recipients and normal hearing adults. *J Music Theory*. 2003;40:78–112.

49. Gfeller K, Turner C, Mehr M, et al. Recognition of familiar melodies by adult cochlear implant recipients and normal-hearing adults. *Coch Implants Int*. 2002; 3(1):29–53.

50. Fujita S, Ito J. Ability of nucleus cochlear Implantees to recognize music. *Ann Otol Rhinol Laryngol*. 1999;108:634–640.

51. Gfeller K, Woodworth G, Robin DA, Witt S, Knutson JF. Perception of rhythmic and sequential pitch patterns by normally hearing adults and adult cochlear implant users. *Ear Hear*. 1997;18(3):252–260.

52. Kong YY, Cruz R, Jones JA, Zeng FG. Music perception with temporal cues in acoustic and electric hearing. *Ear Hear*. 2004;25(2):173–185.

53. Gfeller K, Lansing CR. Melodic, rhythmic, and timbral perception of adult cochlear implant users. *J Speech Hear Res*. 1991; 34(4):916–920.

54. Gfeller K, Witt S, Woodworth G, Mehr MA, Knutson J. Effects of frequency, instrumental family, and cochlear implant type on timbre recognition and appraisal. *Ann Otol Rhinol Laryngol*. 2002;111(4):349–356.

55. McDermott HJ, Looi V. Perception of complex signals, including musical sounds, with cochlear implants. *Proceedings of the VIII International Cochlear Implant Conference*, Indianapolis, IN: Elsevier; 2004:201–204.

56. Schultz E, Kerber M, eds. Music perception with the MED-EL implants. In: *Advances in Cochlear Implants*. Vienna, Austria; 1994:326–332.

57. Gfeller K, Knutson JF, Woodworth G, Witt S, DeBus B. Timbral recognition and appraisal by adult cochlear implant users and normal-hearing adults. *J Am Acad Audiol*. 1998;9(1):1–19.

58. Donnelly PJ, Limb CJ. Music perception in cochlear implant users. In: Niparko JM et al, eds. *Cochlear Implants: Principles and Practices*. 2nd ed. Philadelphia, PA: Lippincott Williams & Wilkins Publishers; 2000.

59. Grasmeder ML, Lutman ME. The identification of musical instruments through nucleus cochlear implants. *Coch Implants Int*. 2006;7:148–158.

60. Kang R, Nimmons GL, Drennan W, et al. Development and validation of the University of Washington Clinical Assessment of Music Perception test. *Ear Hear*. 2009; 30(4):411–418.

61. Nimmons GL, Kang RS, Drennan WR, et al. Clinical assessment of music perception in cochlear implant listeners. *Otol Neurotol*. 2007;29(2):149–155.

62. Firszt JB, Koch DB, Downing M, Litvak L. Current steering creates additional pitch percepts in adult cochlear implant recipients. *Otol Neurotol*. 2007;28(5):629–636.

63. Koch DB, Downing M, Osberger MJ, Litvak L. Using current steering to increase spectral resolution in CII and HiRes 90K users. *Ear Hear.* 2007;28(2 suppl): 38–41.

64. Brendel M, Buechner A, Krueger B, Frohne-Buechner C, Lenarz T. Evaluation of the harmony soundprocessor in combination with the speech coding strategy HiRes 120. *Otol Neurotol.* 2008;29(2):199–202.

65. Drennan W, Won J, Nie K, Jameyson E, Rubinstein J. Sensitivity of psychophysical measures to signal processor modifications in cochlear implant users. *Hear Res.* 2010;262:1–8.

66. Nogueira W, Buchner A, Lenarz T, Edler B. A psycho-acoustic "NofM"—type of speech coding strategy for cochlear implants. *EURASIP J Appl Signal Process.* 2005;18:3044–3059.

67. Lai W, Dillier N. Investigating the MP3000 coding strategy for music perception. In: *Jahrestagung der Deutschen Gesellschaft für Audiologie.* Vol 11. Kiel, Germany: Deutsche Gesellschaft für Audiologie e.V; 2008:1–4.

68. Kosaner et al. *Music for young CI users.* Presented at 9th European Symposium on Paediatric CI, 14–17 May, 2009; Warsaw, Poland.

69. Magnusson L. Comparison of the fine structure processing (FSP) strategy and the CIS strategy used in the MED-EL cochlear implant system: speech intelligibility and music sound quality. *Int J Audiol.* 2011; 50(4):279–287.

Chapter 17

Cochlear Implantation: Reliability and Reimplantation

ROBERT D. CULLEN AND CRAIG A. BUCHMAN

INTRODUCTION

Cochlear implants (CIs) are electrical pulse generators with electrodes that are positioned within the cochlea to provide neural stimulation of the peripheral auditory nerve in response to a variety of specific acoustic signals. Cochlear implantation has become a common form of (re)habilitation for individuals with severe to profound sensorineural hearing loss. For nearly all hearing-impaired individuals, CIs improve environmental sound awareness and lip reading. More importantly, these devices can significantly enhance speech perception abilities, even in the absence of visual cues. For hearing-impaired children, CIs can allow for the development of spoken language, thereby improving educational achievement and ultimately, employment opportunities.[1-3] For adults with later onset hearing loss, these devices frequently restore communication abilities, consequently avoiding social isolation and improving quality of life.[4-6]

Structurally, a CI is composed of an internal, receiver-stimulator and an externally worn device that communicates across the intact skin by way of a radio-frequency (RF) signal. The internal and external device antennas remain aligned for transmission using magnets. The external device consists of a microphone, speech processor, and a transmitter. The speech processor includes filter banks that partition the acoustic signals into various frequency bands. Today, feature extraction algorithms produce an encoded signal consisting mostly of spectral information whereas the temporal components remain somewhat poorly delineated for processing and delivery. The internal device includes a receiving antenna, a complex computer chip for further processing, current source generator(s), and a multiple electrode array for intracochlear stimulation. The intracochlear electrode array is composed of silicone rubber and platinum electrodes of varying sizes, shapes, and number. Moreover, some arrays are curved to conform to the inner cochlear wall or modiolus whereas others track the outer cochlear wall. The computer hardware and current source generators are contained within a titanium can that is in close proximity to the antenna. Clearly, delivering electrical current from the source generators within the hermetically sealed titanium can, along the various wires, to the electrodes within the aqueous environment of the cochlea requires significant design, engineering and know-how.[7]

In 1984, the United States Food and Drug Administration (FDA) approved the 3M/House unit for use in adults and by 1985 the Nucleus/Cochlear Corporation's implant was approved. In 1989, the first child received the Nucleus multi-channel CI. Advanced Bionics first came onto the scene in 1991 and was FDA approved in 1996. MED-EL was founded in 1989 and was FDA approved for use in adults and children in 2001.

Although CIs have been remarkably successful, the fact that they are composed of an implanted electrical pulse generator and a speech processor that are constantly being exposed to adverse environmental conditions both within and outside the human body portends a finite life expectancy. As with all implanted devices, biocompatibility remains a significant issue for device retention and long-term use. As an example, inside the body, devices are constantly under the influence of immune exposure, as well as electrochemical, microbial, and mechanical insults. Surely, a variety of host factors can serve to further modify these conditions as well. Moreover, electrical devices can wear out over time, again resulting in a loss of function.

Revision CI surgery can be indicated when: (1) the device stops functioning (ie, hard failure), (2) there is a suspected

device malfunction despite the fact that auditory percepts are still present (ie, soft failure), (3) medical/surgical issues arise (infection, etc), or (4) when a technology upgrade is considered. This chapter discusses revision CI surgery and device reliability with an emphasis on clinical presentation of device-related issues, surgical replacement and outcomes. Shortcomings of our current evaluation and management paradigms will be discussed. By way of a preamble, the evolution of CI technology is discussed and the current device structures described.

EVOLUTION OF COCHLEAR IMPLANTS

The first electrical stimulation of the inner ear probably occurred by Count Alessandro Volta at the end of the 18th century when he placed 2 metal rods in his ears and connected them to the terminal of 30 or 40 electrolytic cells (~50 volts). He reported the sensation of: "une secousse dans la tate" or a blow on the head followed by a sound like "the boiling of a viscid liquid."[8] Modern inner ear stimulation, for the purposes of auditory perception occurred in 1925 when radio engineers discovered that tones could be produced by electrodes near the ears. Subsequently, 32 articles were published between 1930 and 1946 regarding various types of electrical stimulation in the outer and middle ear and auditory perceptions.[9] Djourno and Eyries are credited with the first intralabyrinthine implantation of an electrical stimulating prosthesis. This was placed through a labyrinthine fistula in a patient with chronic otitis media and cholesteatoma in 1957. Djourno was a French neurophysiologist and Eyries an established otologist. Upon stimulation, the patient described high-frequency sounds that resembled the "roulette wheel of a casino" and "crickets." Their patient was able to discern the words "pap," "mamm," and "allo."[10–12]

In 1957, a patient in Los Angeles, CA brought William House, MD a news article detailing the apparent success of Djourno and Eyries. By 1960 and 1961, House with his colleague Doyle experimented with electrical stimulation of the inner ear. House performed promontory and vestibule stimulation of patients undergoing stapedectomy surgery.[13] Similarly, Blair Simmons, MD with the assistance of Epley at Stanford (1964) implanted 6 electrodes in the modiolus portion of the eighth nerve near the basal cochlear fibers under local anesthesia.[14] In both cases, electrical stimulation resulted in some auditory percepts. Following these initial experiments, House and Doyle implanted 2 adult patients with single gold electrodes for short-term stimulation of hearing. One additional patient received a 5-electrode device. All 3 of these devices were later removed because of compatibility issues.[13] Specifically, the wires were tracked through the skin and resulted in local wound infection and irritation.

Although it became obvious that a hermetically sealed container would be needed to house the electronics for reliable long-term stimulation, the percutaneous connection was not totally abandoned since it was needed to rapidly explore a variety of stimulation strategies for hearing. At the University of Paris as well those at the University of Utah, and University of California at San Francisco (UCSF), percutaneous stimulation was being carried out with great advances.[15–17] Ultimately however, similar to the experiences of House and Simmons, these devices required removal because of local infection. Nonetheless, these studies served a necessary purpose and limited use of this approach has continued in recent times.

The standards required to produce a device that would be strong and impervious to the fluids, enzymes, immune response, and mechanical insults of the human body were very high. Moreover, the absence of a percutaneous connection required an alternative method for energy and data transfer. House later teamed with engineer Jack Urban to produce the first wearable, "take-home" CI, implanted in Chuck Graser in 1972.[13,18–20] This was possible through the use of newer, biocompatible materials first developed for pacemaker utilization. His initial device was a six-wire electrode grounded through the footplate of the stapes. He was ultimately fit with a speech processor/stimulator that had a carrier wave (16 kHz). Although this implant as well as the one used by Michelson (1971)[21] failed to produce open-set speech perception, these devices proved that simple transcutaneous, inductive coupling was possible and that a percutaneous connection was not needed.[21] Dobelle et al[22] later proposed a single RF link for both data and power transfer.[22] In 1974, the University of Melbourne produced an electromagnetic dual link for data and power transfer that was highly efficient. This method allowed for transcutaneous, efficient transfer of power and data and is currently used in the FDA-approved systems that are clinically available today in the U.S.[23,24]

Creating a hermetically sealed device was a major challenge for early investigators. In the earliest devices in Melbourne (1974), glass was melted onto the wires that exited a Kovar steel container that housed the circuitry.[7] Unfortunately, this was unsuccessful as fluid leakage persisted.

In the pacemaker industry as referenced above, epoxy resin was also being tried but penetration and corrosion remained an issue. K. Kratochivil at Telectronics, a pacemaker company in Australia, discovered that when a blend of ceramics was sintered, it would bond to both wires and the metallic container to produce an impermeable seal. For Cochlear Corp in Australia, this technology when used in combination with a titanium package for strength produced the hermetically sealed device that is in use today. However, this construct required moving the data transmission antenna to a remote site, creating an elongated device with a susceptible antenna connection.[7]

For Advanced Bionics Corp (Sylmar, California, USA) and MED-EL Corporation (Innsbruck, Austria), a ceramic housing was chosen so the antenna and electronics were included in the same package. Unfortunately, ceramic was more brittle and susceptible to cracks in response to external trauma. The welding of ceramic to the metal header also created a relative weak point for the hermetic seal. Over time, the ceramic construct of these devices has given way to the Silastic-titanium devices that are in use today by all 3 implant manufacturers producing FDA approved CIs in the United States today.[7]

ELECTRODE ARRAYS

Intracochlear electrode arrays have also evolved over time. The 3M/House and later the 3M/Vienna devices both employed a single electrode placed through the round window membrane, in to scala tympani. The concept was to modulate a carrier wave to convey temporal information (ie, temporal coding). Although over

1,000 devices were placed in to primarily adults, only limited speech perception was possible and, thus, the approach was ultimately abandoned after data generated in adults using the multiple electrode (University of Melbourne and University of Utah), "place-coding" devices demonstrated superior results.[25-31] From this time forward, place-coding using multiple electrodes situated longitudinally along the course of scala tympani to stimulate the tonotopic organization of the cochlear nerve became the preferred approach.[32-34] Speech processing and stimulation paradigms were then further explored to optimize speech understanding.

Creating the multiple electrode array for place coding remains a work in progress and requires electrode carrier and contacts that are atraumatic and produce localized stimulation. The ideal number and spacing of the contacts as well as the extent of cochlear coverage remains a hotly debated topic among the industry. Historically, a variety of electrode contacts and carrier shapes, as well as stimulation paradigms have been devised to achieve these results. House and Simmons placed multiple wires with electrodes in to or through the inner ear.[13-14] Others developed the concept of the "multiple electrode array" as a single carrier of multiple contacts.[7] Today, the individual electrodes are laid down in molds by hand and silicone is poured to achieve the finished array. Some arrays have been curved to conform to the cochlear shape, thereby moving the contacts closer to the neural elements for stimulation specificity. Unfortunately, these devices are susceptible to surgical mishaps that can result in tip rollovers and unwanted device coiling and trauma within the scala tympani. Moreover, some modiolar conforming arrays required an extra-intracochlear positioner that was later associated with the development of meningitis. By contrast, free-form arrays are straight, compliant arrays that are designed to avoid intracochlear trauma by conforming to the cochlear out wall. With these devices, traumatic insertion usually results from deep insertion into the cochlear apex, with resulting: (1) damage at the tipwhere cross-sectional dimensions are inadequate or (2) in the base as a result of force-induced buckling. The perfect electrode array remains to be developed. Avoiding trauma and achieving stimulation specificity remain highly desirable goals as placement of these devices in patients with greater degrees of residual hearing becomes more common.

In summary, receiver-stimulator and electrode array design, materials, and assembly continue to evolve as more is learned about these devices and their interaction with patients. In general, device compatibility issues are very uncommon amongst patients with the most recently implanted devices that are in clinical usage today. We owe a great deal to the scientists, engineers, surgeons, and pioneers of cochlear implantation for developing these devices.

COCHLEAR IMPLANT RELIABILITY

Device reliability is a very important aspect of cochlear implantation and depends upon the robustness of the external speech processor and internal receiver-stimulator construct within the complex environment of the human body. The fact that CIs have a finite life expectancy (in years) that is well below the life expec-

tancy of most young adults and children implies that cochlear re-implantation will be required at some point in many patients' lifetime. Although revision surgery carries with it a group of risks that are presumably unavoidable, this also provides an opportunity for technological upgrade with possible improvements in performance. First-time patients must be counseled about these risks as well as the need (and potential benefits) of future re-implantation.

The current standard for reporting on the performance of electrical pulse generators such as the implantable cardiac pacemakers is ISO Standard 5841-2:2000. This standard has been adopted by the CI manufacturers for reporting internal device reliability using cumulative survival curves. The International Consensus Group for Cochlear Implant Reliability Reporting was formed on November 27, 2005 with the mission to create a clinically relevant reliability standard to be used by all manufacturers as they comply with reporting requirements to their respective governmental authority. An additional goal was to create a minimal reporting guideline for editors of journals who publish results of research related to reliability.[35] After Battmer and colleagues,[35] the following principles should guide the reporting of device reliability:

1. When a device is explanted, it should be immediately returned by the CI Center to the appropriate manufacturer to be analyzed and assigned to one of the reporting categories.
2. All explanted devices (category C) that test out of specification are considered internal device failures. These devices are to be included in the calculation of cumulative survival

rate (CSR). Calculating and reporting of the CSR will be in accordance with the methodology outlined in ISO standard 5841-2:2000.

3. Manufacturer's reports of device reliability should indicate the sources of data, the sample size, and the time interval over which the data were collected. There must be no device exclusions.

4. Reports of CSR should give complete historic data of a given device, describing any technical modifications (that can be integrated into historic data by starting at time 0).

5. The complete data set for internal device reliability of the "mother" product should always be supplied when presenting data on subsequent device modifications.

6. A "new internal device" can be attributed when there has been a change in the case and/or the electrodes that has been labeled by its own mark with a competent authority.

7. The overall CSR is reported and then further divided to separate adults and children (patients younger than 18 yr) and should be reported separately and with 95% confidence intervals as appropriate.

8. Survival time begins with closure of the wound at internal CI device surgical placement.

9. The manufacturer is required to notify, in writing, the CI center caring for the patient within 60 days of receipt of an explanted device as to whether the internal component was "in" or "out" of specification. Once root cause analysis is completed, which may take significant time to complete depending on the particular issue, the CI center should be notified within 60 days, in writing, to inform the patient of the outcome of device analysis.

10. At the 6-month interval from receipt of the explanted CI to the manufacturer, a device remaining under study for reliability should be reported as a Category C and included in CSR reporting until final analysis is completed. If the device is found to be "in specification" and no improved clinical performance is documented after internal device replacement (Category B2), than the device can be removed by the manufacturer from CSR reporting. The competent authority and the CI center should be notified in writing within 60 days of the change in category.

11. Devices determined to be "out of specification" by both clinical testing and reduced clinical benefit (resulting in device nonuse) and are not surgically removed at patient request are required to be reported as Category C and in CSR statistics.

12. Devices damaged due to trauma are categorized with all other explants. If the device is shown to be "out" of specification, they are categorized as C devices and will be listed in the CSR. If ipsilateral reimplatation produces improved clinical benefit, then the device would be listed as Category C and included in CSR reporting. If shown to be within specification, they are classified as Category D and not included in the CSR report.[35] Figure 17–1 was adapted from Battmer et al[35] and shows the device reliability categories in accordance with the ISO standard.

Device reliability metrics are available for all 3 implant manufacturers that produce CIs for usage in the United

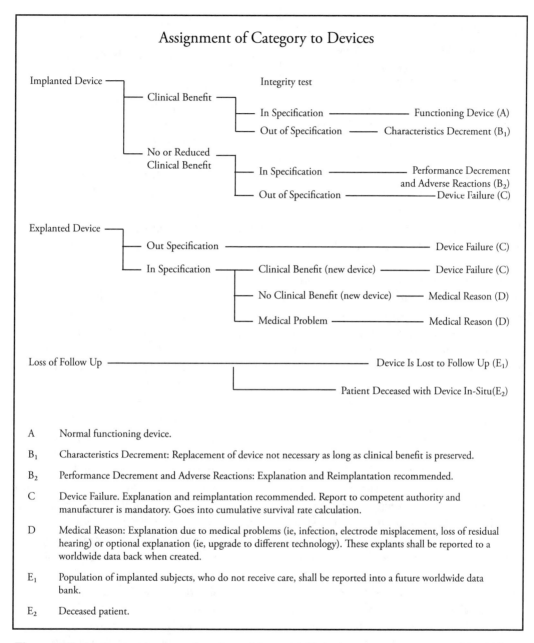

Assignment of Category to Devices

Implanted Device
— Clinical Benefit
Integrity test
— In Specification ———————— Functioning Device (A)
— Out of Specification ———— Characteristics Decrement (B_1)
— No or Reduced Clinical Benefit
— In Specification ———————— Performance Decrement and Adverse Reactions (B_2)
— Out of Specification ———————— Device Failure (C)

Explanted Device
— Out Specification ————————————————————— Device Failure (C)
— In Specification
— Clinical Benefit (new device) ———————— Device Failure (C)
— No Clinical Benefit (new device) ——— Medical Reason (D)
— Medical Problem ——————————— Medical Reason (D)

Loss of Follow Up ———————————————————————— Device Is Lost to Follow Up (E_1)
— Patient Deceased with Device In-Situ (E_2)

A   Normal functioning device.

B_1 Characteristics Decrement: Replacement of device not necessary as long as clinical benefit is preserved.

B_2 Performance Decrement and Adverse Reactions: Explanation and Reimplantation recommended.

C   Device Failure. Explanation and reimplantation recommended. Report to competent authority and manufacturer is mandatory. Goes into cumulative survival rate calculation.

D   Medical Reason: Explanation due to medical problems (ie, infection, electrode misplacement, loss of residual hearing) or optional explanation (ie, upgrade to different technology). These explants shall be reported to a worldwide data back when created.

E_1 Population of implanted subjects, who do not receive care, shall be reported into a future worldwide data bank.

E_2 Deceased patient.

Figure 17–1. *Categorization of explanted internal CI device components as adapted from Battmer et al.[35] Battmer et al adapted the figure from Figure A1 (p. 6) of ISO 5841-2:2000(E). This figure is not considered an official ISO figure nor was it authorized by ISO. Copies of the ISO 5841-2:2000(E) can be purchased from ANSI (http://webstore.ansi.org).*

States and worldwide (see individual Web sites). In general, implant reliability is very good. For all the manufacturers, the 5-year device reliability is well above 95% for the most recent device models produced.

REASONS FOR REVISION COCHLEAR IMPLANT SURGERY

Failure of a CI can occur at three possible levels. First, the CI itself may fail to work. Complete device failure is easy to diagnose, as a patient with a device failure receives no auditory input from the device, and auditory evaluation confirmed that no connection could be made with the device by external means. This has also been referred to as a *hard failure*. In some cases, complete device failure may be preceded by fluctuating or gradually increasing impedance or a progressive loss of electrodes. Second, patient factors may also result in physical or medical contraindications to continued device use. Examples of such a situation might include intractable seizures, sensory integration disorder, autism, or multiple handicaps among others. Medical and surgical factors such as device extrusion through the skin or tympanic membrane or magnet displacement might also fall into this group. Third, despite the presence of auditory percepts, the device may produce aversive symptoms such as pain, shocking, atypical tinnitus or a decrement in function. This suspected device malfunction (also called a *soft failure*) is defined as a clinical failure of the CI.[35]

The decision to reimplant a patient with a CI involves a careful evaluation of the mechanism of failure. For complete device failure, this often involves an evaluation by representatives from the manufacturer of the device to confirm the failure of the device. Once this failure mechanism is confirmed, reimplantation should proceed without delay. Magnet displacements should be addressed in a timely manner, as skin necrosis may develop over the magnet due to the irregular contour that is created by the displaced magnet.

Infections involving a CI deserve special attention. If the internal receiver site becomes infected, biofilm formation may make clearance of this infection difficult. As with most implanted material that is involved with an infection, removal of the device may be required to clear the infection. Reimplantation should not be performed in the setting of active infection, but should be delayed until the infection has completely resolved. If the electrode within the mastoid and middle ear are not involved in the infection, attempts should be made to leave the electrode inside the cochlea in order facilitate later reimplantation. Once an electrode is removed from the cochlea, fibrosis and ossification may hinder the insertion of a new electrode.

Patients with symptoms of a soft failure or suspected device malfunction require a high index of suspicion and thorough evaluation over time. Patients with adverse symptoms such as pain with device use should be considered for immediate reimplantation. Gradual performance decline coupled with changes in impedances or loss of functioning electrodes should be considered suspicious for a soft failure. Reimplantation should be considered if performance with such a device declines consistently below a level previously attained and maintained for a significant period of time. Patients should be carefully counseled regarding the expected benefits of reimplantation in this setting. Although the previous level of performance can usually be attained, this outcome is not universal and may take months to accomplish.[36] As with all explantations, device analysis and performance measurements after reimplantation will be crucial in the final determination of the mode of failure in these cases.

CONSIDERATIONS PRIOR TO EXPLANTATION

Prior to explantation, the patient with a suspected or a confirmed device failure should undergo a thorough evaluation to identify medical surgical reasons for the decline in performance or the aversive symptoms that may exist. This evaluation should include a thorough history and physical examination with careful attention to the details surrounding the onset of the change in their previous condition. Consideration should be given to CT imaging of the temporal bones to assess electrode array location as well as to identify any pathologic changes that might explain such dysfunction. As an example, stimulation of an electrode array that is located outside the cochlear lumen can result in pain, shocking, and a decrement in function that might otherwise be attributed to device malfunction. Moreover, changes in cochlear structure have been identified years following implantation that may result in a gradual decrement in performance.[37] The degree of ossification around the array can also be assessed by CT imaging.

Evaluation of the patient with a suspected device malfunction should include a thorough assessment of the device electronics. First and foremost, the external equipment should be changed out to insure that a speech processor, head piece, or cable connector does not explain the problem. Internal device integrity can be assessed to some extent using the manufacturer's equipment. For instance, electrode impedances and 8th nerve compound action potentials can measured with most of the modern systems. More extensive measurements such as field voltages and spread of excitation are possible using research platforms. The manufacturer should also be given the opportunity to evaluate the patient to see if other factors might be identified while the device remains in situ. Unfortunately, the tools that exist today for evaluating the internal circuitry remain somewhat limited. In many instances, device anomalies can only be identified following removal and careful diagnostic testing by the manufacturer. Thus, device failure or suspected device malfunction remains a clinical diagnosis.

Ultimately, the decision to reimplant the patient with a new device requires careful consideration of the patient's symptoms and performance with the CI. When the device is functionless, the decision is rarely challenging. By contrast, when the patient is experiencing aversive symptoms such as pain, shocking, and atypical tinnitus, attributing these symptoms to a potentially malfunctioning CI, especially in the presence of preserved performance should be done with caution. When a performance decrement is present or diagnostic testing reveals a device abnormality, these can support the decision to reimplant.[36]

SURGICAL CONSIDERATIONS IN REVISION SURGERY

Revision surgery accounts for ~5 to 10% of adult and pediatric CI surgeries in many centers. The reasons for revision fall into the categories listed above. Performance has been shown to be good following revision surgery, including those that require replacement of the CI.[36,37,39] Attaining these results might take some time however, making the decision to consider reimplantation in patients with functioning device complex.

Special precautions must be taken during revision CI surgery. The primary goal in revision surgery for device failure is to safely remove the implanted device and replace it with a functional implant. A secondary goal should be to remove the device as intact as possible for evaluation by the device manufacturer in order to assess the cause of failure. Monopolar cautery should not be used during the procedure as this may further damage the device as well as conduct high electrical current into the cochlea.

If there are no wound complications, the same incision that was used for primary implantation may be utilized. For patients implanted utilizing a large-flap type incision, a smaller, postauricular incision may be used. When contemplating a different incision line, the old incision should be taken into account to maintain an adequate blood supply to the intervening skin.

A previously infected operative site may leave behind thin, macerated skin. If possible, this skin should be avoided in planning the incision as well as the placement of the new implant. Placing any portion of the implant beneath this thin skin risks further wound complications.

The implant will be covered with a fibrous sheath, which must be incised to remove the device. It is not essential, nor desirable, to completely remove this sheath from around the receiver-stimulator. If the same model device is being reimplanted, this sheath can help stabilize the device. Every effort should

be made to preserve the integrity of the device for device analysis. However, the main goal is to safely remove and reimplant a new device for the patient. Cutting the electrode array may be required to accomplish this goal. Dehiscence of bone may exist around the dura mater, sigmoid sinus and the facial nerve. Dense fibrous adhesions may also be present between the device and these structures. Dissection along the medial surface of the device must take these potential complications into account. For this reason, facial nerve monitoring is recommended for all revision CI procedures.

Although every effort should be made to remove the internal receiver and the proximal electrode intact, the intracochlear portion of the electrode should not be removed with the rest of the device. There is often a thick fibrous sheath that surrounds the electrode and extends from the facial recess to the cochleostomy. If the electrode is removed prematurely, this fibrous pathway may be lost, making re-insertion very difficult or impossible. For this reason, we recommend severing the electrode array at the facial recess. The fibrous sheath surrounding the electrode should be dissected away or longitudinally split from the electrode to the level of the cochleostomy. Only after the new device is seated and the electrode is ready to be inserted should the original electrode be removed. In this way, the new electrode may be passed immediately into the original cochleostomy. Sealing of the cochleostomy and wound closure is then performed in the same manner as the initial procedure.

Removal of the original electrode should be performed slowly, as rapid removal may result in excessive negative hydraulic forces being delivered to the cochlea. The ability to atraumatically remove and replace CI electrodes has also been established in patients with hearing preservation.[40] Occasionally, it may not be possible to remove the electrode due to fibrosis or ossification within the cochlea.[41] In this situation, contralateral implantation should be considered.

If a different device is being implanted, the shape and contour of the package and/or electrode array may be quite different and requires consideration. The pocket in which the implant lies will need to be modified to accommodate these differences. Also, a new seat may need to be drilled in the calvarium to appropriately seat the device.

Multiple electrode arrays with unique contours are available across manufacturers. It is very helpful to know which array is in place prior to surgery so that an array with a similar contour can be chosen for reimplantation. CI manufacturers have also made available electrode "depth gauges" or test electrodes. These devices are exact replicas of the electrode array to be implanted, without functioning electrode components. These depth gauges are very useful in determining the appropriate electrode selection without having to insert a functioning device.

PERFORMANCE AFTER REIMPLANTATION

In general, most patients may expect to maintain or improve upon their best preoperative level of performance.[36–38] Exceptions to this generality do occur. Presumably, differences in electrode position or the use of a different device and/or programming strategy may delay the return to the preoperative level of function. This outcome should prompt professionals to use caution when counseling patients regarding expectations following device replacement. Specifically, patients should be counseled that performance after revision surgery is likely to be equal to or better than the best prerevision performance; however, attaining this level of performance may take several months to over a year. In addition, not all patients will attain this goal by one year postrevision.

SUMMARY

Cochlear implants have become the most common form of (re)habilitation for severe-profound sensorineural hearing loss. Great strides have been made over the last 4 decades in improving the biocompatibility and reliability of these devices. However, given the finite lifespan of implantable devices, revision cochlear implant surgery will be necessary in many patients. Special considerations should be made in the selection and counseling of patients who are candidates for reimplantation. Revision surgery can be safely performed and auditory performance can be maintained or re-attained in the majority of patients. Uniform reporting of device failures and explantation data will be essential for continued improvement in device reliability over time.

REFERENCES

1. Niparko JK, Tobey EA, Thal DJ, et al. CDaCI Investigative Team. Spoken language development in children following cochlear implantation. *JAMA*. 2010; 303(15):1498–1506.
2. Moog JS, Geers AE. Early educational placement and later language outcomes

for children with cochlear implants. *Otol Neurotol.* 2010;31(8):1315–1319.

3. Geers AE, Moog JS, Biedenstein J, Brenner C, Hayes H. Spoken language scores of children using cochlear implants compared to hearing age-mates at school entry. *J Deaf Stud Deaf Educ.* 2009;14(3):371–385.

4. Summerfield AQ, Marshall DH, Barton GR, Bloor KE. A cost-utility scenario analysis of bilateral cochlear implantation. *Arch Otolaryngol Head Neck Surg.* 2002; 128(11):1255–1262.

5. Francis HW, Chee N, Yeagle J, Cheng A, Niparko JK. Impact of cochlear implants on the functional health status of older adults. *Laryngoscope.* 2002;112(8 pt 1):1482–1488.

6. Wyatt JR, Niparko JK, Rothman M, deLissovoy G. Cost utility of the multichannel cochlear implants in 258 profoundly deaf individuals. *Laryngoscope.* 1996;106(7): 816–821.

7. Clark G. Engineering and bioengineering. In: Clark G, ed. *Cochlear Implants Fundamentals and Applications.* New York, NY: Springer-Verlag; 2003, 456–536.

8. Volta A. On the electricity excited by mere contact of conducting substances of different kinds. *Trans Roy Soc Phil.* 1800;90: 403–431.

9. Simmons FB. Electrical stimulation of the auditory nerve in man. *Arch Otolaryngol.* 1966;84:2–54.

10. Djourno A, Eyries C. Prothese auditive par excitation electrique a distance du nerf sensorial a l'aide d'un bobinage inclus a demeure. *Presse Medicale.* 1957;65:1417.

11. Blume SS. Histories of cochlear implantation. *Soc Sci Med.* 1999;49:1257–1268.

12. Spenser PE. History of cochlear implants. In: Christiansen JB, Leigh IW, eds. *Cochlear Implants in Children: Ethics and Choices.* Washington DC: Gallaudet University Press, 2002;14–45.

13. House WF, Berliner KI, Crary W, et al. Cochlear implants. *Ann Otol Rhinol Laryngol.* 1976;85(suppl 27):1–93.

14. Simmons FB, Epley JE, Lummis RC, et al. Auditory nerve: electrical stimulation in man. *Science.* 1965;148:104–106.

15. Eddington DK, Dobelle WH, Brackmann DE. Auditory prosthesis research with multiple channel intraochlear stimulation in man. *Ann Otol.* 1978;87:1–39.

16. Atlas LE, Herndon MK, Simmons FB, Dent LJ, White RL. Results of stimulus and speech-coding schemes applied to multichannel electrodes. *Ann NY Acad Sci.* 1983;405:377–386.

17. Pialoux P, Chouard CH, Meyer B. Indications and results of the multichannel cochlear implant. *Acta Otolayrngol.* 1979; 87:185–189.

18. House WF, Berliner KI, Eisenberg LS. Present status and future directions of the ear research institute cochlear implant program. *Acta Otolaryngol.* 1979;87:176–184.

19. House W. Cochlear implants: past, present and future. *Adv Otorhinolaryngol.* 1993; 48:1–3.

20. House WF, Urban J. Long-term results of electrode implantation and electrical stimulation of the cochlear in man. *Ann Otol Rhinol Laryngol.* 1973;82:504–510.

21. Michelson RP. Electrical stimulation of the human cochlea-preliminary report. *Arch Otolaryngol.* 1971;93:317–323.

22. Dobelle WH, Fordemwald JN, Hanson JW, et al. Data processing LSI will help bring sight to the blind. *Electronics.* 1974;47:81–86.

23. Forster IC. Theoretical design and implementation of a transcutaneous, multichannel stimulator for neural prosthesis application. *J Biomed Engineer.* 1981;3: 107–120.

24. Clark GM, Black RC, Forster IC, Patrick JF, Tong YC. Design criteria of a multiple-electrode cochlear implant hearing prosthesis. *J Acoust Soc Am.* 1978;63:631–633.

25. McCabe BF, Tyler RS, Gantz BJ, Lowder MW, Otto SR, Preece JP. Preliminary assessment of the Los Angeles, Vienna and Melbourne cochlear implants. *Acta Otolaryngol Suppl.* 1984;411:247–253.

26. Tyler RS, Lowder MW, Otto SR, Preece JP, Gantz BJ, McCabe BF. Initial Iowa results with the multichannel cochlear implant from Melbourne. *J Speech Hear Res.* 1984; 27(4):596–604.

27. Gantz BJ, Tyler RS. Cochlear implant comparisons. *Am J Otol.* 1985 Nov;suppl:92–98.

28. Gantz BJ, Tyler RS, McCabe BF, Preece J, Lowder MW, Otto SR. Iowa cochlear implant clinical project: results with two single-channel cochlear implants and one multi-channel cochlear implant. *Laryngoscope.* 1985;95(4):443–449.

29. Gantz BJ, Tyler RS, Knutson JF, et al. Evaluation of five different cochlear implant designs: audiologic assessment and predictors of performance. *Laryngoscope.* 1988;98(10):1100–1106.

30. Clark GM, Tong YC, Martin LF. A multiple-channel cochlear implant. An evaluation using open-set CID sentences. *Laryngoscope.* 1981;91:628–643.

31. Cohen NL, Waltzman SB, Fisher SG. A prospective, randomized study of cochlear implants. The Department of Veterans Affairs Cochlear Implant Study Group. *N Engl J Med.* 1993;328(4):233–237.

32. von Békésy G. In: *Experiments in Hearing.* New York, NY: McGraw-Hill; 1960:745.

33. Schuknecht HF. Techniques for study of cochlear function and pathology in experimental animals; development of the anatomical frequency scale for the cat. *Arch Otolaryngol.* 1953;58(4):377–397.

34. Grenwood DD. Critical bandwidth and the frequency coordinates of the basilar membrane. *J Acoust Soc Am.* 1961;33:1344–1356.

35. Battmer RD, Backous DD, Balkany TJ, et al. International Consensus Group for Cochlear Implant Reliability Reporting. International classification of reliability for implanted cochlear implant receiver stimulators. *Otol Neurotol.* 2010;31(8):1190–1193.

36. Buchman CA, Higgins CA, Cullen R, Pillsbury HC. Revision cochlear implant surgery in adult patients with suspected device malfunction. *Otol Neurotol.* 2004;25(4):504–510; discussion 510.

37. Cullen RD, Fayad JN, Luxford WM, Buchman CA. Revision cochlear implant surgery in children. *Otol Neurotol.* 2008;29(2):214–220.

38. Nadol JB Jr, Eddington DK, Burgess BJ. Foreign body or hypersensitivity granuloma of the inner ear after cochlear implantation: one possible cause of a soft failure? *Otol Neurotol.* 2008;29(8):1076–1084.

39. Zeitler DM, Budenz CL, Roland JT Jr. Revision cochlear implantation. *Curr Opin Otolaryngol Head Neck Surg.* 2009;17(5):334–338.

40. Kamat A, Goldin L, Hoffman RA. Unusual electroacoustic device failure and electroacoustic reimplantation with hearing preservation. *Otol Neurotol.* 2011 Apr 28. [Epub ahead of print] PubMed PMID: 21527866.

41. Kang SY, Zwolan TA, Kileny PR, et al. Incomplete electrode extraction during cochlear implant revision. *Otol Neurotol.* 2009;30(2):160–164.

Chapter 18

Auditory Brainstem Implants

HARRISON W. LIN, BARBARA S. HERRMANN, AND DANIEL J. LEE

INTRODUCTION

Otologic surgeons and auditory researchers have successfully developed several implantable prostheses for the habilitation/rehabilitation of pediatric and adult patients with severe to profound hearing loss. These devices bypass nonfunctioning hair cells of the severe to profoundly deafened cochlea or damaged auditory nerve (eg, following bilateral vestibular schwannoma surgery or temporal bone fracture) to stimulate either the peripheral (first-order neurons) or central auditory pathways (second-order neurons), respectively (Fig 18–1). The cochlear implant (CI) represents the most successful attempt to restore function to a special sensory system, with over 200,000 devices placed in children and adults with peripheral deafness worldwide. The CI is inserted into the scala tympani of the cochlea to electrically stimulate neighboring first order auditory neurons (spiral ganglion cells) and provide hearing. CI technology has

matured since its development in the early 1960s, and outcome studies have demonstrated steady improvement of open set word recognition scores over the years, with the largest changes seen with the advent of multichannel systems and refinements in speech processor technology. Today, the majority of pediatric and adult CI users achieve meaningful sound and speech perception abilities.

However, there are a number of deaf individuals who are not candidates for a CI. This more challenging cohort includes patients with neurofibromatosis type 2 (NF2), a devastating autosomal dominant genetic syndrome characterized by bilateral schwannomas of the vestibular nerve as well as other central nervous system (CNS) tumors. Growth and/or treatment of these vestibular schwannomas (VS) will routinely cause bilateral retrocochlear deafness in these NF2 patients.

Cochlear implants, except in rare cases,[1-3] do not work in NF2 patients who are deaf as the auditory nerve is not viable. The auditory brainstem implant

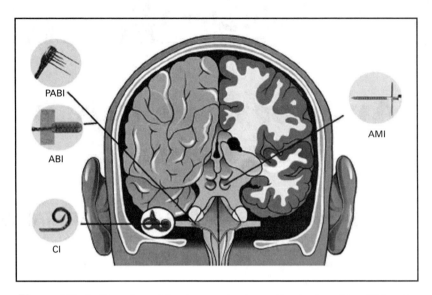

Figure 18–1. *Drawing of the human brain and brainstem identifying the various points along the auditory pathways that are sites for implantable technology. The cochlear implant (CI) is inserted into the cochlea and stimulates the first-order auditory neurons (spiral ganglion cells) that give rise to the auditory nerve. The auditory brainstem implant (ABI) and penetrating auditory brainstem implant (PABI) are placed on or into the cochlear nucleus to access the second-order auditory neurons. The auditory midbrain implant (AMI), currently in clinical trials, is placed into the inferior colliculus to stimulate the auditory pathway at the level of the midbrain prior to its entry into the thalamus and auditory cortex. (Reprinted from Lenarz et al[51] with permission from Lippincott, Williams and Wilkins.)*

(ABI) was developed in the 1970s for NF2 patients who undergo removal of their bilateral VS. Because surgical excision routinely disrupts the auditory nerve, the ABI was designed to stimulate the second order auditory neurons of the cochlear nucleus (CN) with electrical current. Deafness in NF2 patients and others with cochlear or cochlear nerve pathology (eg, ossification of the cochlea, cochlear nerve avulsion due to skull base fracture, or congenital cochlear aplasia) can only be addressed with stimulation of the afferent auditory pathways distal to the cochlear nerve. Approximately 1,000 ABIs have been placed worldwide, and

although the majority of NF2 ABI users derive considerable benefit, performance outcomes have substantially trailed those of CI patients. Most NF2 ABI users will only derive environmental sound awareness and improved lip-reading comprehension but recent data suggests that nontumor ABI users may have better speech outcomes.

Additionally, comparatively poor hearing results from NF2 ABI users relative to nontumor ABI patients have led to speculation that treatment of NF2 tumors may lead to direct damage or devascularization of the cochlear nuclei. As a result, several centers in Europe have directed efforts at targeting the inferior colliculus (IC) with an auditory midbrain implant (AMI).

In this chapter we: (1) discuss the history and development of the ABI, (2) review ABI candidacy and preoperative evaluation, (3) present the two major surgical approaches for ABI placement, (4) outline the intraoperative monitoring techniques used during ABI surgery and provide an overview of ABI activation and maintenance, (5) summarize the results from recent studies on ABI outcomes, and (6) discuss current and future efforts to improve ABI performance.

HISTORICAL BACKGROUND

In 1979, William E. Hitselberger and William F. House of the House Ear Clinic performed the first implantation of a single channel ABI in an NF2 patient following removal of her second VS via a translabyrinthine craniotomy. The ABI was a single ball-type electrode placed on the surface of the cochlear nucleus and provided the patient with useful auditory sensations. In collaboration with researchers at the Huntington Medical Research Institute in Pasadena, California, two- and three-electrode mesh-type array implants were developed and subsequently used in combination with modified cochlear implant processors. Further work in Los Angeles at the House Ear Institute and with scientists at the Cochlear Corporation (Englewood, CO, USA) led to an 8-electrode array implant and then the 21-electrode Nucleus® ABI24 system, which was approved in 2000 by the Food and Drug Administration (FDA). This device is the only ABI in clinical use in the United States.

ABI TECHNOLOGY

COCHLEAR CORPORATION

The Nucleus® multichannel ABI24 system consists of a surgically implanted receiver-stimulator and an externally worn speech processor and headpiece (Fig 18–2). The receiver-stimulator includes an electrode array composed of 21 platinum disk electrodes (diameter = 0.7 mm) aligned on a flexible silicone paddle with a Dacron mesh backing to provide stabilization (see Fig 18–2). The cochlear nucleus is not directly visualized during implantation, and therefore electrophysiologic measurements are needed to aid in placement. Specifically, electrically evoked auditory brainstem responses (EABR) are used to determine the optimal position and orientation of the electrode array within the lateral recess of the fourth ventricle (and to assure close proximity of the electrode to the cochlear nucleus).[4] The Nucleus® system uses the ABI electrode for intraoperative EABR recordings via electrode stimulation using the transcutaneous transmitter coil.

The external components of the ABI consist of a behind-the-ear speech processor with a microphone and a transcutaneous transmitter coil headpiece. The processor uses the Nucleus Spectral Peak (SPEAK) speech coding strategy developed for the Nucleus CI. Although the ABI24 can also accommodate newer, higher rate speech processing strategies, including Continuous Interleaved Sampling (CIS) and Advanced Combination Encoder (ACE), their use has not yet been approved by the FDA.

Because NF2 patients require continuous surveillance of CNS tumors with serial magnetic resonance imaging (MRI),

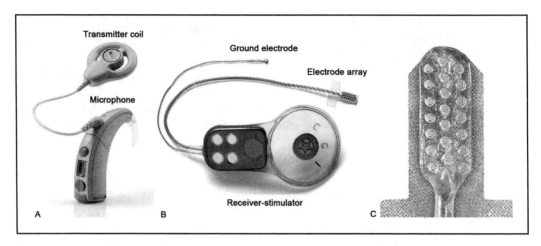

Figure 18–2. *The Nucleus® ABI24 system includes (**A**) the externally worn device, including a behind-the-ear microphone, speech processor, and transmitter coil, and (**B**) the internal portion (receiver-stimulator, electrode array, and ground electrode). The array consists of 21 active platinum electrodes on a Dacron mesh backing (**C**). (Images courtesy of the Cochlear Corporation, Englewood, CO, USA.)*

the receiver-stimulator magnet is replaced by a nonmagnetic metallic spacer prior to implantation (the ABI is packaged with the magnet in a Silastic pocket in the center of the FM coil). Postactivation, the external transmitter coil is attached to the scalp using a removable adhesive magnetic disk. The site of the internal receiver (centered over the nonmagnetic plug) is tattooed on the scalp during surgery to facilitate localization of the receiver-stimulator at device activation (approximately 8 weeks postoperatively). A small area of hair is usually kept shaved to help retention of the adhesive magnetic disk and headpiece coil.

MED-EL

Although not currently approved by the FDA for use in the United States, the MED-EL PulsarCI100® ABI system (Innsbruck, Austria) has been used extensively in Europe. Similar to the Nucleus® device, the MED-EL ABI consists of an internal receiver-stimulator with an active electrode array composed of 12 platinum electrodes (diameter = 0.55 mm) on a Dacron-mesh backing, a ground electrode, and an external microphone, speech processor, and transcutaneous transmitter coil (Fig 18–3). Unlike the Cochlear system, the MED-EL system uses a pared down "placing electrode" to identify the optimal location to generate EABR responses (Fig 18–4) prior to placement of the 12 electrode system. Consisting of only 4 contacts, this placing electrode directly connects with a current stimulator distant to the surgical field which likely reduces the amount of electrical signal artifact often problematic in EABR measurements.[5] The MED-EL ABI user has the option of a behind-the-ear TEMPO+ or Opus-2, or body-worn CIS PRO+ speech processors. The CIS processing strategy is used with this device.

ADVANCED BIONICS

Based on the Clarion 1.2 cochlear implant, the Clarion® ABI (Advanced Bionics Cor-

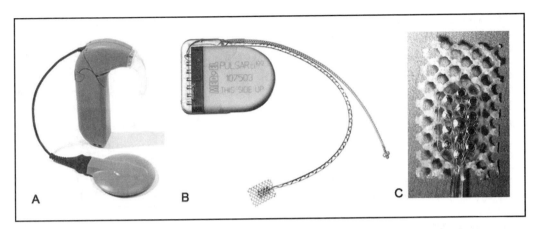

Figure 18–3. *The MED-EL PulsarCI100 ABI System consists of a behind-the-ear microphone, speech processor and transmitter coil (**A**), and a receiver-stimulator, electrode array, and ground electrode (**B**). (**C**) The electrode array consists of 8 active contacts and one central reference contact. The MED-EL ABI system is not currently approved for use in the United States. (Images courtesy of the MED-EL Corporation, Innsbruck, Austria.)*

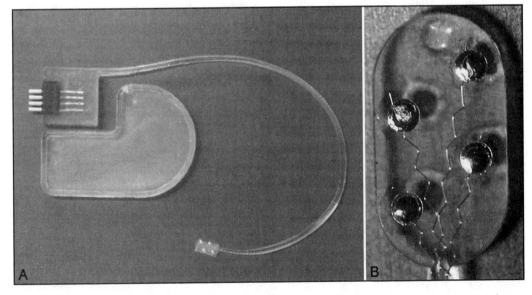

Figure 18–4. *The MED-EL placing electrode (used to find the cochlear nucleus prior to placement of the ABI system shown in Figure 18–3 consists of an 11.28-cm lead with a micro-D-plug interface (**A**) and a four-contact electrode array (**B**). (Images courtesy of the MED-EL Corporation, Innsbruck, Austria.)*

poration, Sylmar, CA, USA) consisted of a Silastic electrode array with 16 platinum-iridium electrode contacts (diameter 1.0 mm) on a Dacron mesh. The device was designed without a magnet and employed a special headset to hold the headpiece in place. The Clarion® ABI allowed its users a choice between different stimulation modes (monopolar and bipolar) and two different speech-processing strategies, including CIS (monopolar) and simultaneous analog stimulation (bipolar). This device was only used in Europe and Advanced Bionics eventually ceased production of the Clarion® ABI.

ABI CANDIDACY

NF2 PATIENTS

Only NF2 patients 12 years or older with reasonable expectations have been FDA-approved to undergo ABI implantation in the United States (Table 18–1). Notably, there are no audiologic criteria. ABI surgery was originally performed following removal of the second VS in patients who would have otherwise been rendered deaf. However, the finding that roughly 8% of patients will fail to derive useful auditory sensation from the ABI has encouraged many centers to perform first-side implantation in the setting of residual contralateral hearing to allow for the opportunity to implant the second side if necessary.[6] Early surgical intervention has been advocated in some centers

Table 18–1. United States Food and Drug Administration (FDA) Criteria for Auditory Brainstem Implantation

1. 12 years of age or older
2. Diagnosis of neurofibromatosis type 2
3. Highly motivated to participate in the rehabilitation process
4. Appropriate expectations

Note that there are no audiologic criteria.

for the first ear to minimize morbidity, ease ABI placement, and provide patients with the opportunity to acclimate to the device while having useful contralateral residual hearing. However, in light of new chemotherapeutic options to prolong or improve hearing and slow down tumor growth, a number of surgeons now favor maximizing the length of useful acoustic hearing time prior to considering VS and ABI surgery. Additionally, NF2 patients whose tumors were initially managed with radiation therapy (formerly a contraindication for ABI placement) have been shown to obtain comparable auditory benefits following surgery.[7]

At the Massachusetts Eye and Ear Infirmary, NF2 patients who are candidates for the ABI are initially evaluated at the multidisciplinary Neurofibromatosis Clinic at the Massachusetts General Hospital. Given the predisposition of NF2 patients for multiple CNS tumors, all newly diagnosed patients undergo a brain and spinal MRI with gadolinium contrast and are seen in the departments of Otolaryngology, Neurology, Neurological surgery, Ophthalmology, and Audiology. NF2 patients with growing tumors and progressive hearing loss at our center are also considered for enrollment into a new clinical trial investigating the use of bevacizumab (Avastin®), a monoclonal antibody directed against vascular endothelial growth factor (VEGF), to reduce VS volume and improve or stabilize residual hearing (http://clinicaltrials.gov/ct2/show/NCT01207687). Preliminary results suggest that bevacizumab may indeed have a significant impact in reducing tumor volume and improving hearing in some NF2 patients.[8] Patients who fail to respond to VEGF inhibitor therapy and elect to undergo either tumor removal and/or ABI placement are not offered surgery at our institution until approximately three months after the end of the treatment trial due to the increased risk of bleeding.

NONTUMOR ABI CANDIDATES

Since 1997, surgeons in Europe have expanded the indications for ABI placement beyond NF2 patients to include profoundly deaf adult and pediatric patients who would not benefit from a cochlear implant due to congenital or acquired cochlear or cochlear nerve pathology. Nontumor ABI users include those with cochlear nerve aplasia, cochlear nerve damage after head trauma, cochlear ossification, auditory neuropathy, or patients with poor CI outcomes.[9–12] Notably, multiple clinical studies have shown better performance in nontumor patients compared with NF2 ABI users.[11,13,14] In 2009, a multinational group of European ABI centers convened in Ankara, Turkey to formulate a consensus statement on the indications for ABI placement in children and non-NF2 patients. The authors concluded that: (1) patients prelingually deafened from inner ear malformations and cochlear nerve hypoplasia/aplasia and (2) patients postlingually deafened from meningitis and labyrinthitis ossificans, temporal bone fractures with cochlear nerve avulsion, otosclerosis with gross cochlear ossification, or intractable facial nerve stimulation with a CI are potential candidates for ABI surgery via the retrosigmoid approach. Moreover, pediatric candidates should be implanted between the ages of 18 months to 3 years to optimize surgical safety as well as to take advantage of the neural plasticity of the central auditory pathways.[15] Children less than 1 year of age will have relatively less blood and cerebrospinal fluid volume and have a smaller window to the lateral recess of the fourth ventricle, increasing the risks of a retrosigmoid craniotomy and ABI placement.

PREOPERATIVE EVALUATION

The preoperative evaluation for ABI candidates at the Massachusetts Eye and Ear Infirmary is similar to that used for cochlear implant candidates. At our center, it consists of a complete head and neck, otologic and neurotologic examination, updated radiology, an audiologic and speech assessment, and a psychosocial evaluation. All patients undergo routine pure tone and speech perception testing and assessment of current use of amplification and/or assistive devices. Patients with residual hearing also undergo acoustic ABR testing in the clinic; if ABRs are present then cochlear nerve function can be monitored under general anesthesia during tumor resection. At our center, if we can preserve acoustically evoked ABRs during VS surgery of the only hearing ear in NF2 patients then we will not place the ABI.

The patient and family are also counseled regarding the expectations of hearing with an ABI, the commitment needed for device use and programming postoperatively, the expected need for auditory rehabilitation services, and care and use of the device. Alternative means or supplements to spoken communication such as sign language and the use of technology (eg, computerized voice to text software) are also reviewed.

Naturally, each patient considering ABI surgery will bring a unique outlook and set of expectations often influenced by the preoperative hearing status. For example, an NF2 patient may be facing a loss of near normal acoustic hearing in exchange for sound detection and an aid to lip-reading provided with ABI use in the setting of rapidly growing or large VS in an only hearing ear. Other NF2 patients have already lost all residual hearing and, having experienced substantial periods of deafness, have learned to communicate and lip-read with minimal auditory cues. Nontumor ABI candidates are similar to cochlear implant candidates in that their decision to proceed with implantation is not precipitated by other medical factors that face NF2 patients with large or growing schwannomas. That is, unlike many NF2 patients, a nontumor candidate is electing to have ABI surgery solely to perceive sound. As will be discussed later, nontumor ABI users have a greater range of performance than NF2 ABI users and for postlingually deafened patients with no other rehabilitative options the benefits of craniotomy surgery for restoring hearing may outweigh the risks of meningitis, CSF leak, cranial neuropathies, and brainstem stroke.

SURGICAL APPROACHES

TRANSLABYRINTHINE CRANIOTOMY

The translabyrinthine craniotomy can provide access to and visualization of the lateral recess of the fourth ventricle and adjacent structures.[16] Requiring minimal cerebellar retraction, this approach provides a wide angle of view posterior to the cochlear nerve and the lateral recess, allows for complete tumor removal

from the fundus of the internal auditory canal, and early identification of the facial nerve.[17] Optimal visualization and access to the facial nerve permits grafting of the facial nerve should transection occur. Monitoring of both the facial and glossopharyngeal nerves is performed at many centers not only to minimize excessive nerve traction and injury during tumor dissection but also to identify inappropriate stimulation of these nerves following placement and stimulation of the electrode array. Recording electrodes are also placed on the scalp to monitor EABRs (as well as acoustically evoked responses in the setting of residual hearing and attempts to preserve the cochlear nerve). Following tumor resection, a bony seat is created into the external surface of the skull above and behind the auricle for placement of the receiver-stimulator and electrode leads. Attention is then turned toward indirect identification of the cochlear nucleus (CN) using the landmarks shown in Figure 18–5 and placement of the electrode array in the lateral recess of the 4th ventricle.

The CN is located on the dorsolateral brainstem at the pontomedullary junction (Fig 18–6) and has an estimated visible area of only 1.0 to 1.28 cm^2.[18–20] Containing roughly 100,000 cells,[21] the CN is consists of the dorsal cochlear nucleus (DCN) and the ventral (accessory) cochlear nucleus (VCN). The DCN, also referred to as the *tuberculum acousticum*, resides on the dorsolateral surface of the inferior cerebellar peduncle and is believed to have a role in the processing of complex auditory stimuli, enhancement of behaviorally important sounds in noisy environments, and in filtering sound localization cues.[22] The VCN is situated between the vestibular and cochlear divisions of the eighth cranial nerve on the ventral aspect of

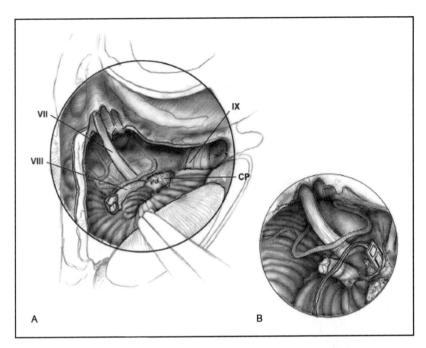

Figure 18–5. A. *Drawing of the operative field following translabyrinthine craniotomy and excision of a right-sided vestibular schwannoma. The facial nerve (VII), remnant of the cochlear nerve (VIII), choroid plexus (CP), and glossopharyngeal nerve (IX) are labeled.* **B.** *The electrode array is pictured in the superior aspect of the lateral recess of the fourth ventricle adjacent to the cochlear nerve remenant. (Reprinted from Schwartz et al[56] with permission from Springer.)*

the inferior peduncle and is further subdivided into the posteroventral cochlear nucleus (PVCN) and the anteroventral cochlear nucleus (AVCN) (see Fig 18–6). The tonotopic organization of the cochlea and cochlear nerve is preserved within the cochlear nucleus, as axons from the apical spiral ganglion cells (low frequency) project to the ventrolateral portions of the DCN and AVCN, whereas more basal (high frequency) neuronal processes synapse with the dorsal portion of the AVCN and the dorsal-medial portions of the DCN. That is, isofrequency lamina (sheets of neurons that have the same characteristic frequency) are distributed from dorsal to ventral across each major cochlear nucleus subdivision and are also seen in higher auditory nuclei. Thus, the spatial representation of frequency-specific information in the cochlea is preserved in the cochlear nucleus. In addition, the temporal and spectral features of sound originating in the ear are processed in the cochlear nucleus; and the cochlear nucleus is the origin of parallel pathways. These pathways that project to the auditory brainstem, midbrain and cortex integrate information from the ear to determine: (1) the identity of the sound source, (2) the intensity of the sound source, and (3) the location of the sound source.[23]

The VCN contains a number of neuronal cell types including both spherical and

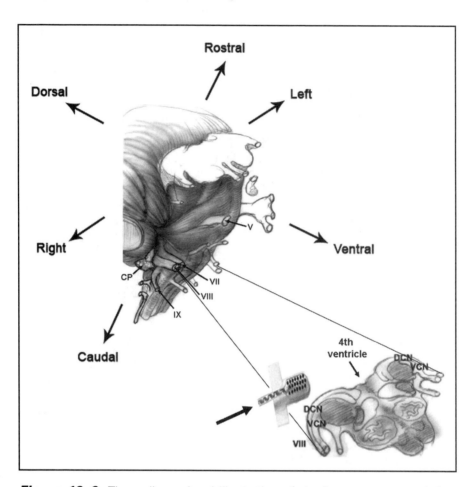

Figure 18–6. *Three-dimensional illustration of the human pontomedullary junction demonstrating the relationships among the anatomic landmarks using during ABI placement (upper left). The choroid plexus (CP) and glossopharyngeal nerve (IX) are used to identify the foramen of Luschka (lateral recess of the 4th ventricle). Magnified section through the brainstem at the level of cochlear nucleus (lower right) showing placement of the electrode paddle of the ABI in close proximity to the right dorsal cochlear nucleus (DCN) and ventral cochlear nucleus (VCN). As shown in this magnified section, neurons of the DCN are closer to the surface electrodes than the VCN. V-trigeminal nerve, VII-facial nerve, VIII-vestibulocochlear nerve. (Modified from Schwartz et al[56] with permission from Springer.)*

globular bushy cells. Bushy cells are second order auditory neurons that receive large terminals from the cochlear nerve and contain multiple synaptic specializations called endbulbs of Held. The exten-

sive contact allows bushy cells to have primary-like responses to action potentials from the cochlear nerve, preserving both temporal and spectral information that is sent to higher auditory brainstem nuclei, the thalamus, and, ultimately, the auditory cortex. Sound perception from ABI stimulation is believed to be result of electrical activation of the VCN, however, given the small size and anatomic relationships as shown in Figure 18–6 it is felt that the current surface electrodes are placed in closest proximity to the DCN and that current spread allows for activation of axons or cell bodies within the VCN. Ultimately, it is not clear which subdivision conveys the sound percept as a result of ABI stimulation.

The CN can be accessed at the foramen of Luschka, which constitutes the terminus of the lateral recess of the fourth ventricle. Extension of the choroid plexus from the fourth ventricle and through the foramen reveals the lateral recess, which can also be defined superiorly by the roots of the seventh and eighth cranial nerves and inferiorly by the root of the glossopharyngeal nerve (see Fig 18–5). Egress of cerebrospinal fluid with a Valsalva maneuver confirms the location of the foramen of Luschka and lateral recess.[24] The electrode is then essentially blindly placed within the lateral recess adjacent to the presumed location of the CN. Intraoperative electrophysiology is performed to confirm the presence of EABRs and to detect any undesired stimulation of adjacent cranial nerves or any consequent hemodynamic instability. Based on the results of the stimulation, the array can be repositioned to a more optimal location. Once established, a small piece of fat or Teflon felt is placed around the array to secure it in position. The receiver-stimulator, with the magnet removed, is then placed into the bony well drilled in the lateral skull and secured. The redundant coils of the electrode array lead are gently tucked within the mas-

toid cavity, whereas the ground electrode is placed deep to the temporalis muscle. The mastoid cavity is then packed with fat harvested from the abdominal wall, and the wound is closed using a watertight closure, followed by a pressure dressing (Fig 18–7). It is important to bear in mind that monopolar cautery cannot be used following ABI placement, similar to CIs.

RETROSIGMOID APPROACH

The retrosigmoid (suboccipital) craniotomy is also used for ABI implantation and is more commonly performed outside the United States in both NF2 and nontumor ABI cases. This surgical approach offers the patient and surgeon the possibility of acoustic hearing preservation and avoidance of ABI placement in the event that the tumor is successfully excised without loss of EABRs (when the patient has both residual hearing AND acoustically evoked ABRs prior to surgery). Advocates of the retrosigmoid craniotomy believe that this surgical approach allows for dissection of larger tumors under direct vision, more direct access to the foramen of Luschka and visualization of the lower cranial nerve roots, improved control of bleeding, and reduced operative times.[25,26] Compared to the translabyrinthine craniotomy, the retrosigmoid approach also avoids the need for harvest of abdominal fat (although some surgeons do use fat to obliterate the IAC) as well as potential contamination of the wound by tympanomastoid cavity flora. The approach begins with a retrosigmoid craniotomy, incision of the dura, cerebellar retraction, and partial tumor resection, followed by identification of the root entry zones of the seventh and eighth cranial nerves and lower cranial nerves. The posterior wall of the internal auditory canal is drilled out to identify the facial nerve, and the tumor is completely

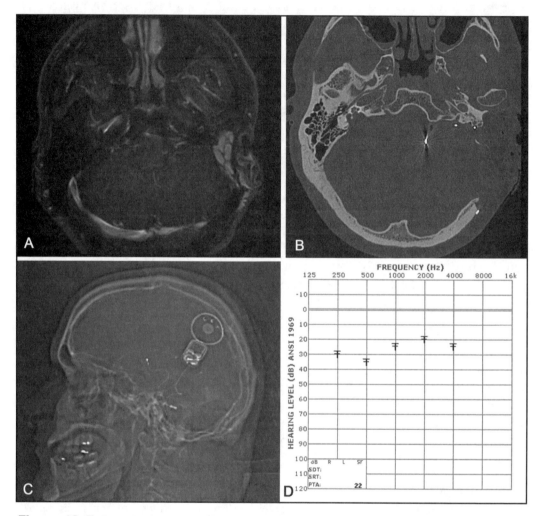

Figure 18–7. *Radiologic and audiologic images from the case of a 35-year-old NF2 patient who had previously undergone VS surgery via retrosigmoid craniotomies on the left side in 2000 and on the right side in 2002 at our institution, leaving him completely deaf bilaterally. In 2009, we placed a left-sided ABI through a translabyrinthine approach. In the postoperative T1-weighted axial MR image (**A**), abdominal fat can be seen obliterating the mastoid cavity and the void represents the electrode cable in the pontomedullary junction. In the axial CT image (**B**) the electrode array can be seen near the region of the lateral recess of the 4th ventricle and left cochlear nucleus. The location of the receiver-stimulator, electrode array and ground electrode can be seen in the postoperative skull film (**C**). Three months following activation, the patient scored Category 1 (sound detection) on the Early Speech Perception test and had sound field thresholds as shown (**D**).*

resected. Following completion of tumor removal in the cerebellopontine angle, a bony well to seat the receiver-stimulator is drilled in the skull of the temporoparietal region, cephalad to the craniotomy. The receiver-stimulator is placed under the pericranial flap, seated into the well and then fixed against the skull. The ground electrode is placed against the skull and under the muscle flap. Microdissection in the plane between the cochlear nerve root and the choroid plexus will then lead to the entrance of the lateral recess of the fourth ventricle. The electrode array is placed gently into the lateral recess, and EABRs are obtained to optimize the position of the array (Figs 18–8 to 18–11). Following electrode placement, soft tissue is placed to stabilize the array, and then a water tight dural closure around the electrode is performed followed by cranioplasty.

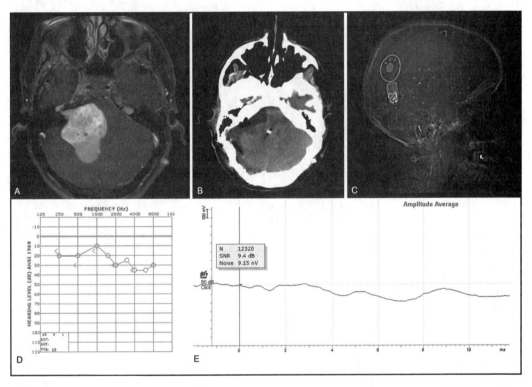

Figure 18–8. *Radiologic and audiologic images from the case of a 23-year-old NF2 patient who had previously undergone a left-sided VS removal via retrosigmoid craniotomy in 2000 at our institution. A preoperative T1-weighted axial MR image demonstrates a bulky VS on the right side (**A**). Postoperative CT (**B**) and skull film (**C**) images again show the location of the right-sided electrode array, receiver-stimulator, and ground electrode. The patient had a mild to moderate pure-tone average and a word recognition score (CNC) of 50% in her only hearing ear (**D**). However, a preoperative ABR was not robust (**E**), likely from the severity of the retrocochlear lesion. As a result, ABRs could not be followed intraoperatively and an attempt at preserving the cochlear nerve and acoustic hearing could not be done based on visual inspection of the eighth nerve alone given the large size of the tumor.*

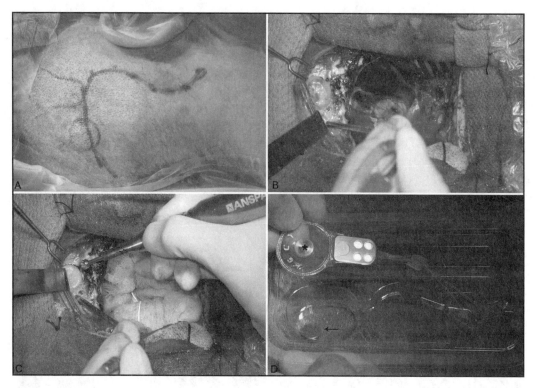

Figure 18–9. *Surgical images from the patient described in Figure 18–8.* **A.** *A curvilinear incision is drawn out in preparation for a right-sided retrosigmoid craniotomy. The ovoid outline superior to the incision defines the approximate location of the bony well for the receiver-stimulator. The circular outline represents a cutaneous schwannoma that was excised following skin incision. Following excision of the tumor* (**B**), *a bony well is drilled into the temporoparietal skull just above the craniotomy* (**C**). *A wet gauze is placed into the defect to minimize entry of bone dust into the cranial defect.* **D.** *The magnet of the ABI* (arrow) *is removed and replaced with a nonmagnetic metal spacer* (asterisk).

INTRAOPERATIVE ELECTRICALLY EVOKED AUDITORY BRAINSTEM RESPONSES

Given the complexity of the brainstem anatomy, distortion of landmarks from tumor growth and removal, and the blind approach to the CN, intraoperative EABRs are essential in confirming optimal placement of the ABI electrode array to maximize the likelihood of useful postoperative auditory sensations while minimizing nonauditory stimulation. Surface recording electrodes are placed at the vertex (positive electrode), over the seventh cervical vertebrae on the neck (reference electrode), and a ground electrode at the base of the neck to minimize contamination from electrical signal artifact.[27] Electrical auditory brainstem responses are obtained by signal-averaging the ongoing EEG with an evoked potential system

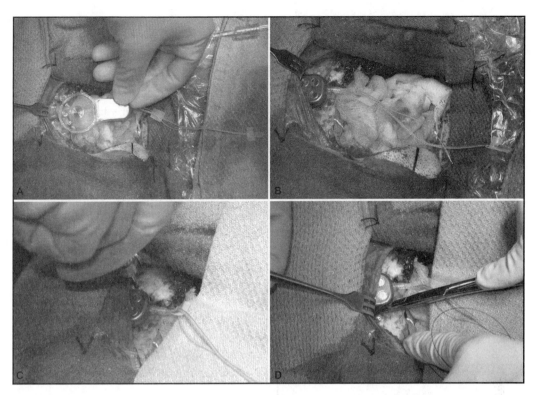

Figure 18–10. *Surgical images from the patient described in Figure 18–8. The receiver-stimulator is brought into the field and inserted into the subperiosteal pocket and bony well (**A**, **B**). It is secured to the skull with two 1.5 × 4.0-mm self-tapping and self-drilling titanium screws on opposite ends of the well (**C**) around which a 3-0 nylon suture is tied (**D**), as described in Lee and Driver.[57]*

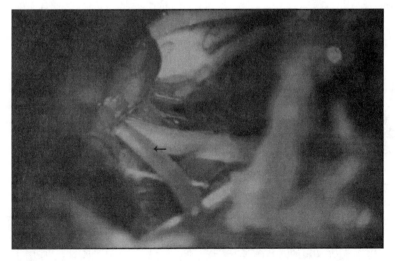

Figure 18–11. *An electrode lead is seen in place (arrow) following a retrosigmoid approach to the brainstem in this microsurgical image provided by the MED-EL Corporation, Innsbruck, Austria.*

triggered by the single electric biphasic pulses delivered to either a pair of electrodes (bipolar) or a single electrode (monopolar). Following the placement of the ABI electrode array near the CN (Fig 18–12), responses or absence of responses to electrode pairs from different regions of the electrode pad provide information regarding the location of the array. With this information the electrode can be moved to optimize responses from all areas of the pad. Adjustments to the array position should be performed delicately to minimize iatrogenic trauma to the CN. The anesthesiologist should be alerted prior to electrode stimulation in the event of inadvertent activation of vasoactive centers and cranial nerves.

Because the cochlear nerve is bypassed by the ABI to directly stimulate the CN, the EABR waveform will lack wave I and have different amplitudes and latencies when compared to the ABR of a normal hearing patient or that of a CI patient (Fig 18–13). Figure 18–14 demonstrates an example of an intraoperative EABR obtained following placement of the ABI electrode array at our center. Also shown is a postoperative EABR recording to stimulation of the same electrode pair obtained after ABI activation in the awake subject. Responses have similar waveform morphologies and the slightly longer latencies seen in the awake patient were likely due to the lower current levels used.

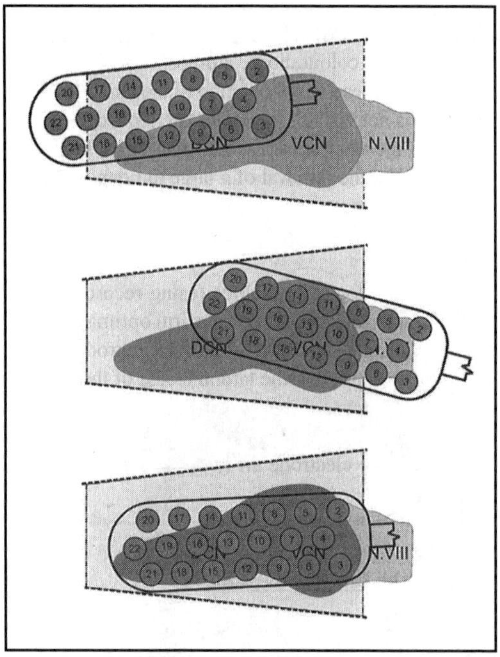

Figure 18–12. *An illustration of the theoretical effect of variable positioning of the electrode array within the lateral recess of the fourth ventricle on the number of electrodes contacting the cochlear nucleus. (Reprinted from Nevison[4] with permission from Karger.)*

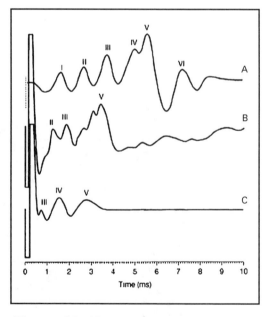

Figure 18–13. *A representation of ABR and EABR waveforms from (**A**) a normal, acoustically hearing individual, (**B**) a CI recipient, and (**C**) an ABI user. (Reprinted from Nevison[4] with permission from Karger.)*

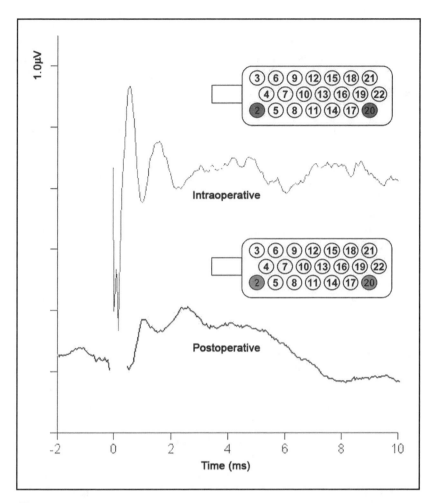

Figure 18–14. *Electrical auditory brainstem responses recorded from the case described in Figure 18–7. Evoked responses were generated by stimulating bipolar electrode pair E2 and E20 with single biphasic pulses (pulse width = 150 microseconds). The top trace was recorded intraoperatively during ABI placement and the bottom trace was recorded 3 months following ABI activation while the patient was resting quietly on a stretcher without anesthesia. The current level used intraoperatively was 220 microA; the current level used postoperatively was 130 microA, which was just below the patient's uncomfortable loudness level for stimulation.*

COMPLICATIONS

Surgery for VS excision alone using the discussed approaches carries a small but clinically significant number of complications. Since its reintroduction as an option for VS excision by William F. House in the 1960s,[28] the translabyrinthine approach has been regarded as a safe and effective method to remove tumors in patients with nonserviceable hearing. In a review of 258 patients who underwent VS surgery via the translabyrinthine approach, Mass and colleagues[29] found that perioperative complications included CSF leak (7.8%), bacterial meningitis (1.6%), failure of complete tumor removal (1.6%), neurovascular compromise (1.1%), and a House-Brackmann facial nerve outcome of grade V or VI (6%).[29] At our institution, we routinely occlude the eustachian tube with muscle or bone wax and obliterate the mastoid cavity with an abdominal fat graft, which has minimized our rate of CSF leak with the translabyrinthine approach for VS surgery.

Charalampakis et al[30] recently reviewed the available literature on the postoperative complications following excision of VS via the retrosigmoid approach and found that comparatively higher rates of CSF leak (2 to 30%), meningitis (up to 2.9%), and postoperative headache (up to 54%) continue to be reported, although the incidence of these complications can be reduced with refinements in surgical technique.[30] In contrast, the retrosigmoid approach has been reported to exhibit the best postoperative facial nerve function results when compared to middle fossa or translabyrinthine approaches for VS excision.[31]

Although the addition of ABI surgery following VS surgery adds additional operative time, further manipulation of the brainstem, and the introduction of hardware into the central nervous system, the overall rates of complications related to tumor excision following VS and ABI surgery have thus far not been reported to be significantly different to those of VS surgery alone. In a review of their 114 adult and pediatric ABI patient experience over eleven years, Colletti and colleagues[32] divided their complications into three categories, including major complications (14%), minor complications (64%), and nonauditory side effects (45%) (Table 18–2). Among major complications, three ABI patients died of unrelated causes, whereas other patients experienced pseudomeningoceles, cranial nerve lesions, hydrocephalus, and meningitis, among others. Minor complications included balance disturbance, temporary facial weakness, headache, transient hydrocephalus, and cerebrospinal fluid leak, among others. All minor complications except for headache were completely resolved with conservative measures or minor interventions. Finally, nearly half of their patients experienced nonauditory sensations, such as ipsilateral body tingle, facial nerve stimulation, dizziness, and throat tickle, with stimulation following ABI activation. Interestingly, many of these side effects diminished over time in the majority of these patients, allowing for the activation of additional stimulating electrodes.[32]

Importantly, the authors found that the complication rates observed for this series of ABI patients were comparable to those of other reported NF2 VS surgery-only institutional experiences. They concluded that the placement of an ABI system in an NF2 patient imparts no significant additional risks over those seen in standard VS surgery. Moreover, the authors assert that the complication rate of ABI placement in nontumor patients and that of CI placement are comparable and that the differences in complication rates lack statistical significance. Given these reasonably low complication rates (in nontumor ABI candidates) that rival more well-established temporal bone and cerebellopontine angle procedures,

Table 18–2. A List of Major and Minor Complications for Patients

	Neurofibromatosis Type 2	Nontumor	
Major complications	Ad	Ad	Ch
Mortality (deaths unrelated to auditory brainstem implantation surgery)	3	0	0
Cerebellar contusion	1	0	1
Permanent facial palsy	1	0	0
Meningitis	1	2[a]	1[a]
Lesions of the lower cranial nerves	2	0	
Hydrocephalus	1	1	0
Pseudomen ingocele	2	0	0
Minor complications	**Ad**	**Ad**	**Ch**
Cerebrospinal fluid leakage	6	1	0
Transient hydrocephalus	7	1	0
Wound seroma	4	2	4
Minor infections	2	2	1
Balance problems	11	2	1
Infection around implant	2	2	0
Infection surgical flap	2	1	0
Transient facial palsy	8	0	0
Temporary dysphonia, temporary difficulties in swelling	0	0	1
Headache	8	3	0
Flap problems	2	0	0
Nonauditory side effects	28	16	7

[a]Approximately 2 years after brainstem impantation activation.

Ad: adults; Ch: children.

Data retrieved from the study by Colletti et al[32] with permission from Lippincott, Williams and Wilkins.

including CI placement, vestibular neurectomy, and microvascular decompression, the authors support the use of ABIs for non-NF2 deaf patients who are not CI candidates.[32]

In their review of 61 patients who underwent VS and ABI surgery via the translabyrinthine approach at the House Ear Clinic, Otto and colleagues[33] reported a 3.3% rate of CSF leak and a 1.6% rate of meningitis. The authors also discussed their rates of implant-specific complications, including failure to provide useful auditory sensations (9.8%) and electrode migration (1.6%). In addition, they found that 24% of individual electrodes on implanted ABI arrays could not be used as a result of intolerable nonauditory sensations, which included dizziness and sensory side effects (tingling, pulling sensations, visual jittering) of the head and body.[33] Such side effects have been observed in as many as 69% of ABI recipients.[12]

FUTURE DIRECTIONS IN ABI SURGERY

In the past decade, cadaveric studies on endoscopic-assisted approaches to the lateral recess and cochlear nucleus have hinted at the potential for endoscopy in neurotologic surgery, including ABI placement. Advantages over the conventional operating microscope include improved visualization of the lateral recess with all surgical approaches (translabyrinthine, retrosigmoid, and middle fossa), higher magnification that provides finer definition of perforating blood vessels, cranial nerves, and neural structures, and the ability to look around corners and behind anatomic structures (Fig 18–15).[34–36] Moreover, the authors propose that the use of endoscopes would make the opera-

tive procedure shorter and less invasive, reducing perioperative morbidity. However, this approach is currently hindered by the lack of a three-dimensional image as well as instruments designed specifically for endoscopic posterior fossa/neurotologic surgery. Moreover, bimanual surgery would require an endoscope holder or a co-surgeon. Continued research on endoscopic-assisted neurotologic technology will provide further insight into the safety and efficacy of this novel approach.

ABI ACTIVATION AND PROGRAMMING

DEVICE ACTIVATION

Approximately 8 weeks following implantation, the ABI is activated using the external speech processor and the manufacturer's programming system. Unlike insertion of the CI electrode, placement of the ABI array on the cochlear nucleus can vary a great deal among patients and there is no clear correspondence of electrode position to the tonotopic organization of the CN. Consequently, the relationship between each electrode and psychophysical sensations must be meticulously explored (to eliminate unpleasant or nonauditory stimulation) and programmed into the device. The initial activation events involve providing monopolar and in some cases bipolar stimulation to the electrode array and collecting and obtaining feedback from the patient regarding the quality, level and pitch of the auditory sensation, the extent of the nonauditory sensations, and the setting of threshold and maximum comfort levels.

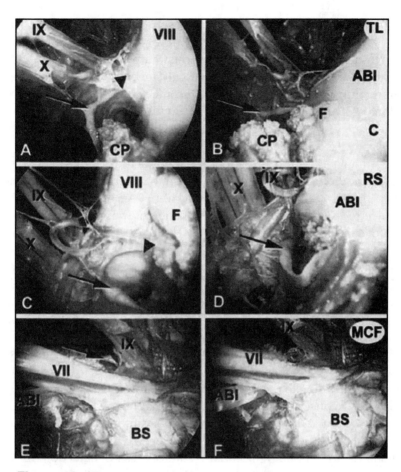

Figure 18–15. *Endoscopic view of the lateral recess of the fourth ventricle in cadaveric specimens with a 30-degree endoscope and using three different surgical approaches. The arrowheads in (**A**) and (**C**) designate the region of the cochlear nucleus as seen in translabyrinthine and retrosigmoid approaches, respectively. The ABI electrode array is seen in place through these approaches in (**B**) and (**D**). The middle fossa craniotomy approach to the brainstem and ABI electrode placement are also demonstrated in (**E**) and (**F**). The authors note that the brainstem surface at the implantation site cannot be visualized with this approach. (Reprinted from Friedland and Wackym[34] with permission from Wiley-Blackwell.)*

Stimulation parameters of each electrode are adjusted to optimize sound quality and minimize stimulation of adjacent cranial nerves. Given the possibility of activating vasoactive centers in the brainstem during this process, the initial stimulation at our center is always conducted with ready availability of emergency medical services and crash cart in the Audiology treatment room, but is no longer performed in an inpatient hospital setting or intensive care unit except in rare circumstances.

PROGRAMMING

Once the electrodes that elicit useful auditory sensations are identified for inclusion in the programming map, the patient provides additional detailed feedback on the pitch value of each electrode using pitch ranking. In this process, two electrodes successively are stimulated, and the patient indicates to the audiologist which of the two is higher in pitch. Ranking of all the serviceable electrodes creates a tonotopic arrangement for stimulation, and once pitch order is determined, a processor map is developed and downloaded into the speech processor for daily use. Audiologic follow-up appointments for measuring speech perception performance, reassessing electrode sensation and reprogramming of the processor occur at progressively longer intervals that usually vary from institution to institution and according to the patient's needs. At the Massachusetts Eye and Ear Infirmary, we see an ABI patient one week after initial activation and then at monthly intervals for about 3 months. After that, we often see the patient at 3-month intervals up to about a year and then every 6 months to a year depending on the patient. Neurotologic follow-up is routinely done at 6-month intervals.

AUDIOLOGIC MONITORING FOLLOWING DEVICE ACTIVATION

Even though patients are counseled both pre- and postoperatively regarding the outcomes following ABI surgery, they frequently report a level of disappointment with the quality of their auditory sensation and need to be encouraged that sound quality and undesirable nonauditory stimulations generally improves with time and experience. Because the expected level of speech perception with an ABI is lower than for a CI is helpful to use a series of tests that measure increasingly more difficult levels of speech perception. For instance, at our institution we use sound-field thresholds for warble tones as a sound detection measure, and the recorded Early Speech Perception Test[37] and, if the patient achieves an unusually high level of speech perception, the open-set monosyllable CNC test (House Ear Institute) to document speech perception performance at follow-up appointments. By starting with sound detection only and then increasing the difficulty of the tasks until the patient is unable to achieve a criterion score we can scale an individual's auditory performance from sound detection to open-set monosyllable word recognition. This sequence allows the audiologist to administer tests that the ABI user can "succeed" on while not frustrating the patient with tests that he or she does not have enough auditory information to obtain any correct answers. By progressing from the easiest auditory task of detection through successively more difficult auditory tasks of pattern perception, closed-set word recognition and perhaps open-set word recognition, the patient is less likely to become discouraged and can therefore be counseled regarding the amount of auditory information they are receiving and how best to use that information during their day to day communication. In addition, we have a level of performance that can be monitored for changes over time.

OUTCOMES

NF2 ABI PATIENTS

The majority of NF2 ABI users achieve auditory sensation, environmental sound detection, and, in some cases, closed-set word recognition. Only rarely do NF2 ABI users achieve open-set speech perception. However, in combination with lip-reading cues, the ABI can significantly improve sentence understanding (Fig 18–16).[33,38–41] Otto et al. reported the House Ear Institute experience with an 8-channel electrode array and found that a great majority of patients were able to perform significantly better than chance on environmental sound discrimination tests and that over 84% of patients scored significantly above chance on several closed-set word identification tests when provided with sound alone. Very few, however, demonstrated sound-only sentence recognition. In combination with lip-reading, however, the ABI clearly provided patients with improved comprehension. Moreover, the authors found considerable

improvements in test performance scores with time and experience with the ABI, even 8 years following implantation.[33] A subsequent report on the House Ear Institute ABI experience demonstrated similar results, again showing that the ABI as an adjunct to lip-reading substantially facilitates oral communication.[41]

A multinational report on the first 27 patients in Europe to undergo ABI placement also demonstrated comparable results, providing 96.2% of their patients, all of whom had NF2, with auditory sensations. Similarly, the authors found the ABI to offer patients improved environmental sound awareness and recognition of speech stress and rhythm patterns that facilitate lip-reading. Again, only a small percentage (7.2%) of patients was able to identify words or sentences in without lip-reading.[40]

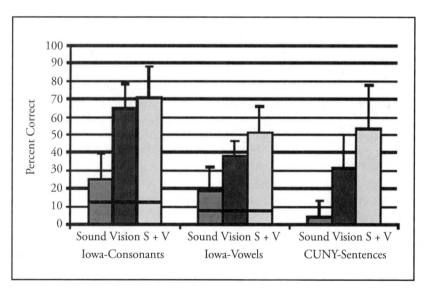

Figure 18–16. *Results of audiologic testing, including closed-set speech (Iowa-consonants, Iowa vowels) and open-set speech (CUNY-sentences) of ABI users demonstrating: (1) improvement over the expected score f or chance (guessing), as indicated by the solid lines, and (2) improvement in comprehension in combination with lip-reading. Error bars indicate standard deviation. (Reprinted from Schwartz[56] with permission from Springer.)*

Encouraging new data, however, suggest that some deaf NF2 patients can achieve reasonable open-set word recognition abilities with a surface electrode ABI system. At the 2010 State of the Art Symposium on ABIs held in Uppsala, Sweden, surgeons at the International Center of Hearing and Speech in Poland have reported open-set speech recognition of single syllable words in four out of five NF2 patients with the MED-EL ABI system placed during a retrosigmoid craniotomy and tumor resection.[42] It is not known why such significant performance differences exist between this small set of patients and the average NF2 ABI user and such observations warrant continued and careful investigation.

NONTUMOR ABI PATIENTS

As more non-NF2 patients with cochlear or cochlear nerve pathology underwent ABI placement in the late 1990s and early 2000s, it became clear to European investigators that mean auditory performance in nontumor ABI users was superior to those of NF2 users. Open-set, sound-only sentence recognition score in 48 non-NF2 patients with an ABI ranged from 10 to 100% with a mean of 59%, whereas 32 analogous NF2 patients scored significantly lower at 5 to 31% with a mean of 10% (Table 18–3).[13,14] Patients who had suffered head trauma resulting in cochlear nerve damage or had altered cochlear ossification achieved the best performance immediately postoperatively and subsequently demonstrated substantial improvement over a 10-year follow-up period, whereas patients with auditory neuropathy or cochlear malformation performed relatively poorly but nevertheless received considerable auditory benefit.[14] In another study, 5 patients who had poor or no speech perception following CI placement achieved more benefit following subsequent ABI placement, with one patient scoring 100% on open-set, sound-only sentence recognition testing.[13] A description of three adult patients with total bilateral cochlear ossification following meningitis reported a mean open-set, sound, and lip-reading sentence recognition of 82%.[43]

In an effort to better understand the performance differences in ABI outcomes between tumor and nontumor patients, Colletti and Shannon carefully evaluated 20 ABI patients (10 with NF2 and 10 without tumors). These subjects underwent an extensive series of psychophysical tests

Table 18–3. Average Performance (percent correct on open-set speech) Over Time for NF2 (T) and Nontumor (NT) Groups.

Group	No. Subjects	Range %	X	Md	SD
T	32	5–31	10	16	21.34
NT	48	10–100	59	53	15.21
T vs NT					
	t-test	*p* = 0.0007			

Data retrieved from the study by Colletti et al[14] with permission from Lippincott, Williams and Wilkins.

to examine electrode placement, stimulation selectivity, modulation detection and speech understanding.[44] Although the results of testing from both groups suggested that both tumor and nontumor patients had sufficient surviving neurons in the CN, optimal electrode placement and minimal interelectrode interference, the authors found that NF2 patients had significantly poorer modulation detection and speech understanding than nontumor patients (Fig 18–17). The authors furthermore speculate that the differences noted among these two groups suggest that a putative subpopulation of specialized CN neurons or neuronal pathway may be important for both modulation detection and speech recognition is disrupted in NF2 patients in the course of the disease or in the surgical excision of the tumor.

NEWER CONCEPTS

Given the relatively low performance level of an NF2 ABI user when compared with a postlingually deafened CI user, researchers have proposed various theories for this discrepancy and investigated ways to address the possible shortcomings of stimulating the CN with a surface electrode. One potential explanation of the poorer performance is that the two-dimensional surface electrode of the ABI fails to make a satisfactory connection to the tonotopically arranged neurons and neural pathways within the three-dimensional volume of the CN.[45] A surface array is believed to be unable to fully access and interface with the tonotopic frequency gradients specifically within the

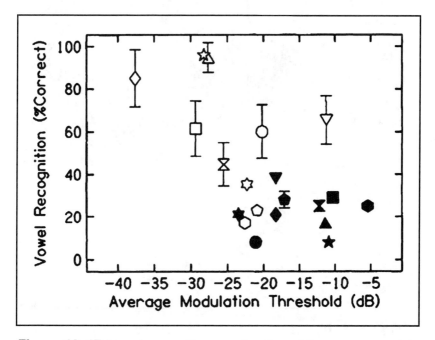

Figure 18–17. *Vowel recognition as a function of the average modulation threshold. Open symbols present data from nontumor patients and filled symbols present data from tumor patients. (Reprinted from Colletti and Shannon[44] with permission from Wiley-Blackwell.)*

VCN, which is composed of various cell types in a layered functional arrangement and less accessible to electrode array contact compared to the DCN. Accordingly, a penetrating electrode ABI (PABI) was developed in a collaborative effort with the National Institutes of Health, Cochlear Corporation (Englewood, CO, USA), and surgeons at the House Ear Institute in an attempt to improve access to the tonotopic organization within the CN (Fig 18–18). In a trial of 10 patients, the investigators found that the penetrating electrodes of the PABI not only retained the capacity to stimulate auditory sensations, but also lowered the electrical stimulation levels required for sensation and enlarged the range of pitch sensation relative to the surface electrodes. However, no significant speech perception benefit was realized, even after more than 3 years of use and experience [46]. Due to a significant adverse effect profile recently reported for the PABI, the trial of this electrode has been discontinued.

Although the promising and consistently superior outcomes of nontumor patients who underwent standard surface electrode ABI placement further dismissed the hypothesis that poor ABI performance was the result of inadequate electrode interface with the CN, recent efforts to improve outcomes in NF2 patients have also been directed at accessing the central auditory pathways beyond the CN to bypass injury due to

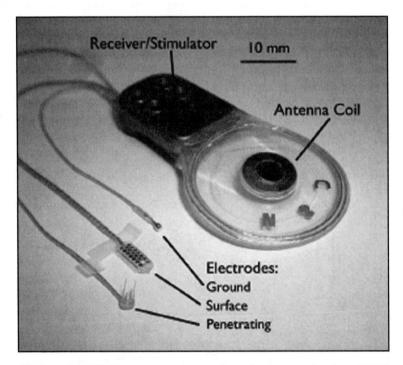

Figure 18–18. *The penetrating auditory brainstem implant (PABI) includes both a penetrating electrode array and a standard surface electrode paddle. (Reprinted from Otto et al[46] with permission from Lippincott, Williams and Wilkins.)*

tumor growth and resection. Injury to the CN is felt to arise from tumor compression and distortion, tumor secretion of as of yet unidentified factors that may cause damage, or ischemia of the second order auditory neurons from tumor excision. Early laboratory[47] and clinical[48] studies have begun on the feasibility and efficacy of placing a stimulating electrode array at the level of the inferior colliculus (IC). The IC is a well-defined structure within the human midbrain that measures roughly 6 to 7 mm in diameter[18] and is surgically accessible following VS excision when using a retrosigmoid cranitomy.[49] Composed of a dorsomedial nucleus, dorsal cortex, lateral nucleus and central nucleus (ICC), the IC is an obligatory synaptic terminus for essentially all ascending auditory pathways. More specifically, the ICC is the main projection center for ascending auditory brainstem projections and consists of a well-defined laminar organization that, based on animal studies, is predicted to tonotopically correspond to different frequency layers.[50] Accordingly, ICC has been proposed as an alternative implantation site for auditory rehabilitation, particularly for NF2 patients.[51]

Using an ABI device with a surface electrode, Colletti and colleagues reported the first successful case of useful auditory sensations obtained with electrical stimulation of the IC. This NF2 patient had multiple tumors bilaterally in the region of the CN and had previously undergone both surgery and gamma-knife radiation therapy for his bilateral AN, and as such, the patient was not considered a viable candidate for ABI placement on the CN. With ABI placement on the IC, the patient attained significant improvements in face-to-face sentence comprehension without any appreciable side effects.[48] Lim and colleagues[53] subsequently published their experience of three patients with AMI placement in Germany using a single-shank, penetrating multielectrode array designed and developed by researchers at the Medical University of Hannover, Germany and at Cochlear Limited (Lane Cove, New South Wales, Australia).[52] The array measures 6.2 mm in length, 0.4 mm in diameter, and consists of 20 platinum ring electrodes linearly spaced at an interval of 200 microns designed with the goal of stimulating the different layers of the ICC (Figs 18–19 and 18–20). The IC is approached via a lateral suboccipital craniotomy,[49] and the array can be positioned along the tonotopic gradient of the ICC (Fig 18–21). Of the three patients who underwent surgery to place the AMI, only one had the array successfully placed into the ICC. This patient exhibited the best performance results that were comparable and in some tests above the average results from NF2 patients with an ABI.[50,52] Although these results are encouraging, additional work on electrode design, accurate surgical array placement, and optimization of array orientation within the ICC will be needed to provide further insight into ways to improve AMI outcomes and to establish AMI as a practical alternative to ABI.

In conclusion, the modern multichannel ABI systems are able to provide most NF2 users with useful auditory sensations but performance continues to lag that of both CI patients and nontumor ABI users. Much work is needed to resolve why such differences exist. What is encouraging is that the inherent design of the ABI appears to be sufficient to provide a high level of auditory performance, including open-set speech understanding, in a number of nontumor ABI patients and

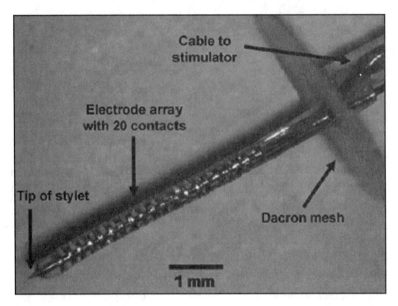

Figure 18–19. *The auditory midbrain implant (AMI) electrode array. (Reprinted from Lenarz et al[51] with permission from Lippincott, Williams and Wilkins.)*

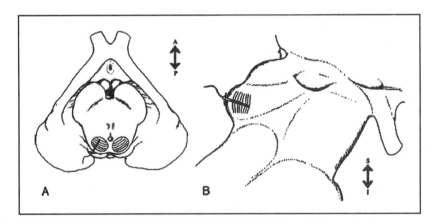

Figure 18–20. *Axial (**A**) and parasagittal (**B**) drawings depicting the orientation of the penetrating electrode array of the auditory midbrain implant across the tonotopic gradient of the inferior colliculus. A, anterior; P, posterior; S, superior; I, inferior. (Reprinted from Samii et al[49] with permission from Lippincott, Williams and Wilkins.)*

more recently, in some NF2 patients as well. That is, electrical stimulation using a surface electrode on the CN can pro-vide some patients who are not CI candidates with meaningful speech perception without lipreading. Both basic and

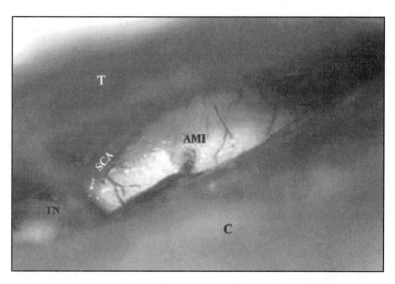

Figure 18–21. *Exposure of the trochlear nerve (TN), superior cerebellar artery (SCA), tentorium (T), and cerebellum (C) through a lateral supracerebellar infratentorial approach allowed for insertion of the auditory midbrain implant electrode array into the inferior colliculus in a fresh cadaver specimen. (Reprinted from Samii et al[49] with permission from Lippincott, Williams and Wilkins.*

clinical investigations are clearly needed to find new ways to improve hearing in NF2 patients. In our laboratory, we are exploring ways to enhance performance by improving the selectivity of CN stimulation in an animal model using (1) conformable electrode designs and (2) optical stimulation.[53,54] Our clinical research aims to correlate electrically evoked responses in awake ABI users with their psychophysical measurements to better improve placement of the electrode in the operating room.[55] Future work will determine: (1) why some patients are able to extract more meaningful auditory input from current ABI technology than others and (2) how we can translate these findings to improve the quality of life and productivity of NF2 patients who already face significant health issues associated with this devastating genetic syndrome.

REFERENCES

1. Lustig LR, Yeagle J, Driscoll CL, Blevins N, Francis H, Niparko JK. Cochlear implantation in patients with neurofibromatosis type 2 and bilateral vestibular schwannoma. *Otol Neurotol.* 2006 Jun;27(4):512–518.

2. Neff BA, Wiet RM, Lasak JM, et al. Cochlear implantation in the neurofibromatosis type 2 patient: long-term follow-up. *Laryngoscope.* 2007 Jun;117(6):1069–1072.

3. Trotter MI, Briggs RJ. Cochlear implantation in neurofibromatosis type 2 after radiation therapy. *Otol Neurotol.* 2010 Feb; 31(2):216–219.

4. Nevison B. A guide to the positioning of brainstem implants using intraoperative electrical auditory brainstem responses. *Adv Otorhinolaryngol.* 2006;64: 154–166.

5. Jackson KB, Mark G, Helms J, Mueller J, Behr R. An auditory brainstem implant system. *Am J Audiol.* 2002 Dec;11(2):128–133.

6. Schwartz MS, Otto SR, Shannon RV, Hitselberger WE, Brackmann DE. Auditory brainstem implants. *Neurotherapeutics.* 2008 Jan;5(1):128–136.

7. Kalamarides M, Grayeli AB, Bouccara D, et al. Hearing restoration with auditory brainstem implants after radiosurgery for neurofibromatosis type 2. *J Neurosurg.* 2001 Dec;95(6):1028–1033.

8. Plotkin SR, Stemmer-Rachamimov AO, Barker FG 2nd, et al. Hearing improvement after bevacizumab in patients with neurofibromatosis type 2. *N Engl J Med.* 2009 Jul 23;361(4):358–367.

9. Colletti V, Fiorino F, Sacchetto L, Miorelli V, Carner M. Hearing habilitation with auditory brainstem implantation in two children with cochlear nerve aplasia. *Int J Pediatr Otorhinolaryngol.* 2001 Aug 20; 60(2):99–111.

10. Colletti V, Fiorino F, Carner M, Sacchetto L, Miorelli V, Orsi A. Auditory brainstem implantation: the University of Verona experience. *Otolaryngol Head Neck Surg.* 2002 Jul;127(1):84–96.

11. Colletti V, Fiorino FG, Carner M, Miorelli V, Guida M, Colletti L. Auditory brainstem implant as a salvage treatment after unsuccessful cochlear implantation. *Otol Neurotol.* 2004 Jul;25(4):485–496.

12. Colletti V, Carner M, Miorelli V, Guida M, Colletti L, Fiorino F. Auditory brainstem implant (ABI): new frontiers in adults and children. *Otolaryngol Head Neck Surg.* 2005 Jul;133(1):126–138.

13. Colletti V. Auditory outcomes in tumor vs. non-tumor patients fitted with auditory brainstem implants. *Adv Otorhinolaryngol.* 2006;64:167–185.

14. Colletti V, Shannon R, Carner M, Veronese S, Colletti L. Outcomes in non-tumor adults fitted with the auditory brainstem implant: 10 years' experience. *Otol Neurotol.* 2009 Aug;30(5):614–618.

15. Sennaroglu L, Colletti V, Manrique M, et al. Auditory brainstem implantation in children and non-neurofibromatosis type 2 patients: a consensus statement. *Otol Neurotol.* 2011 Feb;32(2):187–191.

16. Monsell EM, McElveen JT Jr, Hitselberger WE, House WF. Surgical approaches to the human cochlear nuclear complex. *Am J Otol.* 1987 Sep;8(5):450–455.

17. Brackmann DE, Hitselberger WE, Nelson RA, et al. Auditory brainstem implant: I. Issues in surgical implantation. *Otolaryngol Head Neck Surg.* 1993 Jun;108(6):624–633.

18. Moore JK. The human auditory brain stem: a comparative view. *Hear Res.* 1987;29(1): 1–32.

19. Klose AK, Sollmann WP. Anatomical variations of landmarks for implantation at the cochlear nucleus. *J Laryngol Otol Suppl.* 2000;(27):8–10.

20. Quester R, Schröder R. Topographic anatomy of the cochlear nuclear region at the floor of the fourth ventricle in humans. *J Neurosurg.* 1999 Sep;91(3):466–476.

21. Seldon HL, Clark GM. Human cochlear nucleus: comparison of Nissl-stained neurons from deaf and hearing patients. *Brain Res.* 1991 Jun 14;551(1–2):185–194.

22. Zhang J, Zhang X. Electrical stimulation of the dorsal cochlear nucleus induces hearing in rats. *Brain Res.* 2010 Jan 22;1311: 37–50.

23. Chien W, Lee DJ. Physiology of the auditory system. In: Flint PW, ed. *Cummings Otolaryngology-Head and Neck Surgery.* 5th ed. St. Louis, MO: Mosby; 2010.

24. Toh EH, Luxford WM. Cochlear and brainstem implantation. *Otolaryngol Clin North Am.* 2002 Apr;35(2):325–342.

25. Colletti V, Sacchetto L, Giarbini N, Fiorino F, Carner M. Retrosigmoid approach for auditory brainstem implant. *J Laryngol Otol Suppl.* 2000;(27):37–40.

26. Colletti V, Fiorino FG, Carner M, Giarbini N, Sacchetto L, Cumer G. Advantages of the retrosigmoid approach in auditory brain stem implantation. *Skull Base Surg.* 2000;10(4):165–170.

27. Waring MD. Intraoperative electrophysiologic monitoring to assist placement of auditory brain stem implant. *Ann Otol Rhinol Laryngol Suppl.* 1995 Sep;166:33–36.

28. House WF. Acoustic neuroma. *Arch Otolaryngol.* 1964;80:598–757.

29. Mass SC, Wiet RJ, Dinces E. Complications of the translabyrinthine approach for the removal of acoustic neuromas. *Arch Otolaryngol Head Neck Surg.* 1999 Jul;125(7):801–804.

30. Charalampakis S, Koutsimpelas D, Gouveris H, Mann W. Postoperative complications after removal of sporadic vestibular schwannoma via retrosigmoid-suboccipital approach: current diagnosis and management. *Eur Arch Otorhinolaryngol.* 2011 May;268(5):653–660.

31. Arriaga M, Chen D. Facial function in hearing preservation acoustic neuroma surgery. *Arch Otolaryngol Head Neck Surg.* 2001;127:543–546.

32. Colletti V, Shannon RV, Carner M, Veronese S, Colletti L. Complications in auditory brainstem implant surgery in adults and children. *Otol Neurotol.* 2010 Jun;31(4): 558–564.

33. Otto SR, Brackmann DE, Hitselberger WE, Shannon RV, Kuchta J. Multichannel auditory brainstem implant: update on performance in 61 patients. *J Neurosurg.* 2002 Jun;96(6):1063–1071.

34. Friedland DR, Wackym PA. Evaluation of surgical approaches to endoscopic auditory brainstem implantation. *Laryngoscope.* 1999 Feb;109(2 pt 1):175–180.

35. Wackym PA, King WA, Poe DS, et al. Adjunctive use of endoscopy during acoustic neuroma surgery. *Laryngoscope.* 1999 Aug;109(8):1193–2201.

36. Wackym PA, King WA, Meyer GA, Poe DS. Endoscopy in neuro-otologic surgery. *Otolaryngol Clin North Am.* 2002 Apr; 35(2):297–323.

37. Moog JS, Geers AE. *Early Speech Perception Test.* St. Louis, MO: Central Institute for the Deaf; 1990.

38. Ebinger K, Otto S, Arcaroli J, Staller S, Arndt P. Multichannel auditory brainstem implant: US clinical trial results. *J Laryngol Otol Suppl.* 2000;(27):50–53.

39. Lenarz T, Moshrefi M, Matthies C, et al. Auditory brainstem implant: part I. Auditory performance and its evolution over time. *Otol Neurotol.* 2001 Nov;22(6):823–833.

40. Nevison B, Laszig R, Sollmann WP, et al. Results from a European clinical investigation of the Nucleus multichannel auditory brainstem implant. *Ear Hear.* 2002 Jun;23(3):170–183.

41. Schwartz MS, Otto SR, Brackmann DE, Hitselberger WE, Shannon RV. Use of a multichannel auditory brainstem implant for neurofibromatosis type 2. *Stereotact Funct Neurosurg.* 2003;81(1–4):110–114.

42. Skarzynski H, Behr R, Lorens A, Zgoda M, Mrowka M. *Results after sequential bilateral auditory brainstem implantation* [Abstract]. State of the Art Symposium on Auditory Brainstem Implants, Uppsala, Sweden, 2010.

43. Grayeli AB, Kalamarides M, Bouccara D, Ben Gamra L, Ambert-Dahan E, Sterkers O. Auditory brainstem implantation to rehabilitate profound hearing loss with totally ossified cochleae induced by pneumococcal meningitis. *Audiol Neurotol.* 2007;12(1):27–30.

44. Colletti V, Shannon RV. Open-set speech perception with auditory brainstem implant? *Laryngoscope.* 2005 Nov;115(11): 1974–1978.

45. Kuchta J, Otto SR, Shannon RV, Hitselberger WE, Brackmann DE. The multichannel auditory brainstem implant: how many electrodes make sense? *J Neurosurg.* 2004 Jan;100(1):16–23.

46. Otto SR, Shannon RV, Wilkinson EP, et al. Audiologic outcomes with the penetrating electrode auditory brainstem implant. *Otol Neurotol.* 2008 Dec;29(8):1147–1154.

47. Lim HH, Anderson DJ. Auditory cortical responses to electrical stimulation of the inferior colliculus: implications for an auditory midbrain implant. *J Neurophysiol.* 2006 Sep;96(3):975–988.

48. Colletti V, Shannon R, Carner M, et al. The first successful case of hearing produced by electrical stimulation of the human midbrain. *Otol Neurotol.* 2007 Jan;28(1):39–43.

49. Samii A, Lenarz M, Majdani O, Lim HH, Samii M, Lenarz T. Auditory midbrain implant: a combined approach for vestibular

schwannoma surgery and device implantation. *Otol Neurotol.* 2007 Jan;28(1): 31–38.

50. Lim HH, Lenarz M, Lenarz T. Auditory midbrain implant: a review. *Trends Amplif.* 2009 Sep;13(3):149–180.

51. Lenarz T, Lim HH, Reuter G, Patrick JF, Lenarz M. The auditory midbrain implant: a new auditory prosthesis for neural deafness—concept and device description. *Otol Neurotol.* 2006 Sep;27(6):838–843.

52. Lim HH, Lenarz T, Joseph G, Battmer RD, Samii A, Samii M, Patrick JF, Lenarz M. Electrical stimulation of the midbrain for hearing restoration: insight into the functional organization of the human central auditory system. *J Neurosci.* 2007 Dec 5; 27(49):13541–13551.

53. Lee DJ, Hancock KE, Mukerji S, Brown MC. *Optical stimulation of the central auditory system* [Abstract]. Midwinter Meeting of the Association Research in Otolaryngology. 2009;32(928).

54. Lee DJ, Hancock KE, Mukerji S, Verma R, Brown MC. *Infrared neural stimulation of the cochlear nucleus* [Abstract]. Midwinter Meeting of the Association Research in Otolaryngololology. 2011;33(539).

55. Herrmann BS, Hancock KE, Eddington DK, Brown MC, Lee DJ. *Electrophysiologic response and subject perception in auditory brainstem implant stimulation* [Abstract]. State of the Art Symposium on Auditory Brainstem Implants, Uppsala, Sweden, 2010.

56. Schwartz MS, Otto SR, Shannon RV, Hitselberger WE, Brackmann DE. Auditory brainstem implants. *Neurotherapeutics.* 2008 Jan;5(1):128–136.

57. Lee DJ, Driver M. Cochlear implant fixation using titanium screws. *Laryngoscope.* 2005 May;115(5):910–911.

Chapter 19

Bone-Conduction Hearing Devices

MANOHAR BANCE, ROBERT B. A. ADAMSON, AND ROSS WILLIAM DEAS

INTRODUCTION

Bone-conduction hearing (BCH) has long been recognized as a useful auditory channel, and by the 1700s and 1800s, several types of devices that connected to the teeth or skull to hear environmental sounds or speakers had already been described and manufactured. Berger[1] provides a fascinating and comprehensive history of early development of BCH.

One appeal of BCH is that it accesses the same cochlear structures as air conduction hearing does. Sounds that are transmitted through bone have been shown to be equivalent to those transmitted through air; cancellation experiments have shown that changing the phase and amplitude of a signal delivered through air can lead to nearly complete cancellation of one delivered through bone.[2–4]

The value of this is that the BCH channel is still therapeutically available even when the air conduction route is compromised. BCH has long been used for diagnostic purposes to assess the inner ear during audiometry, but its use therapeutically was initially limited to forms using a steel headband or other static pressure devices (eg, spectacles) to press a vibrator against the skin. Driving head vibrations through the skin is called *transcutaneous* bone conduction, as opposed to more recent *percutaneous* methods in which a fixture is osseointegrated into the bone of the skull and pierces the skin to protrude outside. The fixture is then directly excited by a vibrator on the outside. The transcutaneous method tends to lose about 10 to 15 dB of hearing in the compliance of the skin when compared to percutaneous methods, mostly at the higher frequencies.[5]

Percutaneous BCH was first used in 1977 by Tjellstrom and Hakansson,[6] and became commercially available in Europe in 1984. The main indications in the first decades were subjects with large bilateral conductive losses who could not wear conventional air conduction hearing aids (eg, bilateral canal atresia patients, or patients with severely draining ears). More recently, indications have expanded to include rehabilitation of single sided deafness,[7] and in many centers, this is now the predominant medical indication.

The implantable BCH device market to date has been dominated by the Baha® (Cochlear-BAS). More recently, a similar competing product, the Ponto® (Oticon-Medical) has been introduced. Other products will probably emerge into mainstream markets in the near future. In this chapter, to avoid using proprietary or company specific acronyms, we will term all bone conduction devices based on *implanted fixtures* as bone conduction implanted devices (BCIDs), and bone conduction involving no implanted fixture bone conduction *removable* devices (BCRDs). In more developed countries, BCIDs have almost completely replaced the traditional BCRD bone conduction behind the ear device on a headband, with its attendant pressure, discomfort, cosmetic issues, and skin problems.

Air-conduction hearing aids and BCIDs perform approximately equally, both in temporal and frequency information transfer, provided that sound is equally audible.[8] In the past, air-conduction hearing aids had much more sophisticated signal processing, with wideband multichannel dynamic compression, scene analysis, and so forth, but these features have recently been introduced into the BCID processors, and are no longer a major advantage of air conduction hearing aids. One major advantage of BCIDs over air-conduction hearing aids is that the size of the air-bone gap is irrelevant to them, since it is essentially "invisible" to these devices. Hence, for large air-bone gaps (larger than 30 dB according to Mylanus et al[9]) BCIDs may outperform acoustic hearing aids, which are

working close to their maximum output, with attendant distortion, feedback, and battery life issues. This has led to some centres advocating for the use of BCIDs even for problems traditionally solved with middle ear surgical solutions, for example, for failed surgeries such as stapedotomy, or ossiculoplasty, rather than further revision middle ear surgery.

There are, however, numerous other factors that are unique to bone conduction. First, bone conduction stimulates both cochleae, close to, but not exactly symmetrically. This means a BCH driver placed anywhere on the head will provide a signal to both cochleae. This fact can be used to deliver sound to the contralateral cochlea from a BCH unit on one side of the head, effectively removing the head shadow effect. Sounds arising on one side of the skull are able to cross to the other side's cochlea with little attenuation, and this is the basis for the use of BCIDs for single-sided deafness. The converse of this is that there is less separation of signals to each cochlea in bilateral BCIDs than in air conduction hearing aids, which may impact sound localization or binaural processing.

In air-conduction hearing aids, the sound input to the ear can be measured using real ear measurements, and together with the audiogram this can be used to calculate the actual audibility of an input acoustic signal. A limitation for bone conduction devices is there is no easily available equivalent to measure audibility of bone conducted sound. This is because the skull vibrations that BCIDs elicit cannot be easily measured, although, the output force of the BCID could conceivably be. This makes it difficult, currently, to "fit" a BCID to an audiogram in the same way that an air conduction aid can be fit.

DESIGN OF BONE CONDUCTION TRANSDUCERS

BCH aids require a high-efficiency actuator in a small package capable of operating over a useful auditory frequency range for speech comprehension and appreciation of music. This requires good performance from at least 0.25 to 4 kHz. Historically, variable-reluctance vibrators have been used for this purpose for example, in Cochlear's Baha® devices. In recent years, new devices based on piezoelectric and magnetostrictive materials have also received attention. Although these materials offer the promise of easier manufacturability, higher energy density and smaller size, there are a number of design challenges in obtaining good impedance matching and broadband response from them that have proved stubbornly difficult to address.

In a variable reluctance vibrator, two pieces of soft ferrite, a nonpermanent magnetic material, are separated by a very small air gap. One of the two ferrites (the U-shaped bar in the diagram) has a coil wound around its arms, and when a current flows through this coil, a magnetic field is generated in the ferrite. The second ferrite (the lower bar in the diagram) is in turn magnetized by the magnetic field from the first ferrite in the same way that a steel nail in proximity to a permanent magnet will itself become temporarily magnetized. The two magnetized ferrites then attract each other and the air gap will tend to close. The attraction of the magnets is countered by a suspension system, depicted as a set of springs in the figure, which tends to hold the two magnets apart, maintaining an open air gap (Fig 19–1).

Were this the whole story, the actuator would not respond in a linear way to a driving signal as, regardless of the direction of current flow in the coil, the ferrites would tend to attract, closing the air gap. What is desired instead is that one direction of current flow cause attraction and the other repulsion so that the force output of the vibrator is proportional to the driving current. This is achieved by applying a bias to the system so that a magnetic field exists in the ferrites even when no voltage is applied. One direction of current flow then increases this field, further closing the air gap and the other direction decreases it, decreasing the attraction and hence effectively repelling the magnets and opening the gap. Although such a bias could be achieved with a constant DC current in the coils, it is much more efficient to use a permanent magnet, seen in the centre of the diagram, to apply the bias since a permanent magnet does not dissipate any energy.

To drive force into the skull, a post is attached to one of the two ferrites, whereas the other one (along with the coils and other masses attached to it) is allowed to move independently, forming a "floating mass." When the coil is energized, the two ferrites attract or repel, and a force is generated between the ferrites. The free floating one accelerates away from the head, and according to Newton's third law, it causes an equal and opposite force into the implanted abutment which then moves the head. The presence of the suspension system creates a restoring force to bring the mass back to its equilibrium position.

When driving such a system sinusoidally, at most frequencies the inertia of the mass and the stiffness of the spring will tend to limit the amount of motion that the mass experiences (and hence the

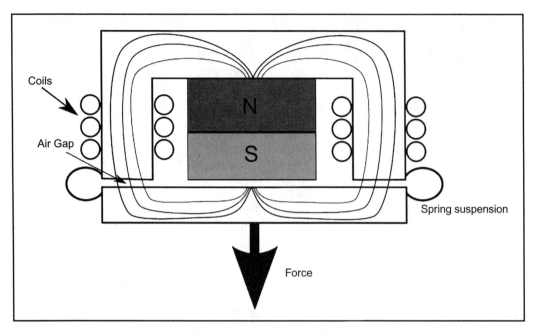

Figure 19–1. *A cartoon of the internals of a variable reluctance motor taken from Berger.[1] N and S denote the north and south poles of the permanent bias magnet. Coils are shown in cross-section as a grid of circles. The two ferrites are the U-shaped bar and the rectangular bar.*

amount of force that the transducer generates), but at a special frequency called the resonance frequency, the spring force resisting motion exactly cancels the mass inertia, and the motion of the mass will grow until it is limited by friction or nonlinear effects like the ferrite hitting the end of its range of motion. As a result, floating mass systems tend to have pronounced resonances that can be detrimental to the usually desired flat frequency response. Often, extra damping is added to such systems in order to increase friction and limit the effect of the resonance. The frequency at which resonance occurs can be engineered by tuning the spring stiffness and by adding extra mass to the ferrite. A resonance that's too high in frequency makes it hard to achieve good low frequency response, and a persistent challenge in small-package devices like BCIDs

is to arrive at a good combination of a large mass and a weak spring sufficient to produce good low-frequency resonance. As can be seen in the Figure 19–2, the Baha® Divino (R) achieves a resonance of around 770 Hz.

Although it has been in use for over four decades, the variable reluctance motor for bone conduction continues to see innovation. For instance, a new design from the Hakansson[10] group called the Balanced Electromagnetic Separation Transducer (BEST) uses two air gaps instead of one in a clever design that nearly eliminates the nonlinear behavior of the classic single air-gap design while improving the low-frequency response and introducing a second resonance for flatter high-frequency response. Other groups have been examining completely different paradigms for transducers, relying on piezo-

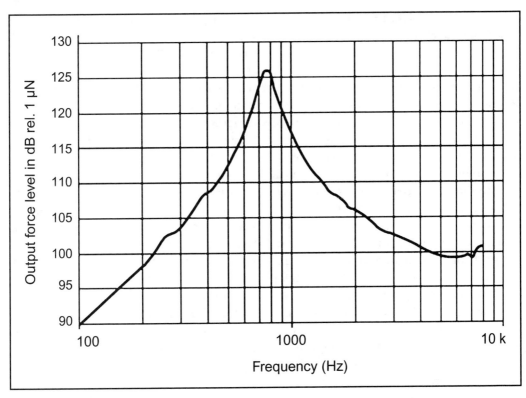

Figure 19–2. *The output force level of the Baha® as a function of frequency. The resonance at 770 Hz causes a sharp increase in the force at that frequency.*

electric and magnetostrictive materials that change their shape under the application of an external electric or magnetic field, respectively. Piezoelectrics have the advantage of naturally producing linear deformation and so do not require biasing whereas magnetostrictives require a biasing permanent magnet to achieve a linear response. In either case, the lack of a need for an air gap or a spring suspension greatly eases manufacturability. The issue with both materials is that vibrations are produced at a high mechanical impedance (ie, a large force but a small displacement), making it difficult to achieve good low-frequency performance in the above classic floating mass design.

One approach to addressing this is to try to improve mechanical matching using "gearbox" schemes that trade off force for displacement such as the piezoelectric cantilever. Another is to make use of ultra-high-strain materials such as terfenol-D[11] in the case of magnetostrictives and single crystal relaxor-ferroelectrics like PMN-PT[12] in the case of piezoelectrics. Still another approach is to do away with the need for a floating mass altogether by bonding a transducer to the skull in such a way that deformation of the transducer directly deforms the bone. Such devices, although requiring a large surface area, can be quite thin, and are a promising direction for fully implanted BCH devices.[13]

BONE-CONDUCTION MECHANICS

Over the past century, a large number of experiments have been undertaken in animal, dry skull and human cadaver models to try to understand the nature of mechanical vibrations propagating in the skull and to ascertain the mechanisms by which they transmit sound to the cochlea. In one famous experiment, von Békésy[2] showed that sound arriving from the air conduction pathway and from the bone-conduction pathway can be made to cancel each other at a particular phase difference. This showed that the cochlear mechanism for conversion of sound into a neural signal is the same for bone-conducted and air-conducted sound, namely the vibration of the hair cells in response to a traveling wave along the basilar membrane. Tonndorff[14] proposed seven distinct mechanisms by which bone conducted sound might excite basilar membrane motion and lead to hearing. These were: the inertia of the middle ear ossicles, the compliance of the middle ear cavity, the compression of the cochlear ducts, relative mobility of the round window and the oval window, the inertia of the cochlear fluids, and the effective compliance of the cochlear aqueduct via the cerebrospinal fluid pathway. In an extensive review paper, Stenfelt and Goode[15] systematically examined the experimental evidence supporting each of these mechanisms. Their conclusion was that at low frequencies (below 1 kHz) the inertia of the cochlear fluid seems to be the dominant contributor to bone-conducted sound. At the middle frequencies middle ear inertia plays a greater role and at frequencies above 4 kHz the compression of the otic capsule of the cochlea is dominant.

The transmission of vibrations across the head is important in understanding binaural BCH and in the application of bone conduction to lifting the head shadow effect for single-sided deaf patients. Hakansson et al[16] conducted an experiment on six patients equipped with bilateral titanium abutments in which a vibrator excited bone vibration at one abutment and the motion of the contralateral abutment was measured with an accelerometer. Using this method, Hakansson[17] was able to establish that the transmission of sound across the skull is a linear process that did not cause any measurable level of distortion. He was also able to measure a number of resonances in both the input point impedance on the driven side, and the transmitted motion on the contralateral side in these patients. A key feature in his data is the presence of antiresonances (sharp drops in motion for a given force input at a given frequency range) in the motion at both sides of the head. These antiresonances (which have also been noted in cadaveric data[18] can be understood as arising from destructive interference of vibrations taking different paths to the measurement point. In Hakansson's study they give rise to up to 20 dB drops in response level over a range of frequencies as short as roughly a tenth of an octave. Although Hakansson did not attempt to audiometrically confirm that the antiresonances increase actual hearing thresholds, it is consistent with the large variability in transcranial attenuation noted by a number of authors.[19] Although Hakansson's data only gave acceleration in one direction, later experiments measured all three directions[18] and found that antiresonances occurred at differed frequencies in the three directions. Consequently, the antiresonances in the vector sum of all directions are not as pronounced as the antiresonances in the motion in any particular direction. It remains unclear as to whether the vector sum or the projection along some particular direction is most strongly correlated with excitation of the basilar membrane.

FITTING AND PREOPERATIVE COUNSELING

As with any rehabilitation device, a major component of candidate selection is managing and developing appropriate expectations. It goes without saying that fitting is a multidisciplinary process, involving audiologists and surgeons, and in children, often speech language and education professionals. Expectations are important to elucidate. If the main problem is audibility of sound, and the problem is primarily a bilateral conductive hearing loss, almost all candidates are happy with BCIDs.[20] If the main problem is drainage from mastoid cavities, BCIDs can also help with this, by not occluding the ear,[21] but these patients may also be helped by mastoid obliteration surgery followed by an air-conduction hearing aid. However, if the patient has single sided deafness, and wants to develop good binaural hearing with a BCID, or has severe mixed hearing loss and wants to hear normal conversational speech, this is unlikely to happen.

For purely audibility issues, the limiting factor for usefulness of the BCIDs is their limited ability to compensate for the sensorineural component of mixed hearing losses. Because of this limitation, the Baha BP100® or Intenso® are recommended by Cochlear Corporation for mixed losses where the sensorineural

component of the loss does not exceed 45 to 50 db HL (at an average 0.5, 1, 2, and 3 kHz), and the Cordelle II® (bodyworn aid) up to 65 dB HL loss.

In essence, BCIDs are very good at closing the air-bone gap, but have difficulty raising thresholds much beyond the audiometric bone curve. Power output of BCIDs is limited by head radiation of sound causing feedback, and the limited current capacity of the small batteries they carry compared to the power required to excite the whole skull. The Cordelle II® from Cochlear BAS has a body worn processor, with a large battery, with the microphone at body level to limit feedback, but there are significant issues with patient acceptance of this kind of body worn device. In general, our experience is that at 40 to 45 dB hearing loss in the bone curve, patients begin to notice lack of power from current BCIDs.

In almost all patients, we recommend a soundfield test of aided thresholds with the BCID worn on a steel spring headband. Alternatively, the "test rod" (Cochlear BAS) can be fitted with the BCID processor and placed on the teeth. We have found that this is not as good in the higher frequencies, unless it is placed on the molars, which is difficult (Fig 19–3).

The headband gives a reasonable approximation of final thresholds, except at higher frequencies[22] (Fig 19–4).

In single-sided deafness patients (SSD, we reserve this term for subjects with single-sided severe to profound sensorineural deafness), the head shadow effect is small for low frequency sounds (see Fig 19–8 below), and ideally only high frequency sound should be transmitted by the BCID, which is currently not an option in processors, although a "low cut" setting can be used. In our center,

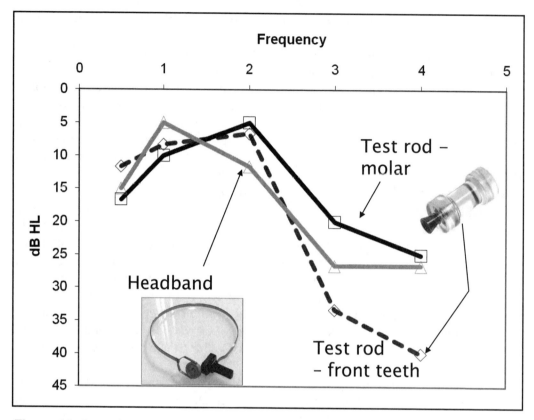

Figure 19–3. *Comparing hearing thresholds for four subjects using a test rod on front teeth, molars, and on headband.*

all patients undergo a trial with a headband for SSD for 2 weeks, with specific instructions about various complex listening environments that they should try the headband in. After this, about 70% of patients will elect for surgery, which is similar to other published reports.[21]

SURGICAL ASPECTS

The names of the different portions of the implants can be confusing, especially with more than one company manufacturing them, and some nomenclature is carried over from a period when the implants were made up of many discrete components in contrast to the composite implant used today in single-stage surgery. Figure 19–5 shows the main components of the two main BCID systems currently used.

The "screw" portion with threads, with a small flange, is called the fixture or "flange fixture." The portion which fits into this, and penetrates the skin to receive the processor in its snap coupling, is called the abutment. In single-stage surgery, these are already fitted together and are implanted as one unit. In two-stage surgery (such as in children), the flange fixture is implanted first, osseointegration achieved, and the abutment added

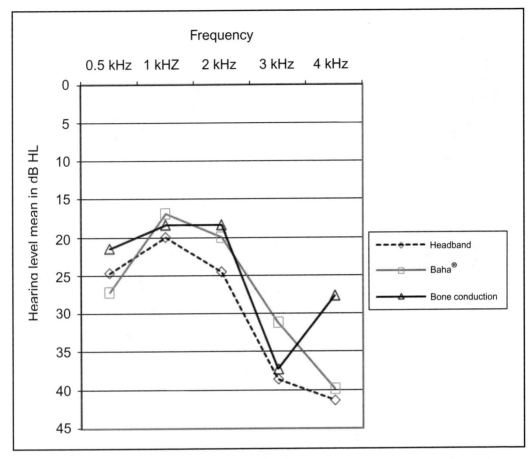

Figure 19–4. *Soundfield thresholds in 31 conductive hearing loss subjects, prior to surgery with Baha® on a headband (Headband), heir audiometric bone conduction hearing level (bone conduction), and final thresholds following surgery, using the Baha® on an abutment (Baha®).*

later. Newer implant designs have been specifically engineered to prevent a large subcutaneous pocket, and because bone often gets resorbed up to the first screw thread in the implant, with more closely spaced "microthreads" at the apical surface of the screw.

SURGICAL PRINCIPLES

There are two main considerations for successful BCID integration in percutaneous devices. The first is achieving osseo-integration with the skull (ie, forming a direct interface between the implant and bone without intervening soft tissue). Good osseointegration creates a rigid, stable fixation of the implant which transmits vibrations without loss from vibrator to skull. Titanium is one of few materials that can integrate with bone, and this requires that titanium oxide surfaces not become contaminated by other materials. Most titanium used for osseointegrated bone conduction devices is 99.75% or more pure, although alloys are used in dental implants for greater strength. From

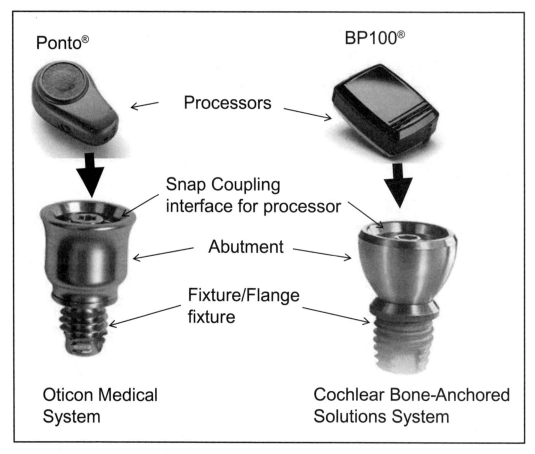

Figure 19–5. *Abutment/fixtures and processors from Oticon Medical and Cochlear BA.*

the dental implants experience, it appears that a rough surface achieved by grit blasting and/or acid etching may be more successful in attracting osteoblasts and other cellular components important for osseointegration, although any exposed rough surface can also be a harbor for bacteria.

Another component necessary for successful osseointegration is the presence of healthy cells in the bone matrix, particularly osteoblasts. Osteoblasts can be damaged by excessive heating during implant insertion, so copious cooling must be applied and slow speeds of insertion used. For instance, Eriksson and Albrektsson[23] showed that heating of rabbit tibia to 47 deg C for even 1 minute reduced bone formation around implants. Some centers emphasize preservation of periosteum for bone nutrition, and also to allow healing of any skin breakdown occurring through secondary infection, whereas other centers routinely remove periosteum around the site of the implant with equally good results.

The second main factor is a tight seal between the skin and the protruding abutment. Pockets, or loose tissue here, or excessive mobility may harbor infection, cause granulation tissue, or stimulate skin overgrowth. To achieve this, several factors have been thought to be important. These are:

1. Adequate subcutaneous debulking next to the abutment site, and seating of skin dermis onto periosteum. This prevents soft tissue mobility next to the abutment, and possibly reduces the incidence of problems with the abutment. Although this has been a mainstay of surgical technique, and is still highly recommended, there have been recent reports of little or no subcutaneous thinning,[24] with seemingly acceptable early results, long-term follow-up is needed before this can be adopted.

2. Removal of hair and hair follicles close to the abutment. These may be a source of granulation tissue and skin overgrowth.

SURGICAL STEPS

Most adult surgery is carried out under local anesthesia, using 1% xylocaine with 1:100,000 epinephrine, 5 to 10 mL. Younger pediatric surgery obviously requires a general anaesthetic.

The common types of skin incision used currently are shown in Figure 19–6, and the surgical steps are shown schematically in Figure 19–7.

1. In adults, the implant is usually placed at 45 degrees from the external ear canal, at least 5.5 cm from the external ear canal. This site might be modified if the patient wears a safety or other helmet, and in children with atresia/microtia, the ears are often lower than they should be, and the implant may be placed higher than

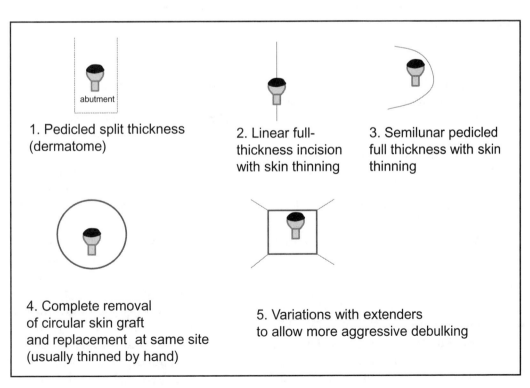

1. Pedicled split thickness (dermatome)

2. Linear full-thickness incision with skin thinning

3. Semilunar pedicled full thickness with skin thinning

4. Complete removal of circular skin graft and replacement at same site (usually thinned by hand)

5. Variations with extenders to allow more aggressive debulking

Figure 19–6. Types of skin incision for BCID insertion.

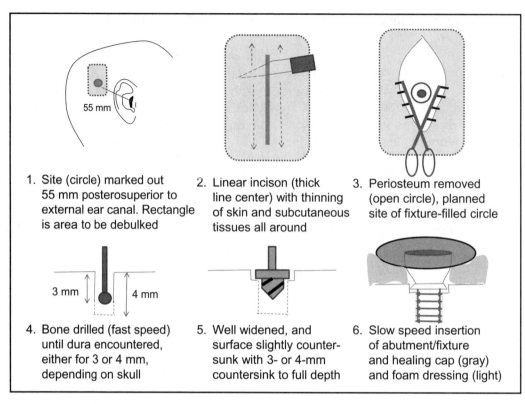

1. Site (circle) marked out 55 mm posterosuperior to external ear canal. Rectangle is area to be debulked

2. Linear incison (thick line center) with thinning of skin and subcutaneous tissues all around

3. Periosteum removed (open circle), planned site of fixture-filled circle

4. Bone drilled (fast speed) until dura encountered, either for 3 or 4 mm, depending on skull

5. Well widened, and surface slightly countersunk with 3- or 4-mm countersink to full depth

6. Slow speed insertion of abutment/fixture and healing cap (gray) and foam dressing (light)

Figure 19–7. *Surgical steps.*

the ear remnant location would indicate. If auricular atresia repair surgery is planned, the hearing and aesthetic reconstruction teams should consult prior to placement, allowing enough room for local flaps and tissue transfers.

2. There are multiple skin incisions described (Figure 19–6). The most commonly used are a semicircular incision,[5] a straight-line incision,[25] or by using the dermatome supplied with the Cochlear-BAS system. Various authors have described extensions of these incisions to allow further debulking of soft tissue. Usually, we prefer to place the abutment in the lower half of the incision because,

with time and aging, the soft tissues from superior are more likely to sag. The skin flaps are made very thin in the dermal plane so as to cut across the hair follicles, so that there is an area of hairless skin adjacent to the abutment, typically skin thickness to try to achieve here is about 0.6 mm.

3. The surrounding subcutaneous tissues are extensively debulked for 2 to 3 cm all the way around down to the periosteum. This is particularly important superiorly, and may necessitate removal of temporalis muscle. The edges should feel flat by palpation, and the goal is to have a gently sloping reduction toward the abutment site. Removal of mobile tissue

superficial to the periosteum decreases skin mobility and resultant irritation around the abutment.

4. The periosteum in the intended site of implantation (in lower half of incision) is either cut and reflected or removed in a 5- to 10-mm circle around the planned abutment site.

Using relatively high-speed drilling (2000 rpm), first a 3-mm guide hole is drilled in the calvarium, and then if there is adequate skull depth, and no damage to dura or venous sinuses, a 4-mm depth is drilled. The guide drill is relatively narrow. If bleeding occurs, it is easily controlled by bone wax or periosteum stuffed into the drill hole, and a new site can be selected if bleeding is copious. Mild oozing will be controlled by the flange fixture screw itself. Similarly, CSF leaks, if encountered, can be stopped easily with bone wax. It is important to drill to the full depth of the guide drill, since the subsequent instruments do not have a sharp cutting tip, and the implant may not sit flush with the skull.

Every attempt is made to drill perpendicular to the skull, to avoid a grossly tilted abutment, which may result in the processor touching the skin. This guide-hole is then widened, still using the higher speed, by the countersink, so called because it causes a circular depression in the skull cortex for the flange fixture, as well as widening the guide drill path. It is important not to countersink too much, as this reduces the skull thickness available for the screw portion of the flange fixture. The main purpose of the countersinking is to flatten any irregularities in the skull surface, so that the flange sits flush without torquing or tilting. The countersink is chosen as 3 or 4 mm long, depending on the depth of skull discovered by the guide drill. Our experience is, however, that even in thin skulls where the 3-mm guide drill perforates the whole skull thickness, the dura can be stripped from the surrounding endosteum, and pushed medially. Then, after countersinking, a 4mm abutment can be placed. These are more stable in the long term, especially in children.[26]

In a single-stage surgery, the flange fixture and abutment combination is then inserted using an adapter that fits into the drill, and inserted at slow drill speed (8 to 15 rpm). This is a self-tapping implant. The torque setting on the drill is set to clutch out to 20 to 32 N cm of torque. In children, a lower torque is used to avoid stripping the threads in the bone. Throughout, copious cooling irrigation is used, and titanium components are handled so as to avoid contaminating their surfaces. We prefer to stop frequently during the insertion process to let the bone cool, and remove bone chips from the countersink.

5. Once the implant is seated flush to the skull the skin edges are reapproximated to the abutment. We take particular care to approximate the first sutures around the abutment carefully, so that these are tightly approximated, and so that during closure, the abutment does not "ride up" to the upper half of the incision. Some advocate suturing the thinned skin back down to the periosteum for extra immobilization. The pressure

dressing is applied, and we prefer a soft foam type dressing to wrapped gauze, which can cause pressure necrosis. The healing cap is then placed, followed by a pressure type mastoid dressing for 24 hours.

POSTOPERATIVE CARE

The healing cap is removed at 10 to 14 days, and the sutures, if permanent, removed. Some surgeons will apply a second dressing at this time, but we prefer to leave the wound open, using only antibacterial ointments for 1 to 2 more weeks, to avoid sensitization to components from longer use. At this time, the wound is cleansed with soap and water during showering. We also prefer to use "corn pads" (used to relieve pressure on warts on the foot), on the healing cap to apply pressure at night during this stage. Later, a baby toothbrush is used to clean the sides and inside of the abutment. If there is skin breakdown early on, simple ointment such as Polysporin® can be used daily until it re-epithelializes. If there is granulation tissue then silver nitrate is applied.

Traditionally, the processor is fitted at 3 months. However, newer implants are wider (eg, the Cochlear BI300 is 4.5-mm width versus the older fixture at 3.75 mm) and more stable from the outset. Because of this improvement, many clinics now begin fitting at 6 weeks and experimental trials are ongoing for loading as early as 2 weeks.[27]

PEDIATRIC CONSIDERATIONS

In general, most authors do not recommend surgical implantation of children until the age of 5 or more,[5] although earlier surgery has been advocated by some.[28] Rehabilitation of children younger than this is quite effectively achieved with a transducer on a "softband" that fits the head with an elastic strap held in place with Velcro.[29] It is vital, for language development, to aim for a hearing solution as early as possible.

Children with atresia or chronically draining ears can frequently have other syndromic conditions, and it is important that the anesthesia and surgical teams are cognisant of these at the time of surgery. Most authors would recommend a two-stage procedure in children, perhaps up to the age of 10 in a consensus statement[30] although each case is individualized, and many centres perform single stage surgery at younger ages. Two-stage surgery involves inserting the flange fixture component at the time of the first surgery, and adding the abutment at the time of the second surgery, 3 to 6 months later, depending on age of the child and the thickness of the skull. We prefer to place the abutment without skin thinning or manipulation in the first procedure. The flange fixture is placed with a cover-screw. Some surgeons have advocated for a "sleeper" fixture, in case the first is lost due to trauma; implant loss is much higher in children than in adults.[31] We prefer to perform skin thinning and abutment placement at the second stage, because without the healing cap to apply pressure (which is only available at the second stage), there is the risk of hematoma following skin thinning. This risk is increased in young children who might traumatize or play with their incisions. Others prefer to perform skin thinning at the first stage in older children, because the abutment can then be placed under local anaesthetic in an outpatient setting.

It is important to rehabilitate children early and effectively in educational settings. Personalized FM systems that plug into the Baha® are often beneficial in the classroom. Psychological and educational professionals, along with speech language pathologists play a key role in developing language, speech, and appropriate educational milestones.

POSTOPERATIVE COMPLICATIONS AND MANAGEMENT

Although numerous rare complications have been described, there are only a few common ones. The most common are related to soft tissue complications, although even these occur less than 10% of the time. Soft tissue complications can be graded using Holgers's[32] classification (Table 19–1).

Complications include postoperative breakdown of the skin around the abutment to expose periosteum and bone. This is managed by liberal application of ointment, and protection of the site by

Table 19–1. Holgers's Classification

Grade 0: Reaction free skin around the abutment
Grade 1: Redness with slight swelling around the abutment.
Grade 2: Redness, moistness, and moderate swelling.
Grade 3: Redness, moistness, and moderate swelling with tissue granulation around the abutment.
Grade 4: Overt signs of infection resulting in removal of the implant

dressings. The skin very often will grow back in a nice thin layer. Overgrowth and thickening of the skin can also occur, particularly in adoslescents. Such problems can make it it difficult to snap the processor on, or, in severe cases can even cover the abutment.[33] This can be managed initially with steroid injections into the skin, or steroid creams,[30] but later requires either thinning of the skin (with risk of recurrence) or switching to a longer abutment, which we have found to be a very effective treatment (see also Doshi et al[33]). Other common complications are related to granulation tissue and bleeding around the abutment (managed with antibacterial creams, hygiene, and silver nitrate applications). Scalp numbness or pain have also been described.[35] In our experience, these can sometimes be very long lasting. Occasionally pain can be managed by local infiltration into the greater and lesser occipital nerves. Loss of the osseointegrated fixture is uncommon (on the order of 5% of fewer of implants),[36] but the abutment can become lose in the flange fixture, requiring retightening. Failure rates are doubled or tripled in children, particularly very young children.[37] Even small changes in the snap coupling can cause significant deterioration in sound conduction.[38,39]

PSYCHOACOUSTICS OF BONE CONDUCTION

The aim of any audiologic intervention is to restore audiologic function: specifically to facilitate the detection and localization of environmental sounds and communication in both quiet and more challenging noisy situations. The following sections discuss the performance of BCIDs in achieving this, and briefly describe the challenges in rehabilitating localization and speech.

LOCALIZATION

To derive the location of a sound source the auditory system integrates multiple cues. Salient cues to the location of a sound's position arise from the separation of the ears in space by the solid mass of the skull. Due to the ears' separation in space, the most important cues used are that for low frequencies (<1.5 kHz) the arrival time in the leading ear (closest to the sound) leads that of the lagging ear because it is closer to the source. For high

frequencies (>1.5 kHz) sounds are attenuated by the head (the head shadow effect) and their level is reduced at the lagging ear. These cues are called interaural timing differences (ITD), and interaural level differences (ILD) respectively. This relationship between attenuation and frequency is illustrated in Figure 19–8.

SPEECH PERCEPTION

Perceiving speech requires an analysis of a complex signal that varies rapidly over time. This can be a challenging task for anyone with a hearing loss, even in quiet environments. It is particularly challenging for patients with asymmetric hear-

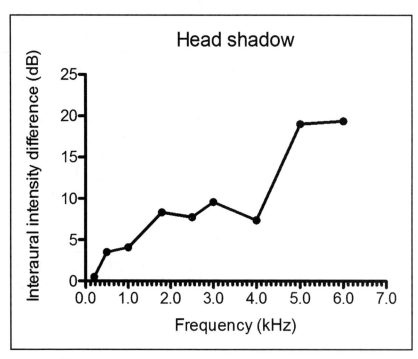

Figure 19–8. *The head shadow effect. The difference in sound pressure level in each ear canal is plotted for a range of frequencies for a signal that is presented to one side of a participant. Level differences increase with stimulus frequency. For frequencies above approximately 1.0 kHz, the head attenuates the signal by 5 to 20 dB, depending on the frequency. Data are replotted from Figure 2, Feddersen et al.*[64]

ing losses or single-sided-deafness (SSD) when the signal originates from their impaired side, owing to the head shadow effect, which attenuates signals differently across frequencies (see Fig 19–8). The head has been shown to attenuate speech signals by 5 dB.[40]

When a speech signal is embedded in noise, comprehension becomes considerably more difficult, owing to spectral and informational masking. Comprehension of the speech signal improves, however, if the speech and the noise are separated in space. There are two reasons for improved speech reception with spatial separation of signal from a noise source. The first is incidental, and is a result of the differing attenuation of a spatially separated speech and noise source by the head, so that one ear has a better signal to noise ratio. The second reason is due to binaural processing, where the brain actively exploits differing interaural differences for the speech and noise to experience less masking from the noise than in situations where there are no interaural cues.[41]

OTHER ISSUES

Although air conduction hearing aids typically only stimulate a single cochlea, hearing aids that operate through bone conduction simulate both cochleae. Thus, with a single bone vibrator, the signal arrives at both ears. However, the signals arriving at each ear are not equal, as the skull both attenuates and delays incoming signals differentially according to frequency.[15,19,42,43] Of particular relevance to fitting BCIDs is transcranial attenuation (and in some cases, transcranial gain). Figure 19–9 illustrates the amount of transcranial attenuation in dB as the

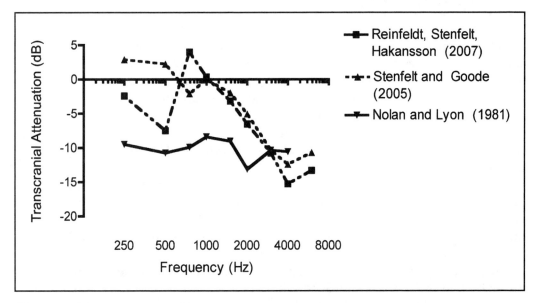

Figure 19–9. *Transcranial attenuation measured for stimulation at the mastoids. Upward triangles and dotted lines: Stenfelt and Goode,[18] measurements taken from the cochlear promontary of cadaveric heads. Upside-down triangles and solid lines: Nolan and Lyon,[19] bone conduction thresholds in hearing participants. Squares and dotted-dashed lines: Reinfelt et al,[44] data from von Békésy audiometry for bone conduction in normal participants.*

signal travels to the contralateral cochlea. The amount of inter-aural attenuation is frequency specific, and participant specific.[15,19,44] It is often cited that the amount of transcranial attenuation is 10 dB, although the standard deviations (not given in Fig 19–9) are large (for example, in Nolan and Lyon's 1981 study[19] on transcranial attenuation, standard deviations at each frequency ranged from 6.6 to 10.75 dB). This is important, as BCIDs are increasingly used for patients with SSD to overcome the head shadow effect (see Fig 19–8) and reroute sounds from the deaf side to the contralateral hearing cochlea. The following section provides a summary for BCID performance for different types of hearing loss, highlighting the success and limitations in rehabilitating localization and speech performance.

UNILATERAL CONDUCTIVE LOSS

A unilateral conductive loss, such as unilateral congenital ear canal atresia, results in a head shadow effect (see Fig 19–8), and impaired binaural processing. Fitting patients with a BCID brings thresholds for signals presented through air to the poorer ear to within 8dB of the good ear,[45] or to levels considered audiologically normal (<25 dB HL).[46] A BCID hence mostly eliminates the head shadow effect, and restores input to the cochlea on the impaired side, and restores true binaural input, although, unlike normal hearing ears, significant signals are also transmitted to the functioning ear for all frequencies and intensity levels. Whether the brain can use this binaural information may be expected to depend to some extent on its previous experience with

receiving sound from the conductive loss ear. Unlike congenital SNHLs, even ears with congenital atresia have received some stimulation by bone conduction, such as own voice, body sounds or loud sounds, from infancy, but never truly participated in binaural processing of spatial sounds.

SPEECH PERCEPTION

Patients with unilateral conductive losses generally have normal speech comprehension unless the speech is presented toward their deaf side. Research shows that improvements for speech in quiet following BCID fitting are fairly participant specific.[45]

Performance improvements are considerably greater when a spatially separated noise source is presented alongside the signal. Studies find fairly consistently that if noise is placed on the functioning side, the addition of a BCID to the poorer ear improves performance.[45,46] When noise is on the impaired side, performance is not significantly altered;[45,46] some individual participants show improvements whereas others show deterioration in performance.

LOCALIZATION

Localization is typically impaired in patients with unilateral conductive losses. The degree of impairment, however, depends on the level of the loss, and the listening experience of the patient (patients with congenital conductive losses typically perform worse than patients with acquired losses). Improvements with the addition of a BCID can be large; one study showed an improvement in error from 74° to 26°,[45] whereas other studies show more modest improvements (eg, an 8° reduction in error; Wazen et al, 2001).[47] The extent of improvements is participant specific, with some participants showing much greater improvements than others.[45-47]

BILATERAL CONDUCTIVE LOSS

Patients with bilateral conductive losses, such as those with bilateral aural atresia can be very successfully rehabilitated with BCIDs. Clinicians have historically fitted one device, due to costs associated with fitting a second device. This approach improves detectability and speech perception from the front and from the aided side. Fitting with a single aid does not overcome the head shadow

effect, or recover binaural processing. Figure 19–10 shows improvements in thresholds for bilateral BCIDs relative to unilateral BCIDs. Data show that, with the addition of a second device, improvements of up to 15 dB are observed on the shadow side.

SPEECH IN QUIET

Unilateral BCIDs restore hearing to that of the bone curve, unless stimuli originate from the impaired side. Bilateral BCIDs yield a 4 to 6 dB improvement in speech comprehension in quiet relative to unilateral BCIDs,[48-50] which is consistent with the doubling in power associated with the addition of a second device.

Improvements in speech comprehension in noise are equivocal and seem

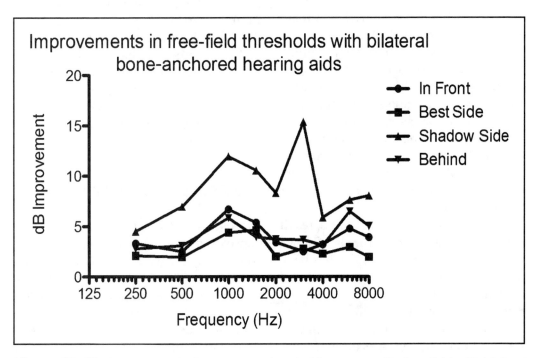

Figure 19–10. *Improvements in pure-tone thresholds measured in free field with bilateral BCIDs relative to unilateral BCIDs. Data are replotted from Priwin et al.[50]*

to depend on the location of the speech and noise signals relative to the aided and unaided sides. For unilateral BCIDs, speech in noise performance improves when the speech signal is presented toward the aided side, or the noise toward the unaided side. The addition of a second BCID device appears to boost thresholds only when the addition the second device overcomes the head shadow.[48,49] If noise surrounds the participant, with the speech in front, performance for bilateral BCIDs improves by 2.8 dB.

LOCALIZATION

Patients with bilateral conductive losses and a single BCID typically demonstrate poor sound localization abilities. In unilateral BCID users, there is a tendency to mislocalise sounds toward the amplified ear.[50] When localization performance for bilateral BCIDs is compared to unilateral BCIDs, bilateral BCIDs outperform unilateral BCIDs.[48–50] Frequency is unimportant, with participants able to localize low frequency and high frequency noise bursts—which suggests that binaural processing is in play as interaural intensity and timing differences are being used.[48–50] Note that localization performance is not at normal levels—participants do not have normal spatial acuity, although it is improved significantly.[48]

Whether improvements are a result of binaural processing, or simply of alleviation of the head shadow effect has been probed by scientists who measured binaural masking level differences. Binaural masking level difference is an effect where detection of a signal in noise when presented to one ear, improves through routing either the signal or the noise through both ears, but inducing a phase offset to either the signal or the noise. Through air, when phase offsets are applied to the signal or the noise, signal detection thresholds improve by up to 15 dB. There is significant release from masking using bilateral BCIDs; however, the effect is small compared to air conduction (6 dB improvement; Bosman et al, 2001).[48] This suggests that although some binaural processing is restored, binaural processing is not entirely rehabilitated.

UNILATERAL SENSORINEURAL LOSS (SINGLE-SIDED DEAFNESS; SSD)

Unilateral sensorineural losses handicap patients in two ways: due to the head shadow effect, and due to the loss of binaural processing. Because of this, unilateral sensorineural losses are associated with a number of handicaps such as impaired localization, impaired speech in noise performance, and reduced quality of life.[51–55] Unlike patients with unilateral conductive losses, patients with SSD cannot restore binaural function.

SPEECH PERCEPTION

The use of a BCID in patients with SSD improves performance of speech perception in quiet.[47,56] Where a spatially separate noise source is added, the addition of a BCID improves performance in situations where the alleviation of the head shadow effect increases the level of the speech signal relative to the level of the noise signal.[40,47,56,57]

LOCALIZATION

Not surprisingly, the addition of a BCID does not improve localization.[40,56,57]

ALTERNATIVE REHABILITATION STRATEGIES

It should be remembered that standard air conduction hearing aids are improving all the time, and for SSD, for instance, newer wireless types of contralateral routing of sound (CROS) aids are emerging that may show increased patient acceptance. With SSD on one side, and hearing loss on the contralateral side, a BiCROS (bilateral CROS) aid may be more appropriate, since it allows amplification on the more intact hearing loss side as well as contralateral routing of sound.

In some patients, cosmetic acceptance, or skin complications are an issue with BCID acceptance. In others, the sensorineural hearing loss component of the mixed hearing loss is too severe to be ameliorated by BCIDs. In both cases, alternate methods have been espoused, particularly the use of middle ear implants. The MED-EL Vibrant Soundbridge® has been reported placed on the round window membrane in ears with no other ossicles, and may give more "over-closure" of the bone curve than a standard BCID in mixed hearing loss cases.[58] It has also been successfully used, placed on the incus in atretic ears.[59] Middle ear drivers placed on the ossicular chain, rather than the round window, can also provide far more power to the cochlea than a BCID placed distally on the skull, and so may be an intermediate step between BCIDs and cochlear implants. With new electroacoustic stimu-lation strategies, short electrode cochlear implants can be place in the basal turn, with residual low frequency hearing stimulated with conventional acoustic hearing aids. For SSD, there are recent reports of successful implantation and acceptance of a cochlear implant on the deaf side.[60]

In general, particularly in malformed ears, it should be remembered that the closer to the cochlea that a device is placed, the greater is the risk to the facial nerve and inner ear, and such risks are far higher for middle ear placement than the relatively safe location of the BCID. All these developments make candidate selection even more complex, with significant overlap at the boundaries of where one technology is effective to where the next is more effective. This has to be balanced with the incremental cost and risk of moving between technologies.

FUTURE DIRECTIONS

Future directions are trending toward either a fully implantable device (eg, Hakansson, 2011),[61] or removable devices that are comfortable to wear. These include alternate placement methods (eg, Otomag Alpha®, which uses an implanted magnet as a retainer for a transcutaneous driver),[62] or on teeth (Soundbite®, Sonitus Medical).[63] We have reported on a new fully implantable piezoelectric technology that launches bending waves into the skull, a fundamentally new mode of bone conduction compared to all the other the inertial drivers.[13] Many more devices are expected in the next decade. It is unlikely that bone conduction devices will achieve, by themselves, enough power to rehabilitate severe sensorineural hearing losses.

It is interesting to note that bone-conduction devices are starting to cross into consumer applications, for music or cell phone use, currently in niche markets such as swimmers. These are likely to spur another wave of innovation in BCH applications.

REFERENCES

1. Berger KW. Early bone conduction hearing aid devices. *Arch Otolaryngol.* 1976 May;102(5):315–318.
2. von Békésy G. Zur Theorie des Horens bei der Schallaufnahme durch Knochenleitung. *Ann Physik.* 1932;13:111–136
3. Khanna SM, Tonndorf J, Queller J. Mechanical parameters of hearing by bone conduction. *J Acoust Soc Amer.* 1976; 60:139–154.
4. Stenfelt S. Simultaneous cancellation of air and bone conduction tones at two frequencies: extension of the famous experiment by von Békésy. *Hear Res.* 2007;225: 105–116.
5. Tjellström A, Hakansson B, Granström G. Bone-anchored hearing aids: current status in adults and children. *Otolaryngol Clin North Am.* 2001;34:337–364.
6. Hakansson B, Tjellström A, Rosenhall U, Carlsson P. The bone-anchored hearing aid. Principal design and a psychoacoustical evaluation. *Acta Otolaryngol.* 1985; 100:229–239.
7. Baguley DM, Bird J, Humphriss RL, Prevost AT. The evidence base for the application of contralateral bone anchored hearing aids in acquired unilateral sensorineural hearing loss in adults. *Clin Otolaryngol.* 2006 Feb;31(1):6–14.
8. Bance M, Abel SM, Papsin BC, Wade P, Vendramini J. A comparison of the audiometric performance of bone anchored hearing aids and air conduction hearing aids. *Otol Neurotol.* 2002 Nov;23(6):912–919.

9. Mylanus EA, van der Pouw KC, Snik AF, Cremers CW. Intraindividual comparison of the bone-anchored hearing aid and air-conduction hearing aids. *Arch Otolaryngol Head Neck Surg.* 1998 Mar;124(3):271–276.
10. Hakansson B. The balanced electromagnetic separation transducer. *J Acoust Soc Am.* 2003;113(2):818–825.
11. Moffett MB, Clark AE, Wun-Fogle M, Linberg J, Teter JP, McLaughlin EA. Characterization of Terfenol-D for magnetostrictive transducers. *J Acoust Soc Am.* 1991;89:1448.
12. Zhang S, Shrout T. Relaxor-PT single crystals: observations and developments. *IEEE Trans Ultrason Ferroelectr Freq Control.* 2010 Oct;57(10):2138–2146.
13. Adamson RB, Bance M, Brown JA. A piezoelectric bone-conduction bending hearing actuator. *J Acoust Soc Am.* 2010 Oct; 128(4):2003–2008.
14. Tonndorf J. Bone conduction: studies in experimental animals. *Acta Otolaryngol.* 1966;213:1–132.
15. Stenfelt S, Goode RL. Bone-conducted sound: physiological and clinical aspects. *Otol Neurotol.* 2005b Nov;26(6):1245–1261.
16. Håkansson B, Brandt A, Carlsson P, Tjellström A., Resonance frequencies of the human skull in vivo. *J Acoust Soc Am.* 1994 Mar;95(3):1474–1481.
17. Håkansson B, Carlsson P, Brandt A, Stenfelt S. Linearity of sound transmission through the human skull in vivo. *J Acoust Soc Am.* 1996 Apr;99(4 pt 1):2239–2243.
18. Stenfelt S, Goode RL. Transmission properties of bone conducted sound: measurements in cadaver heads. *J Acoust Soc Am.* 2005a Oct;118(4):2373–2391.
19. Nolan M, Lyon DJ. Transcranial attenuation in bone conduction audiometry. *J Laryngol Otol.* 1981;95:597–608.
20. Arunachalam PS, Kilby D, Meikle D, Davison T, Johnson IJM. Bone-anchored hearing aid quality of life assessed by Glasgow Benefit Inventory. *Laryngoscope.* 2001; 111:1260–1263
21. Hol MKS, Bosman AJ, Snik AFM, Mylanus EAM, Cremers CWRJ. Bone anchored

hearing aid in unilateral inner dear deafness: a study of 20 patients. *Audiol Neurotol.* 2004a;9:274–281.

22. Verstraeten N, Zarowski AJ, Somers T, Riff D, Offeciers EF. Comparison of the audiologic results obtained with the bone-anchored hearing aid attached to the headband, the testband, and to the "snap" abutment. *Otol Neurotol.* 2009 Jan;30(1): 70–75.

23. Eriksson RA, Albrektsson T. The effect of heat on bone regeneration: an experimental study in the rabbit using the bone growth chamber. *J Oral Maxillofac Surg.* 1984;42:705–711.

24. Weber PC. *Minimally invasive approach for Baha surgery.* Abstracts of 3rd International Symposium Bone Conduction Hearing and Craniofacial Osseointegration, Sarasota, Florida. March 23–26, 2011.

25. De Wolf MJF, Hol MKS, Huygen PL, Mylanus EAM, Cremers CWRJ. Clinical outcome of the simplified surgical technique for BAHA implantation. *Otol Neurotol.* 2008;29:1100–1108.

26. Granström G, Bergström K, Odersjo M, Tjellström A. Osseointegrated implants in children: experience from our first 100 patients. *Otolaryngol Head Neck Surg.* 2001;125:85–92.

27. Green K. *First experiences of loading a BAHA sound processor at 2 weeks following surgery.* Abstracts of the 3rd International Symposium on Bone Conduction Hearing and Craniofacial Osseointegration, Sarasota Florida. March 23–26 2011.

28. Davids T, Gordon KA, Clutton D, Papsin BC. Bone-anchored hearing aids in infants and children younger than 5 years. *Arch Otolaryngol Head Neck Surg.* 2007 Jan; 133(1):51–55.

29. Hol MK, Cremers CW, Coppens-Schellekens W, Snik AF. The BAHA Softband. A new treatment for young children with bilateral congenital aural atresia. *Int J Pediatr Otorhinolaryngol.* 2005 Jul;69(7):973–980.

30. Snik AF, Mylanus EA, Proops DW, et al. Consensus statements on the BAHA system: where do we stand at present? *Ann Otol Rhinol Laryngol Suppl.* 2005 Dec; 195:2–12.

31. Zeitoun H, De R, Thompson SD, Proops DW. Osseointegrated implants in the management of childhood ear abnormalities: with particular emphasis on complications. *J Laryngol Otol.* 2002 Feb;116(2):87–91.

32. Holgers KM, Tjellström A, Bjursten LM, Erlandsson BE. Soft tissue reactions around percutaneous implants: a clinical study of soft tissue conditions around skin-penetrating titanium implants for bone-anchored hearing aids. *Amer J Otol.* 1988 Jan;9(1):56–59.

33. Doshi J, McDermott AL, Reid A, Proops D. The 8.5mm abutment in children: the Birmingham bone-anchored hearing aid program experience. *Otol Neurotol.* 2010 Jun;31(4):612–614.

34. Falcone MT, Kaylie DM, Labadie RF, Haynes DS. Bone-anchored hearing aid abutment skin overgrowth reduction with clobetasol. *Otolaryngol Head Neck Surg.* 2008;139:829–832.

35. Mylanus EA, Johansson CB, Cremers CW. Craniofacial titanium implants and chronic pain: histologic findings. *Otol Neurotol.* 2002 Nov;23(6):920–925.

36. van der Pouw CT, Mylanus EA, Cremers CW. Percutaneous implants in the temporal bone for securing a bone conductor: surgical methods and results. *Ann Otol Rhinol Laryngol.* 1999 Jun;108(6):532–536.

37. McDermott AL, Williams J, Kuo M, Reid A, Proops D. The Birmingham pediatric bone-anchored hearing aid program: a 15-year experience. *Otol Neurotol.* 2009 Feb;30(2):178–183.

38. Majdalawieh O, Van Wijhe RG, Bance M. Is there loss of vibration amplitude across the snap coupling of the bone-anchored hearing aid? *Otol Neurotol.* 2006 Apr; 27(3):342–345.

39. Majdalawieh O, Van Wijhe RG, Bance M. Output vibration measurements of bone-anchored hearing AIDS. *Otol Neurotol.* 2006 Jun;27(4):519–530.

40. Bosman AJ, Hol MKS, Mylanus EAM, Cremers CWRJ. Bone-anchored hearing aids in unilateral inner ear deafness. *Acta Otolaryngolica*. 2003;123:258–260.

41. Freyman RL, Helfer KS, McCall DD, Clifton RK. The role of perceived spatial separation in the unmasking of speech. *J Acoust Soc Amer*. 1999;106:3578–3588.

42. Hurley RM, Berger KW. The relationship between vibrator placement and bone conduction measurements with monaurally deaf subjects. *J Aud Res*. 1970;10:147–150.

43. Stenfelt S, Hakansson B, Tjellstrom A. Vibration characteristics of bone conducted sound in vitro. *J Acoust Soc Amer*. 2000;107:422–431.

44. Reinfeldt S, Stenfelt T, Good, Hakansson B. Examination of bone-conducted transmission from sound field excitation measured by thresholds, ear-canal sound pressure, and skull vibrations. *J Acoust Soc Amer*. 2007;121:1576–1587.

45. Snik AFM, Mylanus EAM, Cremers CWRJ. The bone-anchored hearing aid in patients with unilateral air-bone gap. *Otol Neurotol*. 2002;23:61–66.

46. Kunst SJW; Leijendeckers JM, Mylanus EAM, Hol MKS, Snik AFM, Cremers CWRJ. Bone-anchored hearing aid system application for unilateral congenital conductive hearing impairment: audiometric results. *Otol Neurotol*. 2007;29:2–7.

47. Wazen JJ, Spitzer JB, Ghossaini SN, et al. Transcranial contralateral cochlear stimulation in unilateral deafness. *Otolaryngol Head Neck Surg*. 2003;129:248–254.

48. Bosman AJ, Snik AM, van der Pouw CTM, Mylanus EAM, Cremers CWRJ. Audiometric evaluation of bilaterally fitted bone-anchored hearing aids. *Int J Audiol*. 2001;40:158–167.

49. van der Pouw KTM, Snik AF, Cremers CWRJ. Audiometric results of bilateral bone-anchored hearing aid application in patients with bilateral congenital aural atresia. *Laryngoscope*. 1998;108:548–553.

50. Priwin C, Stenfelt S, Granström G, Tjellström A, Håkansson B. Bilateral bone-anchored hearing aids (BAHAs): An audiometric evaluation. *Laryngoscope*. 2004;114:77–84.

51. Newman CW, Sandridge SA, Wodzisz LM. Longitudinal benefit from and satisfaction with the Baha system for patients with acquired unilateral sensorineural hearing loss. *Otol Neurotol*. 2008;29:1123–1131

52. Welsh LW, Welsh JJ, Rosen LF, et al. Functional impairments due to unilateral deafness. *Ann Otol Rhinol Laryngol*. 2004;113:987–993.

53. Newman CW, Jacobson GP, Hug GA, Sandridge SA. Perceived hearing handicap of patients with unilateral or mild hearing loss. *Ann Otol Rhinol Laryngol*. 1997;106:210–214.

54. Newman CW, Weinstein BE, Jacobson GP, Hug GA. The Hearing Handicap Inventory for Adults: psychometric adequacy and audiometric correlates. *Ear Hear*. 1990;11:430–433.

55. Chiossoine-Kerdel JA, Baguley DM, Stoddart RL, Moffat DA. An investigation of the audiologic handicap associated with unilateral sudden sensorineural hearing loss. *Amer J Otol*. 2000;21:645–651.

56. Lin LM, Bowditch S, Anderson MJ, May B, Cox KM, Niparko JK. (2006). Amplification in the rehabilitation of unilateral deafness: speech in noise and directional hearing effects with bone-anchored hearing and contralateral routing of signal amplification. *Otol Neurotol*. 2006;27:172–182.

57. Hol MK, Spath MA, Krabbe PF, et al. The bone-anchored hearing aid: quality-of-life assessment. *Arch Otolaryngol Head Neck Surg*. 2004b Apr;130(4):394–399.

58. Colletti V, Soli S, Carner M, Colletti L, Treatment of mixed hearing losses via implantation of a vibratory transducer on the round window. *Int J Audiol*. 2006;45:600–608.

59. Frenzel H, Hanke F, Beltrame M, Steffen A, Schönweiler R, Wollenberg B. Application of the Vibrant Soundbridge to unilateral osseous atresia cases. *Laryngoscope*. 2009;119:67–74.

60. Vermeire K, Van de Heyning P. Binaural hearing after cochlear implantation in subjects with unilateral sensorineural deafness and tinnitus. *Audiol Neurotol.* 2009;14(3):163–171.

61. Hakansson B. The future of bone conduction hearing devices. *Adv Otorhinolaryngol.* 2011;71:140–152.

62. Siegert R: Magnetic coupling of partially implantable bone conduction hearing aids without open implants. *Laryngorhinootologie.* 2010;89:346–351.

63. Popelka GR, Derebery J, Blevins NH, et al. Preliminary evaluation of a novel bone-conduction device for singlesided deafness. *Otol Neurotol.* 2010;31:492–497.

64. Feddersen WE, Sandel TT, Teas DC, Jeffress LA. Localisation of high-frequency tones. *J Acoust Soc Am.* 1957;29:988–991.

Chapter 20

Baha® Surgery: Evolution, Techniques, and Complications

DAVID A. GUDIS AND MICHAEL J. RUCKENSTEIN

INTRODUCTION

The implantation of a Baha® device is a relatively simple procedure that yields gratifying results in the vast majority of cases. That said, strict adherence to certain key principles is required to ensure that this positive result is obtained. This chapter reviews the evolution of the surgical techniques for Baha® implantation, the authors' recommendations for surgical technique, and the management of complications of Baha® surgery.

OSTEOINTEGRATION

Osteointegration (or *osseointegration*), first described by Brånemark and colleagues in the 1960s in Sweden, is the process by which native vital bone forms a direct structural and functional interface with a prosthetic implant without any intervening connective tissue or sur-

rounding inflammation.[1,2] In his initial canine studies of titanium dental prostheses, Brånemark noted on histology that bone "appeared to grow into all the minute pits and impressions" of his implants. Today the principle of osteointegration still governs the design and surgical technique for implantable bone-anchored hearing aids. Titanium continues to be the material of choice for bone anchored hearing aids, as it is generally resistant to erosion by biologic tissues or fluids, and the oxide layer which forms on its surface tends to favor integration and prevent inflammatory rejection by native tissue. Additionally, titanium's compatibility with magnetic resonance and computed tomography imaging becomes invaluable in a population for whom serial imaging of the temporal region may be necessary.

INDICATIONS FOR BAHA®

The Baha® is indicated for patients with unilateral or bilateral conductive hearing loss or in patients with mixed hearing loss (bone conduction pure-tone average <45 dB at 0.5, 1, 2, 3 kHz). It is also indicated in patients with unilateral severe to profound sensorineural hearing loss.

SURGICAL TECHNIQUE

THE DEVICE

The Baha® system consists of three components: a titanium implant, a percutaneous abutment, and an external sound processor. The titanium implant is surgically embedded into the cortex of the mastoid bone ipsilateral to the hearing-impaired ear, and the percutaneous abutment is affixed to the implant. Sufficient time postoperatively must then be allowed for adequate osteointegration to occur. The osteointegration of the implant not only creates a firm structural bond to the skull to support the connected sound processor, but the direct osseous interface with the metal also facilitates efficient mechanical conduction of sound without the dampening effect of intervening soft tissue observed in transcutaneous bone-conduction amplification devices. After a designated period of time to allow for osteointegration the sound processor is snapped onto the percutaneous abutment.

EVOLUTION OF BAHA® SURGERY

The Baha® device and its surgical implantation were introduced by Tjellström and colleagues in 1977 as a two-stage procedure, and since its inception the surgery has become progressively more efficient with lower risk of complications. The prin-

ciples of osteointegration had been established by Brånemark[1] in his studies with titanium dental implants and subsequent development of percutaneous abutments for reconstructive facial prosthetics. However, the management of the soft tissue surrounding an implanted bone conduction amplification device required refinement. As complications involving this soft tissue became apparent from early Baha® techniques, the procedure underwent several modifications (Fig 20–1).

It was noted early on that a thinner and hairless soft tissue flap overlying the implant and surrounding the abutment was less likely to become inflamed. Therefore, during the 1980s the first stage of the procedure involved removing a circular composite of skin and soft tissue down to periosteum from the hear-bearing scalp overlying the mastoid bone. The periosteum was incised and elevated. A guided drill was then used to create a well for the implant, and the implant was then drilled into place. A free full-thickness skin graft was harvested ipsilaterally from the hairless postauricular sulcus. The free graft, thinner than the native soft tissue that was removed, was placed over the implant and closed circumferentially. The skin graft harvest site was closed primarily. The second stage of the procedure, performed after a period of three to four months to allow time for adequate osteointegration, involved incising the flap to remove a circular section of skin and expose the implant, and attaching the percutaneous abutment. The sound processor would then be attached several weeks later. However, the free skin graft was found to undergo partial necrosis in 15.7% of patients and total necrosis in 0.9% of patients.[3,4] Several attempts were made to refine the free-flap technique, with mixed results.[5–7]

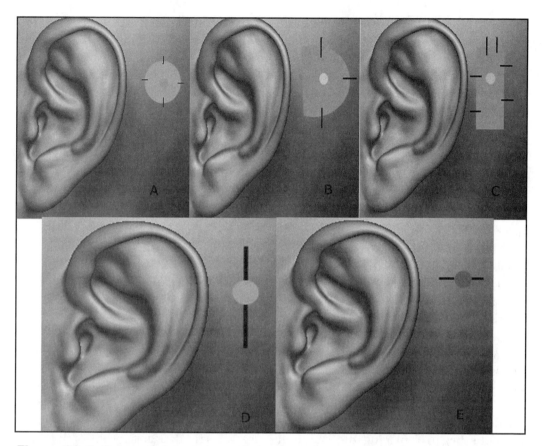

Figure 20–1. *The evolution of the techniques employed for Baha® implantation is illustrated.* **A.** *The original technique employed a full-thickness skin graft harvested from the postauricular crease. The graft was used to cover a circular region that had been denuded of skin and subcutaneous tissues to the level of the periosteum. The implant was placed 55 to 65 mm posterior-superior to the external auditory meatus and brought through the center of the graft.* **B.** *An anteriorly based full-thickness skin flap was elevated, with excision of the subcutaneous tissues to the level of the periosteum. The skin flap was then replaced and sutured in place.* **C.** *A specialized dermatome is used to elevate a split-thickness skin graft. The soft tissues are excised to the level of the periosteum with undermining and excision of the soft tissues around the perimeter of the graft site. The implant is brought through the center of the graft and the graft is sutured in place and tacked to the underlying periosteum.* **D.** *A linear vertical excision is made of approximately 3.5 cm to 4.0 cm is made. Subcutaneous tissues anterior and posterior to the incision are undermined and excised. The implant is brought through the incision line.* **E.** *The "Weber" approach currently utilized by the senior author. A 1.5-cm horizontal incision is made centered 55mm to 65 mm posterior to the external auditory meatus. Subcutaneous tissues are undermined and excised and the implant is brought through the incision line.*

To preserve adequate blood supply to the overlying soft tissue, an anteriorly based skin flap was subsequently developed instead of a free graft for the first stage of the procedure. This technique involved a semicircular incision made in the hear-bearing scalp over the mastoid bone after shaving the region. A skin flap pedicled anteriorly was then raised and thinned with a blade to remove the hair follicles. The subcutaneous tissue was elevated to expose bone, and after similarly drilling the implant into place the subcutaneous tissue was removed. The incision was undermined circumferentially and tacked to underlying periosteum, and the overlying skin flap was laid down and closed primarily. The incidence of partial necrosis of the skin flap decreased to 9.8% and total necrosis to 0.6% of patients, and periodic resultant inflammation was thought to be secondary to remnant hair follicles. Further refinement of these techniques led to a reduction in incidence of adverse skin reactions, but the procedure remained time consuming and results were inconsistent among practitioners.[3-5,8]

In 1989, with the observed decreased incidence of skin flap necrosis, some surgeons began replacing the standard two-staged procedure with a single-stage procedure in adults.[4] In the single-stage procedure, the percutaneous abutment was placed at the same time as the initial implant procedure. Studies confirmed the safety and efficacy of the single-stage Baha® in adults, yet for several more years, the Baha® was still placed in a two-stage procedure in children to allow for osteointegration of younger bone. More recently, however, some studies suggest that the single-stage procedure is safe in the pediatric population as well.[8,9] The single-stage procedure added the use of a healing cap that clipped to the abutment and provided protection to the underlying skin.

The procedure was modified further with the introduction of a specially designed dermatome in 2001 compatible with the drill equipment. This device formalized the practice utilized by a number of surgeons of creating a split thickness skin graft taken from the implant site, removing the underlying soft tissues, and then replacing the graft. After the postauricular region was shaved, the dermatome was used to raise a skin flap of 0.6-mm thickness and 25-mm width, leaving the hair follicles in the subcutaneous tissue. Again, after placement of the implant, the subcutaneous tissue including hair follicles was removed and the skin flap was laid down upon the implant and closed primarily. The Baha® skin punch, designed in conjunction with the implant, was then used to bring the abutment through the skin.

Although decreased in incidence, soft tissue complications including skin flap necrosis remained present with the dermatome technique. The procedure has since been further simplified to a single-stage simplified implantation without the use of a skin flap, and results of the safety and efficacy have been positive. Although some surgeons were refining the pedicled flap and dermatome techniques, a group in Nijmegen, Netherlands, in the 1990s began reducing the approach to a simplified single-stage technique with a curvilinear incision closed around the protruding abutment.[10] In 2007 Bovo and others refined the technique further.[11,12] Bovo reported a simplified Baha® implantation technique without the use of a skin flap that was a more rapid procedure with a very low risk of infection or necrosis of the overlying soft tissue. The technique, reported in a small series of 5 patients, described a vertical 4- to 5-cm incision through a circle approximately 4 cm in diameter, representing the site of the implant centered 5.5 cm posterior-superior to the external auditory canal.

After removing the periosteum of the region corresponding to the circle on the skin, the implant was placed into the bone in the traditional fashion. The skin on both sides of the incision was then undermined, and the subcutaneous tissue and muscle was removed circumferentially around the implant to create a circular lodging site. The incision was then sutured closed on both sides of the abutment, protruding through its center, and ointment gauze was packed under the healing cup. Using a similar simplified and efficient technique in a much larger series of patients, the Nijmegen group also reported encouraging results in 2008.[12]

The postoperative healing period traditionally recommended by the Baha® manufacturing company and pioneers of the technique to allow for adequate osteointegration was 3 months for adults and 4 to 6 months for children. Even when loading the titanium implant with the abutment in the single-stage technique, it was believed that a shorter waiting period would fail to allow sufficient maturation and strength of the biological bond between the titanium oxide and bone to support the weight and function of the sound processor. As the surgical implantation technique was revised for safety and efficiency, so too was the postoperative course for patients. Studies have since shown that a shorter waiting period of 6 weeks in adults is safe for patients, with enhanced patient satisfaction and no increase in failure of osteointegration or implant extrusion.[13] In children, some investigators have adjusted the waiting period based on the thickness of bone at the time of implantation.[14]

More recently, Weber has described an even further simplification in the technique involving a small horizontal incision (1.5 cm) with minimal undermining (personal communication). The senior author has utilized this technique successfully, described in detail below.

PROCEDURE IN DETAIL AS PERFORMED BY SENIOR AUTHOR

The procedure is performed in an outpatient ambulatory setting. The majority of cases in adults can be performed under local anesthesia. In some patients the addition of parenteral analgesia and sedation (MAC) is required. Pediatric patients require general anesthesia. The patient is supine with head turned away from the surgeon, in standard otologic positioning. The location on the scalp overlying the ultimate position of the implant is marked with a marking pen approximately 5 to 6 cm posterosuperior to the external auditory meatus. A small surrounding region of the scalp, approximately 3 × 3 cm, is shaved, and the patient is prepped and draped in the standard fashion.

The incision line is infiltrated with 1% lidocaine solution with epinephrine 1:100,000 concentration. Incision is made with a No. 15 blade, and sharp dissection is carried down to the periosteum (Fig 20–2). Hemostasis is usually achieved with either monopolar or bipolar electrocautery. The incision line is then undermined approximately 0.5 to 1.5 cm circumferentially, and the undermined subcutaneous tissue and muscle is removed down to periosteum. The diameter of the undermined region depends on the thickness of the scalp, with thicker scalps requiring a wider area undermined. A circular section of periosteum approximately 3 to 4 mm in diameter centered under the incision is removed with the undermined tissue, leaving exposed bone for the titanium implant.

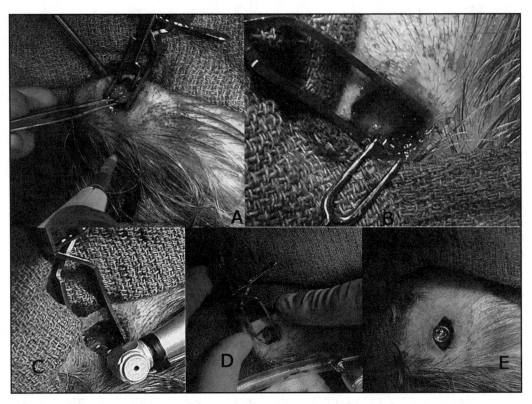

Figure 20–2. A. *A 1.5-cm horizontal incision is made and the subcutaneous tissues are undermined and excised.* **B.** *Dissection is carried down to the periosteum and a circular area of periosteum 4 mm in diameter is excised.* **C.** *A drill hole is made 55 to 65 mm postero-superior to the external auditory meatus.* **D.** *The drill hole is widened using the countersink bit.* **E.** *The implant is inserted.*

Once exposure is complete, the implant may be placed. Copious irrigation must be used throughout the drilling. During the drilling, the bits should be withdrawn periodically to allow for cleaning and irrigation for the bit and drill hole. The drill motor has preprogrammed settings. The drill guide hole and countersink hole are drilled at a speed of 2000 rPM. In general the 4-mm length screw is used. However, patients with thinner bone, such as children, may require a 3-mm implant. If there is any question as to the thickness of the bone in the pediatric patient, a 3-mm guide hole may be drilled initially that can then be deepened to 4 mm if the bone is found to be adequate. In adults, a 4-mm deep guide hole can be drilled initially. The drill countersink is then used to widen the hole at 2000 rpm with adequate irrigation. After the hole has been irrigated and suctioned clear of bone dust, the implant is grasped with the abutment inserter attachment for the drill, with the drill rotating at a low speed at a torque of 50 newtons/m^2. The implant is placed into the hole using a low drill speed, initially without irrigation. Irrigation is begun only when the threads of the implant begin to seat within the bone. Two 3-0 Vicryl sutures are used to close the incision (Fig 20–3).

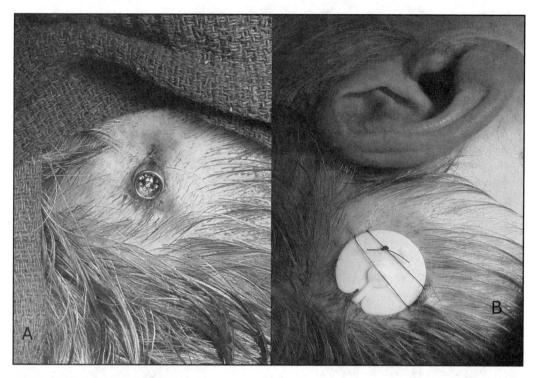

Figure 20–3. A. *Sutures are placed, one anterior and one posterior to the implant. The sutures should include the periosteal layer in order to tack the tissues in place.* **B.** *The healing cap is held in place with a single Prolene 2-0 suture. Xeroform impregnated gauze is placed medial to the healing cap. The dressing is removed 1 week after surgery.*

Xeroform®-impregnated gauze is placed around the abutment and the healing cap is then clipped onto the abutment. The senior author generally places a Prolene suture across the healing cap to secure it in place and prevent it from disengaging when the patient is active. The procedure is generally completed in approximately 25 minutes and the dressing removed one week subsequent to the surgery. It should be noted that for this technique, using the 9-mm abutment coupled to the 4-mm implant often yields a better result in terms of abutment exposure and lack of skin overgrowth when compared to the 6-mm abutment. Final results achieved with this technique are illustrated in Figure 20–4.

COMPLICATIONS AND MANAGEMENT

The complications of Baha® surgery can be broadly divided into failure of osteointegration, bone reaction or overgrowth, and soft tissue reaction, loss, or overgrowth (Table 20–1).

FAILURE OF OSTEOINTEGRATION

Inadequate osteointegration can result in a range of outcomes, from poor bone conduction of sound to complete extrusion of the implant. The thickness of the

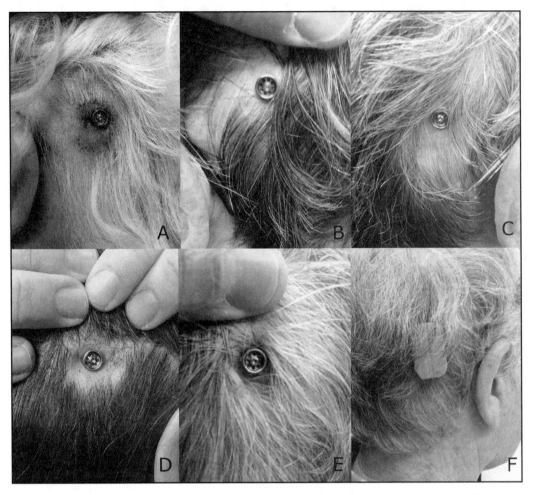

Figure 20–4. A. Baha® implant in place 1 week after surgery. **B through E**. Baha® implant in 4 different patients at least 6 months following surgery. **F**. Same patient as illustrated in F with his Baha® Intenso in place.

Table 20–1. Relative Contraindications to Baha® Implantation

- History of radiation therapy to region
- History of Baha® implantation with failure of osteointegration
- Primary disorders of bone mineralization (such as osteogenesis imperfecta)
- Medical conditions that compromise vascular health (such as diabetes mellitus, tobacco abuse)
- Thin mastoid cortex (less than 3 mm)

bone is a critical factor in the success of osteointegration, which becomes particularly relevant in the pediatric population. In general it has been found that bone thick enough to support a 3-mm implant is more likely to successfully integrate the implant.[15] As such, the current FDA guidelines limit implantation of implantable bone conduction devices to 5 years of age, although several investigators have reported success with implantation in patients as young as one year of age. The traditional two-stage procedure is more likely to be performed in this population, and some investigators have further developed a three-stage procedure to augment the recipient site with bone grafting prior to implantation.[14] The timing of loading the implant with the abutment and subsequently the sound processor may vary by clinical factors including patient age, bone thickness, and presence of any pertinent craniofacial abnormalities.

If the bone is found to be too thin at the time of implantation, the surgeon may elect to abort the procedure and attempt again after the patient has grown. In adults or those for whom a longer waiting period is undesirable, some surgeons have reported an alternative technique whereby the fixture of the implant is only partially drilled into the cortex of the bone, leaving as much as 1 mm of the fixture exposed external to the skull, and packing the gap underneath the flange with bone dust or a synthetic material.[16,17] In these cases, the surgery is performed as a two-stage procedure.

In addition to bone thickness, bone health and vascularity are thought to be vital to successful osteointegration. As Baha® candidates include those who have undergone skull base ablative procedures, many potential recipients may have undergone prior radiation therapy.

Some investigators have found an implantation failure rate as high as 64% in patients who undergo radiation therapy before or after implantation secondary to osteoradionecrosis of the surgical site.[18] However, adjunctive hyperbaric oxygen therapy appears to reduce the failure rates in these patients.[19] Therefore, although prior radiation therapy is not an absolute contraindication to the placement of a bone-anchored hearing aid, the surgeon should strongly consider recommending adjuvant hyperbaric oxygen therapy in this population.

Finally, infection or trauma to the surgical site or the abutment may compromise successful osteointegration.[15,17] Although no intraoperative measures can decrease the risk of postoperative trauma, it should be noted that incidental trauma is more likely in the pediatric population and a staged procedure may be preferable for some of these patients. In patients who are considered to be at risk of failed osteointegration for any reason, some surgeons recommend "banking" a second implant at the time of surgery so that if the primary implant fails, the abutment may be placed on the banked implant.[20]

Treatment

A patient with evidence of a postoperative infection of the soft tissue or bone should be treated aggressively and promptly with topical and systemic antibiotic therapy directed against common skin flora, and any abscess or collection should be drained and cultured. Some practitioners will image the skull with computed tomography after resolution of the infection to assess the health of the bone surrounding the implant.

If the implant feels loose in its well or is found to spin easily, the patient may experience distorted or muted sound conduction. When failed osteointegration is thus suspected and the patient has a second banked implant, then it should be affixed with the abutment and sound processor. If the patient does not have a banked implant, then revision surgery should be considered, where the same technique is applied several millimeters posterior to the original implant.[15] If the patient does have a banked implant but that too has failed to osteointegrate successfully, then the surgeon should consider an alternative amplification therapy, as revision surgery would be more likely to fail as well.

Occasionally in children bony overgrowth under the flange of the implant has been found to interfere with normal seating of the implant, and thus normal bone conduction. In cases in which the bone was too thin for a 3-mm implantation, as discussed above, this bony overgrowth may be beneficial by stabilizing the external component of the fixture. However in the event that it interferes with proper placement of the abutment or optimal bone conduction, a revision procedure may be warranted in which the bone is removed with a drill or curette.

SKIN REACTION AND TISSUE LOSS

As technique has developed, the incidence of complications involving the skin and soft tissue around the implant has decreased considerably. In particular, the use of either linear or horizontal incisions with minimal undermining and no skin graft have virtually eliminated the skin reactions described below (with the exception of skin overgrowth). Key intraoperative principles must be kept in mind by the surgeon, including adequate undermining to thin and to immobilize the tissue surrounding the implant. In 1988 Holgers[21] published a classification system to evaluate skin reactions. Table 20–2 summarizes Holgers' classification system with current treatment recommendations.[12,15,17,21,22]

Any sign of postoperative skin reaction must be treated aggressively with very close continued follow-up regardless of reaction severity. Additionally, the practitioner is advised to maintain a low threshold to obtain imaging of the region by CT or MRI if there are any unusual findings such as therapy resistant infections, neurologic symptoms including headache, or any other concerns. Although rare, intracranial abscesses have been reported to occur as complications even several years postoperatively.[23]

Skin loss has become less frequent with newer Baha® surgical techniques, but still may occur usually within the first six months postoperatively secondary to ischemia and necrosis. Postoperative complications, such as a hematoma or infection, may contribute to tissue ischemia. Additionally, medical comorbidities that compromise normal wound healing may also contribute to tissue ischemia, including vascular disease, diabetes mellitus, smoking, and a history of local radiation. If underlying bone is not exposed, then the wound may be allowed to heal by secondary intention with generally good results.[15] When bone is exposed or conservative measures fail to promote adequate wound healing, then a revision procedure may be required. For a small defect, office-based skin graft procedures with adequate wound care and tissue bolstering may be sufficient. Larger defects may require local rotation flaps, such as with superficial temporal parietal fascia, and split-thickness skin grafting.

Table 20–2. Holgers Classification

Holgers Classification		Recommended Therapy
Grade 0	• Reaction-free skin well-healed around the abutment • Incidence 90 to 95%	• None indicated
Grade 1	• Redness with slight swelling around the abutment • Incidence 3 to 5%	• Application of topical antibiotic ointment
Grade 2	• Redness, moistness, moderate swelling around the abutment • Incidence 1 to 4%	• Application of topical antibiotic ointment • Dressing changes with antibiotic ointment-impregnated gauze and replacement of healing cap
Grade 3	• Redness, moistness, moderate swelling, and granulation tissue around the abutment • Incidence 0.5 to 1.5%	• Oral and topical antibiotic therapy • Local cauterization of granulation tissue • If above measures fail, surgical debridement of infected tissue and placement of skin graft
Grade 4	• Overt signs of infection including severe cellulitis or abscess • Incidence < 0.5%	• Explantation of entire implant • Placement of a skin graft • Repeat implantation in 3 months if region has healed

SOFT TISSUE OVERGROWTH

Continued growth of subcutaneous tissue surrounding the implant is the most frequent indication for revision Baha® surgery.[15] Excessive skin and subcutaneous tissue growth around the implant may interfere with normal placement of the sound processor. Fortunately, the majority of cases of skin overgrowth can be managed with topical high potency steroid creams, such as clobetasol.[24] Local triamcinolone infiltration of the subcutaneous tissues and skin is a useful adjuvant treatment. Local excision of the skin overgrowth is indicated if the implant is mostly or completely covered. Replacement of the Baha® abutment with a longer one to protrude beyond the skin (9.0-mm abutment instead of the standard 6.0-mm abutment) is also very helpful. In extreme cases, surgical revision of the tissue flaps is recommended, whereby all tissue from skin to periosteum is removed circumferentially around the abutment in a circular section of approximately 3 cm in diameter, with a placement of a split-thickness skin graft (Fig 20–5).

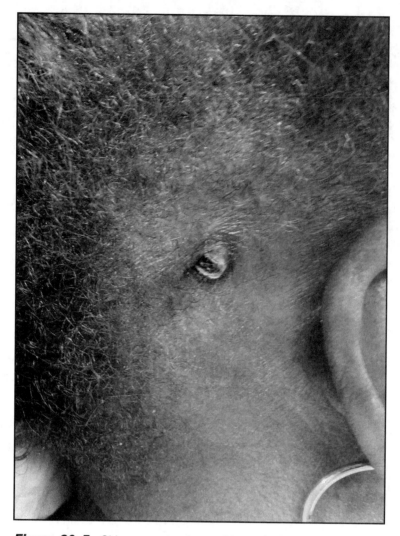

Figure 20–5. *Skin overgrowth requiring minor skin excision performed in clinic.*

REFERENCES

1. Brånemark PI, Adell R, Breine U, Hansson BO, Lindström J, Ohlsson A. Intraosseous anchorage of dental prostheses. I. Experimental studies. *Scand J Plast Reconstr Surg.* 1969;3(2):81–100.
2. Parkin JL, Bloebaum R, Parkin BD, Parkin MJ. Osseointegration and growth effects of temporal bone percutaneous pedestals. *Amer J Otol.* 1996 Sep;17(5):735–742.
3. Tjellström A, Granström G. How we do it: Frequency of skin necrosis after BAHA surgery. *Clin Otolaryngol.* 2006;31:216–232.
4. Tjellström A, Granström G. One stage procedure to establish osseointegration: a zero to five years follow-up report. *J Laryngol Otol.* 1995 Jul;109(7):593–598.
5. Tjellström A. Osseointegrated systems and their applications in the head and neck. *Adv Otolaryngol Head Neck Surg.* 1989;3:39–70.
6. Browning GG. Bone conduction implants. *Laryngoscope.* 1990 Sep;100(9):1018–1019.

7. Mylanus EAM, Cremers CW. A one stage surgical procedure for placement of percutaneous implants for the bone anchored hearing aid. *J Laryngol Otol.* 1994 Dec; 108(12):1031–1035.

8. Kohan, Morris, Romo. Single-stage BAHA implantation in adults and children: is it safe? *Otolaryngol-Head Neck Surg.* 2008 May;138(5):662–666.

9. Ali S, Hadoura L, Carmichael A, Geddes N. Bone-anchored hearing aid: a single-stage procedure in children. *Int J Ped Otorhinolaryngol.* 2009 Aug;73(8):1076–1079.

10. de Wolf M, Myrthe K, Huygen P, Mylanus E, Cremers C. Nijmegen results with application of a bone-anchored hearing aid in children: simplified surgical technique. *Ann Otol Rhinol Laryngol.* 2008 Nov;117(11):805–814.

11. Bovo R. Simplified technique without skin flap for the bone-anchored hearing aid (BAHA) implant. *Acta Otorhinolaryngol Ital.* 2008 Oct;28(5):252–255.

12. de Wolf M, Hol M, Huygen P, Mylanus E, Cremers C. Clinical outcome of the simplified surgical technique for BAHA implanttion. *Otol Neurotol.* 2008 Dec;29(8): 1100–1108.

13. Wazen JJ, Gupta R, Ghossaini S, Spitzer J, Farrugia M, Tjellström A. Osseointegration timing for Baha system loading. *Laryngoscope.* 2007 May;117(5):794–796.

14. Granström G, Bergström K, Odersjö M, Tjellström A. Osseointegrated implants in children: experience from our first 100 patients. *Otolaryngol-Head Neck Surg.* 2001 Jul;125(1):85–92.

15. Battista RA, Littlefield PD. Revision BAHA surgery. *Otolaryngol Clin North Amer.* 2006 Aug;39(4):801–813, viii.

16. Proops DW. The Birmingham bone anchored hearing aid programme: surgical methods and complications. *J Laryngol Otol Suppl.* 1996;21:7–12.

17. Reyes RA, Tjellström A, Granström G. Evaluation of implant losses and skin reactions around extraoral bone anchored implants: a 0- to 8-year follow-up. *Otolaryngol-Head Neck Surg.* 2000;122(2):272–276.

18. Granström G, Tjellström A. Effects of irradiation on osseointegration before and after implant placement: a report of three cases. *Int J Oral Maxillofac Implants.* 1997 Jul–Aug;12(4):547–551.

19. Granström G, Tjellström A, Brånemark P. Osseointegrated implants in irradiated bone: a case-controlled study using adjunctive hyperbaric oxygen therapy. *J Oral Maxillofac Surg.* 1999 May;57(5):493–499.

20. Papsin B, James A. Bone-anchored hearing aid in children. *Oper Techn Otolaryngol-Head Neck Surg.* 2001 Dec;12(4):219–223.

21. Holgers KM, Tjellström A, Bjursten LM, Erlandsson BE. Soft tissue reactions around percutaneous implants: a clinical study of soft tissue conditions around skin-penetrating titanium implants for bone-anchored hearing aids. *Amer J Otol.* 1988 Jan;9(1):56–59.

22. Badran K, Arya AK, Bunstone D, Mackinnon N. Long-term complications of bone-anchored hearing aids: a 14-year experience. *J Laryngol Otol.* 2009 Feb;123(2): 170–176.

23. Schloz M, Eufinger H, Anders A. Intracerebral abscess after abutment change of Baha. *Otol Neurotol.* 2003;24(6):896–899.

24. Falcone MT, Kaylie DM, Labadie RF, Haynes DS. Bone-anchored hearing aid abutment skin overgrowth reduction with clobetasol. *Otolaryngol-Head Neck Surg.* 2008;139(6): 829–832.

Chapter 21

Middle Ear Implantable Hearing Devices: Present and Future

JEFFERY J. KUHN

INTRODUCTION

Hearing loss affects approximately 17% of the population (36 million) in the United States. The prevalence increases with age and over one-third of people age 65 years and older have significant hearing loss. Hearing loss may adversely affect family relationships, self-esteem, and work and school performance. A recent study conducted of over 40,000 households in the United States assessed the relationship between hearing loss and employment status and found that individuals with untreated hearing loss may average as much as $30,000 per year less in income compared to those with normal hearing. Even for those without severe hearing loss, income drops as the degree of hearing loss increases.[1] The annual loss in income for those with untreated hearing loss due to underemployment is estimated at $176 billion, and the societal cost is estimated to be as high as $26 billion in unrealized federal income taxes. The use of hearing aids seems to, at least, mitigate the adverse financial impact of

hearing loss. With these economic data in mind, it would seem reasonable to encourage every hearing impaired individual to entertain the options for amplification. The out-of-pocket expense and relative lack of coverage by private health care insurers have deterred many from even considering the use of hearing aids. For others, the overall benefit must be weighed against the unsightly appearance of an object in the outer ear.

Recent advances in conventional hearing aid technology have resulted in improvements in functionality and cosmesis. The miniaturization of components, advances in digital signal processing, addition of directional microphones, and improvements in the ease of use (eg, selective programming, automatic telecoil, Bluetooth capablities, data logging, remote control) have lead to greater acceptance of these devices by the hearing-impaired consumer. Despite these advances, only approximately 25% of individuals that would benefit from conventional amplification actually own hearing aids. Of hearing aid users, approximately 45% are either dissatisfied or neutral with regard to their experience and about 12% have abandoned their aids to the dresser drawer.[1] Historically, the various reasons for dissatisfaction or noncompliance include acoustic feedback, occlusion, adverse effects on the ear canal such as dermatitis and cerumen buildup, and inherent limitations of the device such as limited amplification above frequencies 4 to 6 kHz, sound distortion, and poor speech intelligibility in noisy environments. Although less problematic in the age of Bluetooth cell phone ear sets, some hearing aid candidates perceive a social stigma associated with hearing aid use.

Implantable hearing device manufacturers have made considerable strides in the past two decades in addressing the problems encountered by hearing aid users with the development of partially and fully implantable middle ear hearing devices. Conventional acoustic hearing aids function by receiving environmental sounds through a microphone and converting the vibratory information into an electrical signal that is processed, amplified, and delivered to the ear canal as acoustic energy. Contrary to conventional hearing aids, middle ear implantable hearing devices (MEIHDs) transmit acoustic energy directly to a mobile structure within the middle ear space (ossicle or round window membrane) through the use of a vibrational transducer, thereby bypassing the external auditory canal. These devices are either partially or totally implantable. The partially implantable devices consist of an external ear level microphone, amplifier, signal processor, and battery similar to that found in a conventional hearing aid. The electrical signals are then transmitted to either a receiver coil close to the tympanic membrane that converts the signal to electromagnetic energy that drives a magnet attached to the ossicular chain (MAXUM System, Ototronix, LLC) or to a subcutaneous receiver-stimulator that decodes the signal and transmits the electrical energy to a transducer attached to the incus (Vibrant Soundbridge, Vibrant MED-EL Hearing Technology GMBH, Innsbruck, Austria) or to a transducer in contact with the incus (Otologics MET™, Otologics, LLC, Boulder, CO). The fully implantable devices consist of an implanted microphone or sensor connected to an internal sound processor that amplifies and filters the signal and transmits the electrical signal to a transducer that converts the signal into mechanical vibration which is then transmitted to either the incus (MET Fully-Implantable Ossicular Stimulator [Carina™], Otologics, LLC, Boulder, CO) or the stapes (Esteem Totally Implantable Middle Ear Hearing System, Envoy Medical Corp, St. Paul, MN).

The impetus for the development of MEIHDs has been centered primarily on the need to fulfill the amplification needs of patients with moderate to severe sensorineural hearing loss (SNHL). This segment of the hearing-impaired population (approximately 7.3 million) have gain requirements in the mid- to high-frequency range that would increase the risks of acoustic feedback and sound distortion with the use of conventional hearing aids. Reducing feedback may necessitate a tighter fitting ear mold, which may lead to discomfort and a more pronounced occlusion effect. Although open-fit/receiver in canal technology has virtually eliminated the problems of occlusion and feedback, this hearing aid design is best suited for individuals with mild to moderate hearing loss. The currently available implantable devices have the advantage of amplifying high frequencies without creating feedback, tend to improve sound fidelity by directly stimulating the ossicular chain, and eliminate discomfort and the occlusion effect by leaving the external auditory canal open.

Conceptually, MEIHDs are niche products that are meant to fill the hearing rehabilitation void between hearing aids and cochlear implants. Because the use of these devices involve surgical risks not associated with the fitting of traditional hearing aids, candidates for middle ear implantable devices should be compelled to first try conventional hearing aids. Unlike with conventional hearing aids, MEIHDs can only be prescribed and placed by a physician. Patients should be free of infection and have a relatively normal middle ear anatomy in order to properly anchor the transducer. Hearing loss should be stable, and word recognition scores should meet the device manufacturer's candidacy criteria. Most importantly, the patient's expectations of benefit should be reasonable. MEIHDs are expensive and the cost is typically not covered by health insurance. The estimated cost for the device, surgery and anesthesia fees, facility fees, and postoperative programming ranges from $9,000 to $37,000 depending on the particular device used.

MIDDLE EAR TRANSDUCER TECHNOLOGY

The currently available MEIHDs in the United States and in the Europe use one of two types of transducers: electromagnetic or piezoelectric. Electromagnetic devices function by transmitting an electrical current through an induction coil that is in proximity to a magnet. The magnetic field that is produced with this configuration will cause the magnet to vibrate resulting in movement of the ossicular chain. The induction coil may be located separate

from the implanted magnet or integrated with the magnet in an assembly attached to the ossicular chain or in contact with the round window membrane (round window application approved for use in the European Union). The implant design that has the induction coil and magnet at a distance from one another requires considerable fitting accuracy as the power delivered from the coil to the magnet will decrease by as much as the cube of the distance between the two components.

Piezoelectric devices function by transmitting an electrical current through a piezoceramic crystal. The ceramic crystal consists of layers of lead, zirconium, and titanium oxide with the property of reversible electromechanical transduction: when a force is applied to the material, a voltage is generated; when a voltage is applied, motion is created. More specifically, by applying a sinusoidal input to a piezoelectric biomorph (two layers of lead-zirconate-titanate crystal on either side of a stiffening material, typically carbon fiber), the tip of the biomorph will oscillate according to the input frequency. Mechanical flexion of the biomorph, at a given rate, produces a characteristic electrical sinusoid. Conversely, by applying a direct current voltage to the biomorph ceramic crystal, one side of the crystal will expand while the other side contracts producing a bending motion. Therefore, attaching a probe or rod to one end of the crystal will serve to either collect sound energy for the purpose of transmitting an electrical signal or to transmit vibrational energy as a result of an incoming electrical signal.

Electromagnetic and piezoelectric technologies have their advantages and disadvantages. Common to both designs, however, is the accuracy required for placement of the transducer. Although the implementation of an extracoil electromagnetic system (induction coil and magnet separate from one another) is relatively simple from a surgical standpoint, the distance between the coil and magnet must adhere to strict guidelines to maintain optimal magnetic field strength. Attaching an electromagnetic transducer to the ossicular chain adds weight and, therefore, may attenuate vibration at high frequencies by a mass loading effect. If the transducer shifts or is placed at an angle relative to the coincident axis of stapes movement, sound energy transfer will be reduced and optimal performance is lost. Coupling the tip of an electromagnetic or piezoelectric transducer to the ossicular chain demands precision. Insufficient pressure at the point of contact with the ossicle will reduce acoustic energy transfer, whereas excessive tension may result in a conductive loss.[2] Electromagnetic transducers tend to have high power consumption and, therefore, require a rechargeable battery for the fully implantable device. Piezoelectric transducers consume less power and are highly sensitive, but generate limited voltage and displacement.[3] Whether electromagnetic or piezoelectric, both types of transducers should be able to generate forces corresponding to acoustic sound pressure levels of at least 110 to 120 dB SPL in order to provide adequate amplification to patients with hearing loss in the 50 to 90 dB HL range.[4]

CURRENTLY AVAILABLE MIDDLE EAR IMPLANTABLE HEARING DEVICES

The middle ear implantable hearing device manufacturing community has evolved rapidly over the past 15 years as new technologies and designs have become

available. Regardless of the specific marketing agenda of a given manufacturing firm, a common goal exists among the various research and development teams that have contributed to the advancement of these devices: amplify sound without sacrificing fidelity and do it with a device that is biocompatible, invisible, and reliable. Although certain middle ear implantable devices are no longer available (partially implantable Rion Ehime [E]-type device; Totally Integrated Cochlear Amplifier [TICA], Implex American Hearing Systems, now owned by Cochlear Corp, Sydney, Australia; partially implantable Soundtec Direct System, formerly marketed by Soundtec, Inc, Oklahoma City, OK) their influence in the hearing rehabilitation marketplace has lead to improvements in later designs. The following section reviews the semi- and fully implantable middle ear hearing devices that are a currently available in the United States and Europe. Although each manufacturer has slightly different audiometric criteria for determining candidacy for their device, in general, these devices have been designed for patients with moderate to severe SNHL with a minimum speech discrimination of 40 to 60%. Expanded criteria have been established within the European Union for the use of certain devices in patients with conductive and mixed hearing loss.

ELECTROMAGNETIC DEVICES

Vibrant Soundbridge

The Vibrant Soundbridge (VSB)(developed and formerly marketed by Symphonix Devices, Inc, San Jose, CA) was the first middle ear implantable hearing device to be FDA approved (received in 2000) for use in patients with moderate to severe SNHL (Fig 21–1). The device was acquired by Vibrant MED-EL (MED-EL Corp, Innsbruck, Austria) in 2003 and has since seen little change in the design of its implantable components. Since commercial release of the device in the Europe in 1998, there have been several upgrades to the speech processor circuitry, however. The first semi-implantable system used a two-channel analog processor with auto-matic gain control, known as the Vibrant P. A three-channel digital processor with automatic gain control (Vibrant D) was then developed and used in the Phase III multicenter clinical trial in the United States (concluded in 2000).[5] Currently, an eight-channel digital processor (Vibrant Signia) is available and has been shown significantly improve functional gain and speech intelligibility in noise as compared

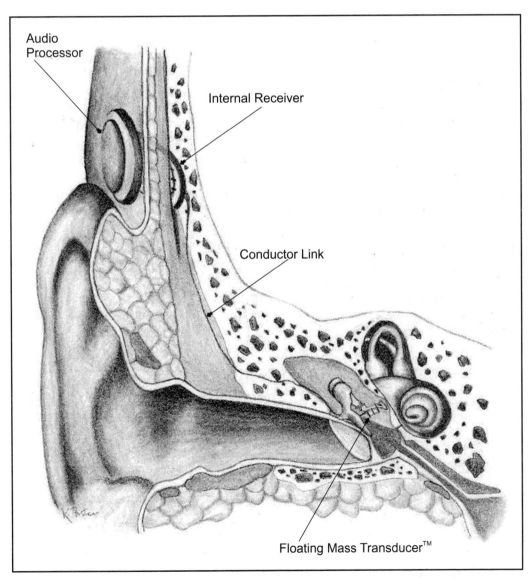

Audio Processor

Internal Receiver

Conductor Link

Floating Mass Transducer™

Figure 21–1. *MED-EL Vibrant Soundbridge®.*

to the preimplant hearing aid condition that used the same eight-channel digital processor circuitry.[6]

The VSB consists of an implanted component, the Vibrating Ossicular Prosthesis (VORP) (Fig 21–2), which contains an internal coil and magnet and receiver module that is connected by a conductor link to the Floating Mass Transducer (FMT) (Fig 21–3), and an externally worn audio processor. The VORP is implanted posterior superior to the pinna on the temporal bone similar to the technique used in cochlear implant surgery. The conductor link exits the VORP and traverses the mastoid cavity and the facial recess opening to the FMT that is attached to the long process of the incus with a titanium attachment clip. The FMT is placed such that its orientation is coincident with the axis of stapes movement. The FMT is an electromagnetic transducer that consists of an electromagnetic coil that encases a small permanent magnet. The design of the FMT takes advantage of the natural vibratory motion of the ossicular chain and provides certain advantages as a "direct drive" system in terms of frequency response and fidelity.[7–10] The external audio processor contains the microphone, signal processor, transmitting coil, centering magnet and battery. It is held in place by transcutaneous magnetic attraction to the magnet in the implanted receiver coil. The auditory signal is collected by the microphone and transmitted via an amplitude-modulated carrier to the implanted internal receiver in the VORP. The signal is then demodulated and sent via the conductor link to the FMT.[5]

Although the VSB has not been shown to be superior to conventional hearing aids in all studies that have assessed benefit in terms of audiometric criteria, many clinical studies have reported overall improved patient satisfaction. Subjective benefit as measured by validated questionnaires has shown reduced problems with feedback, occlusion effect, reverberation and sound distortion, and, at least, equivalent amplification of sound as compared to traditional hearing aids.[11–14] In terms of functional gain and speech recognition in quiet and noise, several studies have demonstrated a significant benefit over conventional hearing aids.[6,11,12,15] This is especially notable given the technologic advances in conventional hearing aid manufacturing within the last 10 years.

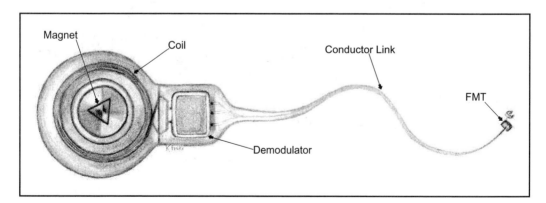

Figure 21–2. *Vibrating Ossicular Prosthesis (VORP).*

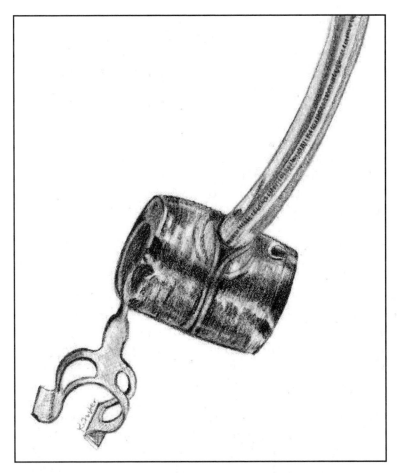

Figure 21–3. *Floating Mass Transducer (FMT).*

Even in those studies that have shown no significant difference with regard to audiometric criteria and standardized or nonstandardized satisfaction surveys,[16,17] the VSB was declared a "good option" for patients with moderate to severe SNHL who could not tolerate a conventional aid and in those with chronic otitis externa. Long-term reliability of the VSB has been demonstrated in two recent studies[18,19] that have shown stability of functional gain and speech recognition. Both studies recognized few long-term problems, such as local skin irritation, and there were no internal devices failures in those patients implanted within the last 10 years. These studies help to confirm the long-term safety and efficacy of the VSB. The device has also been found to be a cost-effective solution for managing SNHL in patients with chronic external otitis media as determined by a quality-adjusted life year outcome measure.[20]

Since 2008, the indications for the VSB have been expanded in the Europe to include treatment of conductive and mixed hearing loss. As a result of considerable research efforts that have included a mathematical middle ear simulation model,[21] cadaveric temporal bone studies,[22–24] and clinical studies,[25–30] the placement of the FMT onto vibratory structures within the middle ear space other than the incus, may be equally efficacious. Previous animal studies have demonstrated that the placement of a transducer against the round window membrane is capable of producing evoked responses equivalent to sound stimulation levels of 85 to 110 dB SPL across a broad frequency range. By modifying the FMT to fit into the round window niche, Colletti, et al[25] were able to demonstrate favorable results in seven patients with severe mixed hearing loss. In this study, the postoperative functional gain ranged from 10 to 40 dB and the aided SRTs at 50% intelligibility were 50 dB HL, with most patients reaching 100% intelligibility at conversation levels. The relatively wide interindividual difference in postoperative audiometric test results may have been attributed to migration of the FMT over time. A more recent study reported favorable results with a similar wide variability in hearing benefit, suggesting either inadequate interface between the FMT and the round window membrane at the time of placement or eventual migration.[29] Cadaveric temporal bone studies using laser Doppler vibrometric measurements of stapes movement with the FMT subjected to various orientations and soft tissue cover conditions, concluded that the best orientation of the FMT was perpendicular to the RWM and that a supporting soft tissue cover was important.[23,24] These studies disagreed, however, as to the benefit of soft tissue interposed between the FMT and RWM. The results in a recent clinical study suggested that the use of soft tissue to facilitate the physical coupling of the FMT and the RWM may reduce the relative coupling efficiency as compared to direct placement of the FMT onto the

RWM.[30] A round window coupler prosthesis (Vibroplasty-RW-Coupler) has been developed by the manufacturer to facilitate placement of the FMT against the RWM. Although the round window insertion technique has been used primarily in patients with chronic otitis media and otosclerosis, favorable results have also been shown in patients with congenital aural atresia.[31,32] Other applications reported include the use of a titanium partial or total ossicular replacement prosthesis coupled to the FMT (Vibroplasty PORP and TORP) for use in patients with moderate to severe mixed hearing loss.[26,33,34] The manufacturer has now made available several titanium Vibroplasty Couplers for this purpose including the Vibroplasty-oval window(OW)-Coupler (Fig 21–4A), Vibroplasty-Bell partial prosthesis(Bell)-Coupler (Fig 21–4B), and Vibroplasty-Clip partial prosthesis(CliP)-Coupler. As a result of the work in Europe, the VSB received the Communauté Européene (CE) mark for conductive and mixed hearing loss in adults in 2008 and for the same indication in children in 2009. The device also received the CE marked for moderate to severe SNHL in children in 2009.

MRI compatability studies in the temporal bone model have demonstrated stability of the ossicular chain with an attached FMT both from a theoretic standpoint[35] and based on direct exposure to a 1.5-T MRI scanner.[36,37] Although magnetization and functional integrity were maintained following 1.5-T exposures, positional changes of the FMT occurred in 5/18 temporal bone specimens when coupled to the incus. This study also reiterated the importance of securing the FMT with a soft tissue cover when placed against the RWM as 5/5 were dislodged in fresh specimens without soft tissue cover. One study reported no changes in

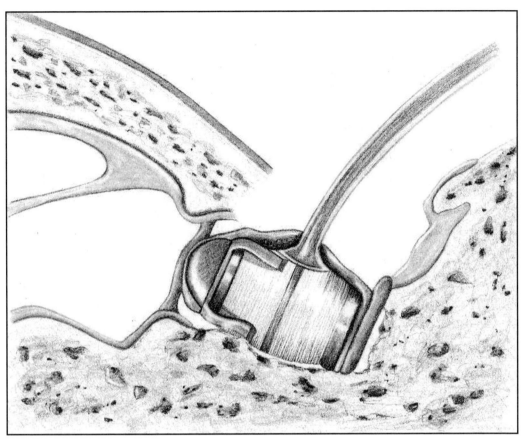

A

Figure 21–4. **A.** *FMT and Vibroplasty-RW-Coupler in position against round window membrane.* continues

hearing or the functional integrity of the device in two patients exposed to a 1.5-T MRI scanner.

Otologics MET Fully Implantable Hearing System (Carina™)

The Otologics Fully Implantable Hearing System (Carina™) (Otologics, LLC, Boulder CO) consists of four primary components: the implant, the programming system, the charger, and the remote control. The implant consists of the electronics capsule that contains the rechargeable battery, digital signal processor, microphone, and transmission coil and is implanted entirely beneath the skin behind the auricle (Fig 21–5A). The electronics capsule is connected to an electromagnetic transducer that is placed in contact with the incus (Fig 21–5B). The programming system consists of a NOAHlink™ programming interface that is worn around the neck. Using the OtoFit™ software, the NOAHlink™ interface receives signals from the computer through a wireless connection and sends the signals to the implant site through a radiofrequency coil that is held in place magnetically. Programming the

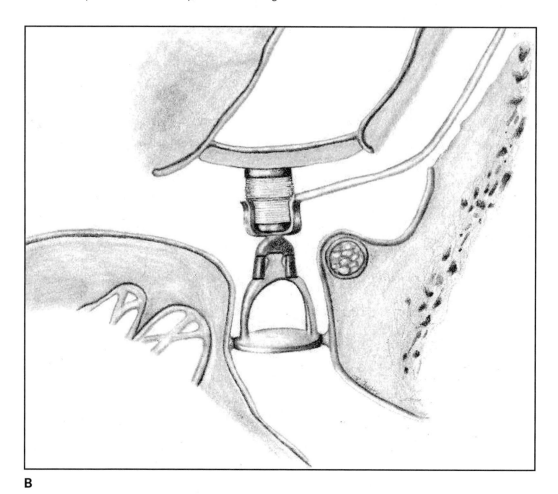

B

Figure 21–4. continued **B.** *FMT and Vibroplasty-Bell-Coupler in position between cartilage block and stapes capitulum.*

implant is similar to the programming techniques used for conventional digital hearing aids. The programming system also provides the means for extensive testing and diagnostics of the MET (Middle Ear Transducer) Fully Implantable Ossicular Stimulator. The charger system consists of a base station, charging coil, and charger body. The charging coil is placed over the implant site and held in place magnetically. Charging time is typically one hour if charging occurs on a daily basis. While charging the implant, the patient may conduct normal daily activities, adjust the volume, and turn the implant on and off. The remote control may be used to adjust the volume and turn the implant on and off by placing the remote against the skin over the implant site. The IS-1 connector between the electronics package (processor) and the MET stimulator allows for the implanted device to be exchanged with a minor surgical procedure. The processor must be exchanged when the rechargeable battery has reached its lifetime of use, which is specified as eight years with daily charging. The implantable microphone is per-

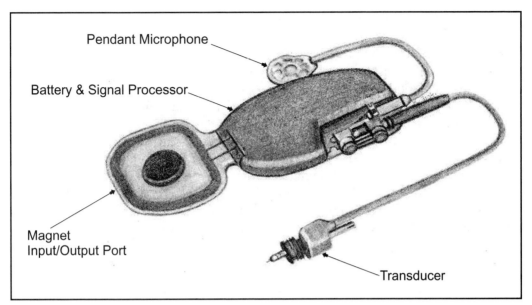

A

Pendant Microphone

Battery & Signal Processor

Magnet
Input/Output Port

Transducer

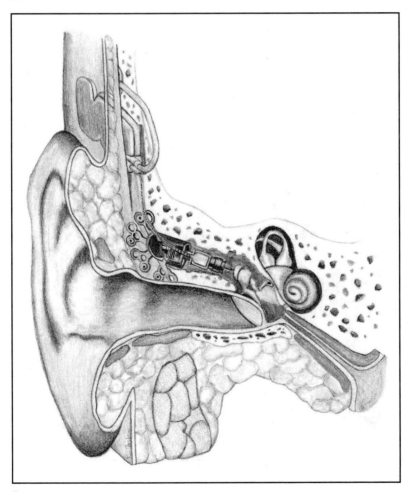

Figure 21–5.
A. *Otologics MET Fully Implantable Hearing System (Carina™) electronics capsule.* ***B.*** *Otologics MET Fully Implantable Hearing System (Carina™).*

B

manently connected to the processor and must be exchanged with the processor.

A semi-implantable version of the device (MET) (Fig. 21–6), further developed by Otologics, LLC from 1996 to 2000, received the CE mark in 2000 for moderate to severe SNHL in adults. FDA approval was not sought for the semi-implantable device in the U.S. in favor of developing and testing the fully implantable version. The semi-implantable device consists of an ear level audio processor (button

processor) that contains the microphone, signal processor, transmitting coil, and battery. The auditory signal is converted to an electrical signal that is transmitted transcutaneously to an internal coil and receiver stimulator. The receiver stimulator is connected to an electromagnetic tranducer that is secured to the body of incus in a similar manner to that of the fully implantable device. Recent studies suggest that there may be no distinct advantage over the best digitally aided

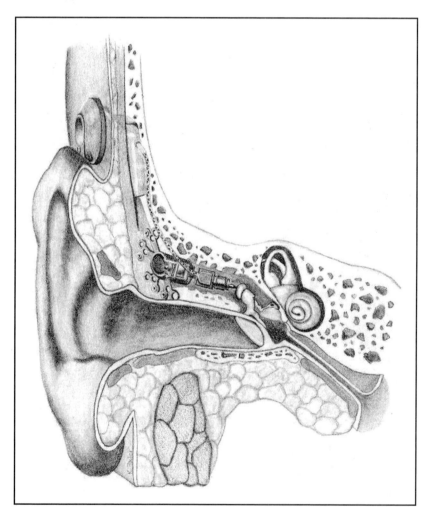

Figure 21–6. *Otologics MET Semi-implantable Hearing System.*

condition as measured by aided thresholds, monaural speech discrimination, and subjective questionnaire.[17,38] Among several factors that may influence outcome is the coupling efficiency between the transducer and the ossicles. Insufficient pressure against the ossicles during transducer placement may limit energy transfer, whereas, excessive pressure may result in a conductive loss. An intraoperative loading instrument (transducer loading assistant) has been developed to provide real-time impedance information to the surgeon during loading of the MET™ Ossicular Stimulator.[2]

The fully implantable MET (marketed as the Carina™) received the CE mark for moderate to severe SNHL in 2006 and for conductive and mixed hearing loss in 2007. Studies conducted in Europe have demonstrated benefit in small groups of patients with placement of the transducer against the round window membrane in those with moderate to severe mixed hearing loss due to either sclerotic disease of the oval window niche or otosclerosis and with placement of the transducer coupled to a partial titanium prosthesis on the stapes capitulum in patients with congenital aural atresia.[39,40] The Phase I clinical trial in the United States, which included 20 patients with moderate to severe SNHL, and speech recognition scores greater than 40%, demonstrated no significant benefit over the preoperative hearing aid condition as measured by monaural and binaural speech discrimination using consonant/nucleus/consonant (CNC) words and phonemes and hearing-in-noise testing (HINT). HINT scores improved substantially, however, after refitting at 12 months. The general perception of benefit as measured by subjective questionnaires (including APHAB)

showed that the implant performed at least as well as, if not significantly better than, the preimplant hearing aid condition in nearly every category.[41] One of several problems identified in the Phase I trial was microphone migration which contributed to the deterioration of speech recognition, feedback, and limited functional gain. Adjustment of the digital processing algorithms to account for tissue thickness or migration resulted in significant improvement. The manufacturer has since modified the implant design by placing titanium straps on both the implant capsule and the microphone in order to anchor the components to the cranium. Although earlier work had been conducted to reduce the potential for transmission of biological noise (eg, skin movement, chewing, voicing),[42] patients had reported this as a minor concern in the Phase I trial. Phase II trials have been completed (10 patients in Phase IIa and 57 patients in Phase IIb) and the manufacturer has since revised the implant design to include a hermetically sealed titanium casing for the transducer, a smaller electronics capsule with modified connector, and new processor algorithms to eliminate feedback and reduce biological noise.

Ototronix MAXUM

The MAXUM System (Ototronix, LLC, Houston, TX) is a partially implantable device with a design based on Soundtec Direct System technology acquired by Ototronix in 2009 (Fig 21–7). The MAXUM middle ear implant consists of a neodymium-iron-boron (NdFeB) magnet encased in a titanium housing, which is attached to the incudostapedial joint at the level of the neck of the stapes. The external processor is available in either a behind-

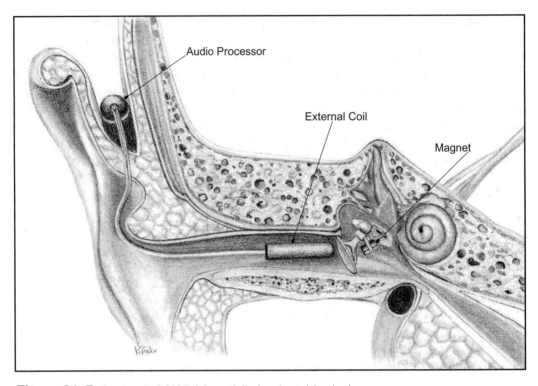

Figure 21–7. *Ototronix MAXUM partially implantable device.*

the-ear (BTE) or in-the-canal (IPC) configuration and consists of a digital sound
processor and electromagnetic coil. The
sound processor receives the auditory signal, amplifies it, and transmits the electrical signal to the transceiver coil located
near the tympanic membrane. The transceiver coil converts the electrical signal
to electromagnetic energy that drives the
middle ear implant, thereby, causing the
ossicles to vibrate. Although the transceiver coil is located in the external auditory canal, energy transfer occurs through
electromagnetic induction and direct drive
of the ossicular chain, therefore, obviating the need for an acoustic seal and the
generation of sound pressure energy in
the canal. This design reduces the potential for occlusion, sound distortion, and
feedback. The BTE configuration contains
an electromagnetic coil embedded in an

acrylic mold that is seated at an optimal distance of 2 mm from the tympanic
membrane. The fully digital sound processor features directional microphones,
noise cancellation capabilities and a wide
dynamic range of compression. The audio
processor and implantable components
were FDA approved in October 2009.
The company has also developed a 3D
computed tomography integrated fitting
protocol that is currently awaiting FDA
review. The proposed protocol should
provide a means for establishing accuracy and consistency in the fitting distance between the transceiver coil and
the implanted magnet. Clinical studies
conducted for the Soundtec Direct device demonstrated statistically significant improvement in various parameters measured including functional gain,
speech discrimination in quiet, and per-

ceived aided benefit (APHAB) compared to the best conventionally aided condition.[43,44] Magnet instability and noise were frequent complaints of implanted subjects, although occlusion and feedback were greatly reduced or eliminated. The interposition of adipose tissue between the neck of the stapes and the collar of the magnet served to reduce the potential for magnet movement in subsequent patients. The MAXUM device has been redesigned to allow for placement of the magnet without separating the incudostapedial joint. Previous MRI compatibility studies conducted with the Soundtec device in cadaveric temporal bone specimens and in patients have demonstrated retained stability and integrity of the implant and the ossicular chain in a 0.3-Tesla open MRI using a modified protocol.[45,46]

PIEZOELECTRIC DEVICE

Envoy Esteem®

The Esteem® Totally Implantable Middle Ear Hearing System (Envoy Medical Corporation, St Paul, MN) consists of three implantable components: the piezoelectric sensor and driver that are implanted in the middle ear and the sound processor that is implanted on the temporal bone behind the auricle (Figs 21–8A and 21–8B). The piezoelectric sensor tip is attached to the incus using a bioactive glass-ionomer cement through a transmastoid atticotomy approach. The sensor "senses" vibrations from the tympanic membrane via its attachment to the incus and converts the mechanical vibrations into electrical signals that are transmitted to the sound processor. The sound processor amplifies and filters the signal,

then sends it to the piezoelectric driver, which is coupled to the stapes capitulum using bone cement. The driver converts the modified electrical signal back to mechanical energy and vibrates the stapes. The incus and stapes are disarticulated and one to two millimeters of the distal aspect of the incus is resected to prevent feedback to the sensor. In short, the device uses the tympanic membrane as the microphone and amplifies acoustic energy delivered through the natural pathway of the external auditory canal.

The Esteem® has three external instruments that are used for programming and testing the device after implantation. The Esteem® Programmer is used by the audiologist to program the settings in the sound processor and the Personal Programmer is used by the patient to adjust volume, select preset environmental modes, and turn the device on or off. The Intraoperative System Analyzer is used to perform diagnostics of system components intraoperatively and to verify proper performance of the implanted system postoperatively. The system contains a nonrechargeable lithium-iodide battery with an average useful life of 6 to 9 years. Battery replacement requires surgical replacement of the sound processor.

The Phase I trial in the United States identified several problems with the original implant design (Envoy System, St. Croix Medical, Minneapolis, MN) including breaches in transducer hermaticity and limited functional gain in the high frequencies.[47] The manufacturer addressed these issues in the development of the second generation of the device (Esteem II) prior to Phase II clinical trials. The Phase II trial enrolled 57 adult patients with mild to severe SNHL and speech discrimination scores greater than 40%.[48] The study

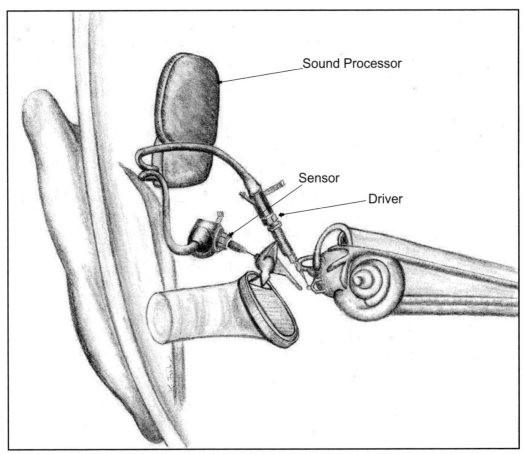

A

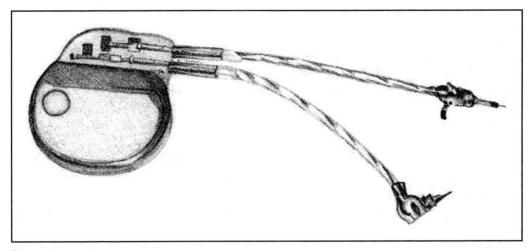

B

Figure 21–8. A. Envoy Esteem® Totally Implantable Middle Ear Hearing System. **B.** Envoy Esteem® sound processor and piezoelectric sensor and driver.

results demonstrated a mean improvement in SRT of 11.4 ± 1.8 dB at 10-months follow-up (52 patients) over the preimplant hearing aid condition. The word recognition score (WRS) at 50 dB was significantly better for 56% of patients and equal to in 37%, as compared to the preimplant hearing aid condition at the 4-month endpoint evaluation (54 patients). The device provided a 27 dB mean improvement in three-frequency pure-tone average (PTA) compared to the unaided baseline condition at both 4 and 10 months. This result was consistent with findings in a previous study that demonstrated an average functional gain (measured against preoperative thresholds) of 26 dB (250 to 4000 Hz) in a small group of implanted patients.[49] Quality of life measures showed a statistically significant improvement in mean benefit with the implanted device over hearing aids on the APHAB assessment. There was no postoperative decline in bone thresholds as compared to the pre-implant condition. The results of the Phase II trial lead to FDA approval of the device for moderate to severe SNHL in adults (age ≥18 years) in March, 2010. The Envoy Esteem® had previously received the CE mark for moderate to severe SNHL in 2006. Notable postoperative adverse events during the Phase II trial included taste disturbance (40%), tinnitus (14%), and transient facial paresis or paralysis (7%). Revision surgery was necessary in three patients due to fibrotic tissue interference at the transducer site. A postapproval study is planned and will include additional patients in order to address the postoperative adverse events. There are currently no studies that address the MRI compatibility of the Envoy Esteem. The manufacturer warns against exposure of the device to an MRI scanner.

INVESTIGATIONAL DEVICES

Direct Acoustical Cochlear Stimulation (DACS)

The DACS system (Phonak Acoustic Implants SA, Sonova Holding AG, Lausanne, Switzerland) is based on the principle of a power-driven stapes prosthesis and, therefore, intended for use in patients with severe mixed hearing loss due to advanced otosclerosis. It consists of an externally worn audio processor, an implanted electromagnetic transducer, a percutaneous plug and fixation system, and an "off-the-shelf" stapes prosthesis.[50] The external audio processor contains two microphones, a digital signal processing unit, and battery. The electrical output of the audio processor is delivered to the transducer via a percutaneous plug secured to the temporal bone. The vibrational energy is transferred to a coupling rod extending from the transducer onto which is placed a stapes wire-piston prosthesis. In order to allow for the natural transmission of sound energy when the device is turned off, a second stapes prosthesis is attached to the incus and placed into the stapedectomy opening. The device was originally developed as a joint venture between Cochlear™ Ltd, Sydney, Australia and Phonak AG, Stäfa, Switzerland. Clinical results in four patients at 2 years postimplantation demonstrated substantial improvements in sound field thresholds and speech intelligibility in quiet and noise (statistically analysis not conducted). Monosyllabic word recognition scores in quiet improved by 40 to 100% at 75 dB SPL. Postoperative unaided air conduction thresholds were improved by 14 to 28 dB pure-tone average (PTA) by virtue of the second stapes prosthesis. Subjective assessment by the Abbreviated Profile of Hearing Aid Benefit (APHAB) in three patients at 12-months postimplantation showed significant improvements in three of four subscales in two patients and in all four in one patient.[4] Because of patient complaints regarding the percutaneous coupling of the external and internal device components, the manufacturer has replaced the percutaneous plug with a transcutaneous radiofrequency transmission component similar to that found in a cochlear implant.

Fully Implantable Hearing System (FIHS)

The Fully Implantable Hearing System (FIHS) (OtoKinetics, Salt Lake City, UT) is an investigational device that is being developed for use in individuals with conductive, mixed or SNHL. The device consists of fully implanted microphone and sound processor that transmits the signal to a piezoelectric microtransducer implanted into the wall of the cochlea. There is currently no clinical outcomes data regarding this device.

CONCLUSION

Improvements in digital signal processing and miniaturization of components in conventional hearing aid design has provided added flexibility in managing the amplification requirements for individuals with SNHL. However, certain limitations still exist in terms of quality of sound and comfort. MEIHDs provide a viable option for patients with moderate to severe SNHL, particularly in those who cannot tolerate a traditional hearing aid due to inherent device-related limitations (feedback, occlusion effect, poor sound quality, physical sensation of an earmold) or because of chronic external auditory canal inflammatory conditions. MEIHDs have seen considerable improvements in design, performance, and reliability in the past two decades. They are expensive, however, and there are additional costs related to surgical implantation that are not associated with the fitting of a conventional hearing aid. As components become smaller, surgical procedures to implant them become less cumbersome, and cost is reduced, MEIHDs will gain wider acceptance by hearing health professionals and become more attractive to the hearing-impaired consumer as an alternative to conventional amplification. Although fully implantable middle ear devices, in particular, may be advantageous to those who would enjoy a safe and unobtrusive means of amplification, technical hurdles still exist such as stability of implanted components, long-term reliability, battery life, and reversibility. Technologic challenges aside, the penetrance of these devices in the marketplace may ultimately hinge on the interpretation of benefit by the health care insurance industry. Even if the audiologic benefit of MEIHDs is no greater than that of conventional hearing aids, they may serve as an important alternative for patients who perceive little benefit from or are intolerant to the adverse affects of conventional hearing aids.

REFERENCES

1. Kochkin S. MarkeTrak VIII: consumer satisfaction with hearing aids is slowly increasing. *Hear J*. 2010;63(1):19–32.

2. Jenkins HA, Pergola N, Kasic J. Intraoperative ossicular loading with the Otologics fully implantable hearing device. *Acta Oto-Laryngologica*. 2007;127:360–364.

3. Javel E, Grant IL, Kroll K. In vivo characterization of piezoelectric transducers for implantable hearing aids. *Otol Neurotol*. 2003;24:784–795.

4. Backous DD, Duke W. Implantable middle ear hearing devices: current state of technology and market challenges. *Curr Opin Otolaryngol-Head Neck Surg*. 2006; 14:314–318.

5. Luetje CM, Brackman D, Balkany TJ, et al. Phase III clinical trial results with the Vibrant Soundbridge implantable middle ear hearing device: a prospective controlled multicenter study. *Otolaryngol Head Neck Surg*. 2002;126(2):97–107.

6. Truy E, Philibert B, Vesson JF, Labassi S, Collet. Vibrant Soundbridge versus conventional hearing aid in sensorineural high-frequency hearing loss: a prospective study. *Otol Neurotol*. 2008;29:684–687.

7. Dietz T, Ball G, Katz B. *Partially implantable vibrating ossicular prosthesis*. Transducers '97: 1997 International Conference on Solid-State Sensors and Actuators. Chicago, IL: 433–436.

8. Frederickson JM, Cotcchia JM, Khosla S. Ongoing investigations into an implantable electromagnetic hearing aid for moderate to sever sensorineural hearing loss. *Otolaryngol Clin North Am*. 1995;28:107–120.

9. Hough J, Vernon J, Himelick T, Meikel M, Richard G, Dormer K. A middle ear implantable hearing device for controlled amplification of sound in the human: a preliminary report. *Laryngoscope*. 1987; 97:141–151.

10. Kartush JM, Tos M. Electromagnetic ossicular augmentation device. *Otolaryngol Clin North Am*. 1995;28:155–172.

11. Todt I, Seidl RO, Gross M, Ernst A. Comparison of different Vibrant Soundbridge audioprocessors with conventional hearing aids. *Otol Neurotol*. 2002;23:669–673.

12. Uziel A, Mondain M, Hagen P, Dejean F, Doucet G. Rehabilitation for high-frequency sensorineural hearing impairment in adults with the Symphonix Vibrant Soundbridge: a comparative study. *Otol Neurotol*. 2003; 24:775–783.

13. Sterkers O, Boucarra D, Labassi S, et al. A middle ear implant, the Symphonix Vibrant Soundbridge: retrospective study of the first 125 patients implanted in France. *Otol Neurotol*. 2003;24:427–436.

14. Fraysse B, Lavieille JP, Schmerber S, et al. A multicenter study of the Vibrant Soundbridge middle ear implant: early clinical results and experience. *Otol Neurotol*. 2001;22:952–961.

15. Boeheim K, Pok SM, Schlogel M, Filzmoser P. Active middle ear implant compared with open-fit hearing aid in sloping high-frequency sensorineural hearing loss. *Otol Neurotol*. 2010;31(3):424–429.

16. Schmuziger N, Schimmann F, àWengen D, Patscheke J, Probst R. Long-term assessment after implantation of the Vibrant Soundbridge device. *Otol Neurotol*. 2006; 27:183–188.

17. Verhaegen VJO, Mylanus EAM, Cremers CWRJ, Snik AFM. Audiological application criteria for implantable hearing aid devices: a clinical experience at the Nijmegen ORL Clinic. *Laryngoscope*. 2008;118: 1645–1649.

18. Mosnier I, Sterkers O, Boucarra D, et al. Benefit of the Vibrant Soundbridge device in patients implanted for 5 to 8 years. *Ear Hear*. 2008;29(2):281–284.

19. Rameh C, Meller R, Lavieille JP, Deveze A, Magnan J. Long-term patient satisfaction with different middle ear hearing implants in sensorineural hearing loss. *Otol Neurotol*. 2010;31:883–892.

20. Snik AFM, van Duijnhoven NTL, Mylanus EAM, Cremers CWRJ. Estimated cost-effectiveness of active middle-ear implantation in hearing-impaired patients with sever external otitis. *Arch Otolaryngol Head Neck Surg*. 2006;132:1210–1215.

21. Bornitz M, Hardtke HJ, Zahnert T. Evaluation of implantable actuators by means of a middle ear simulation model. *Hear Res*. 2010;263(1-2):145–151.

22. Huber AM, Ball GR, Veraguth D, Dillier N, Bodmer D, Sequeira D. A new implantable middle ear hearing device for mixed hearing loss: a feasibility study in human temporal bones. *Otol Neurotol.* 2006;27: 1104–1109.

23. Arnold A, Stieger C, Candreia C, Pfiffner F, Kompis M. Factors improving the vibration transfer of the floating mass transducer at the round window. *Otol Neurotol.* 2009;31:122–128.

24. Pennings RJE, Ho A, Brown J, van Wijhe RG, Bance M. Analysis of Vibrant Soundbridge placement against the round window in human cadaveric temporal bone model. *Otol Neurotol.* 2010;31:998–1003.

25. Colletti V, Soli SD, Carner M, Colletti L. Treatment of mixed hearing loss via implantation of a vibratory transducer on the round window. *Int J Audiol.* 2006;45: 600–608.

26. Hüttenbrink KB, Zahnert T, Bornitz M, Beutner D. TORP-vibroplasty: a new alternative for the chronically disabled middle ear. *Otol Neurotol.* 2008;29:965–971.

27. Linder T, Schlegel C, DeMin N, van der Westhuizen S. Active middle ear implants in patients undergoing subtotal petrosectomy: new application for the Vibrant Soundbridge device and its implication for lateral cranium base surgery. *Otol Neurotol.* 2009;30(1):41–47.

28. Dumon T, Gratacap B, Firmin F, et al. Vibrant Soundbridge middle ear implant in mixed hearing loss: indications, techniques, results. *Rev Laryngol Otol Rhinol.* 2009:130(2):75–81.

29. Beltrame AM, Martini A, Prosser S, Giarbini N, Streitberger C. Coupling the Vibrant Soundbridge to cochlea round window: auditory results in patients with mixed hearing loss. *Otol Neurotol.* 2009;30:194–201.

30. Rajan GP, Lampacher P, Ambett R, et al. Impact of floating mass transducer coupling and positioning in round window vibroplasty. *Otol Neurotol.* 2011;32: 271–277.

31. Frenzel H, Hanke F, Beltrame M, Steffen A, Schönweiler R, Wollenberg B. Applica-tion of the Vibrant Soundbridge to unilateral osseous atresia cases. *Laryngoscope.* 2009;119(1):67–74.

32. Colletti L, Carner M, Mandalà M, Veronese S, Coleti V. The floating mass transducer for external auditory canal and middle ear malformations. *Otol Neurotol.* 2010; 32:108–115.

33. Colletti V, Carner M, Colletti L. TORP vs round window implant for hearing restoration of patients with extensive ossicular chain defect. *Acta Otolaryngol.* 2009;129: 449–452.

34. Shimizu Y, Puria S, Goode RL. The floating mass transducer on the round window versus attachment to an ossicular replacement prosthesis. *Otol Neurotol.* 2010;32:98–103.

35. Jesacher MO, Kiefer J, Zierhofer C, Fauser C. Torque measurements of the ossicular chain: implication on the MRI safety of the hearing implant Vibrant Soundbridge. *Otol Neurotol.* 2010;31:676–680.

36. Todt I, Rademacher G, Wagner F, et al. Magnetic resonance imaging safety of the floating mass transducer. *Otol Neurotol.* 2010;31:1435–1440.

37. Todt I, Seidl RO, Ernst A. MRI scanning and incus fixation in Vibrant Soundbridge implantation. *Otol Neurotol.* 2004;25:969–972.

38. Jenkins HA, Niparko JK, Slattery WH, Neely JG, Frederickson JM. Otologics Middle Ear Transducer™ ossicular stimulator: performance results with varying degrees of sensorineural hearing loss. *Acta Otolaryngol.* 2004;124:391–394.

39. Martin C, Deveze A, Richard C, et al. European results with totally implantable Carina placed on the round window: 2-year follow-up. *Otol Neurotol.* 2009;30: 1196–1203.

40. Siegert R, Mattheis S, Kasic J. Fully implantable hearing aids in patients with congenital auricular atresia. *Laryngoscope.* 2007;117:336–340.

41. Jenkins HA, Atkins JS, Horlbeck D, et al. Otologics fully implantable hearing system: phase I trial 1-year results. *Otol Neurotol.* 2008;29:534–541.

42. Jenkins HA, Pergola N, Kasic J. Anatomical vibrations that implantable microphones must overcome. *Otol Neurotol.* 2007;28: 579–588.

43. Hough JVD, Matthews P, Wood MW, Dyer RK. Middle ear electromagnetic semi-implantable hearing device. *Otol Neurotol.* 2002;23:895–903.

44. Silverstein H, Atkins J, Thompson JH, Gilman N. Experience with the SOUNDTEC implantable hearing aid. *Otol Neurotol.* 205;26:211–217.

45. Dyer RK, Nakmali D, Dormer KJ. Magnetic resonance imaging compatibility and safety of the SOUNDTEC Direct System. *Laryngoscope.* 2006;116:1321–1333.

46. Dyer RK, Dormer KJ, Hough JVD, Nakmali U. Biomechanical influences of the magnetic resonance imaging on the SOUND-TEC Direct System implant. *Otolaryngol Head Neck Surg.* 2002;127:520–530.

47. Chen DA, Backous DD, Arriaga MA, et al. Phase I clinical trial results of the Envoy system: a totally implantable middle ear device for sensorineural hearing loss. *Otolaryngol Head Neck Surg.* 2004;131(6):904–916.

48. Envoy Medical Corp. Esteem PMA P0090018, Sponsor Executive Summary 003905-400 Rev 01 October 2009.

49. Barbara M, Manni V, Monnini S. Totally implantable middle ear devices for rehabilitation of sensorineural hearing loss: preliminary experience with the Esteem® Envoy. *Acta Otolaryngol.* 2009;129:429–432.

50. Hausler R, Stieger C, Bernhard H, Kompis M. A novel implantable hearing system with direct acoustic cochlear stimulation. *Audiol Neurotol.* 2008;13:247–256.

Appendix

Immunization for Cochlear Implant Recipients

Over the past decade, it became apparent that cochlear implant recipients were more prone to develop pneumococcal meningitis than their age-matched cohort who did not receive implants. Children composed the majority of patients affected (64%). Risk factors for developing meningitis after cochlear implantation include:

1. Use of a 2-part implant that incorporates a separate Silastic positioner. These implants were withdrawn from the market by the manufacturer.
2. Inner ear malformations (eg, Mondini, common cavity).
3. Immunocompromise.
4. Implantation at a very young age.
5. The presence of a ventriculoperitoneal or similar shunt.
6. Insertion trauma.
7. Failure to seal the cochleostomy.

As a result of the identified risk, the Centers for Disease Control and Prevention (CDC) developed recommendations for immunization for children undergoing cochlear implantation (see http://www.cdc.gov/vaccines/vpd-vac/mening/cochlear/dis-cochlear-gen.htm and http://www.cdc.gov/mmwr/preview/mmwr html/mm5909a2.htm). A campaign to disseminate the CDC recommendations was conducted. The recommendations are summarized below and on the Web site of the American Academy of Otolaryngology—Head and Neck Surgery Web site (http://www.entnet.org/HealthInformation/Cochlear-Meningitis-Vaccination.cfm).

➤ Children who have cochlear implants or are candidates for them should receive PCV13 (Prevnar 13®). It is now routinely recommended that all infants and children should receive PCV13.

➤ Older children with cochlear implants (aged 2 through 5) should receive 2 doses of PCV13 if they have not received any PCV7 (Prevnar 7®) or PCV13 previously. If they have already completed the 4-dose PCV7 series, they should receive 1 dose of PCV13 through age 71 months.

➤ Children aged 6 through 18 with cochlear implants may receive a single dose of PCV13, regardless of whether they have previously received PCV7 or the pneumococcal polysaccharide vaccine (PPSV) (Pneumovax®).

➤ In addition to receiving PCV13, children with cochlear implants should receive 1 dose of PPSV at age 2 or older, and after completing all recommended doses of PCV13.

➤ Adult patients (19 and older) who are candidates for a cochlear implant, and those who have received a cochlear implant, should be given a single dose of PPSV.

➤ For children and adults, vaccinations should be completed 2 weeks or more before surgery.

REFERENCES

Cohen NL, Hirsch BE. Current status of bacterial meningitis after cochlear implantation. *Otol Neurotol.* 2010;31:1325–1328.

Wei BPC, Shepherd RK, Robins-Browne, RM, Clark GM, O'Leary SJ. Pneumococcal meningitis post-cochlear implantation: preventative measures. *Otolaryngol Head Neck Surg.* 2010;143:S9–S14.

Index